Oxford Medical Publications

A Life Course Approach to Chronic Disease Epidemiology

Tracing the origins of ill-health from early to adult life

A Life Course Approach to Chronic Disease Epidemiology

Edited by

Diana Kuh

Medical Research Council National Survey of Health and Development
Department of Epidemiology and Public Health
University College London Medical School

and

Yoav Ben-Shlomo

Department of Social Medicine
University of Bristol

OXFORD   NEW YORK   TOKYO
OXFORD UNIVERSITY PRESS
1997

Oxford University Press, Great Clarendon Street, Oxford OX2 6DP

Oxford New York
Athens Auckland Bangkok Bogota Bombay Buenos Aires
Calcutta Cape Town Dar es Salaam Delhi Florence Hong Kong
Istanbul Karachi Kuala Lumpur Madras Madrid Melbourne
Mexico City Nairobi Paris Singapore Taipei Tokyo Toronto Warsaw
and associated companies in
Berlin Ibadan

Oxford is a trade mark of Oxford University Press

Published in the United States
by Oxford University Press Inc., New York

A catalogue record for this book is available from the British Library

Library of Congress Cataloging in Publication Data
(Data available)
ISBN 0 19 262782 1

Typeset by Downdell, Oxford
Printed in Great Britain by
Biddles Ltd
Guildford & King's Lynn

Foreword

by Professor Mervyn Susser, Emeritus Professor of Epidemiology and Director of the
Sergievsky Centre, Columbia University, New York

This book stems from a continuing debate, recently revived in Britain, about
chronic disease. The question at issue is what the appropriate overarching
framework of ideas should be. Claims and counter-claims enliven the journals.
The largest such claim is for fetal programming as a paradigm for adult
disease. Historical context might aid readers in evaluating the contribution of
the book to the debate.

As an Anglophile with long and enduring ties to the UK, I might well be
suspected of bias in drawing attention to the signal contributions to modern
epidemiology that have emanated from that country. These stretch from the
beginnings with John Graunt and William Petty in the 17th century to the
present day.

This implied continuity is not without discontinuities. Over the succeeding
three and a half centuries, we can stand witness in retrospect to at least four
turns in epidemiological thought that qualify as paradigm shifts by the criteria
set out by Thomas Kuhn in his book, *The structure of scientific revolutions.* As
his title indicates, changes of this large order are seen as revolutionary. They
supplant the leading scientific ideas of an era with a new ideological
structure, reinterpret past science in that light and, as the new gains
maturity, are ensconced in standard texts and even in new disciplines.

The first period of modern epidemiology was mainly one of exploratory
description, typified by Graunt's analysis of the London Bills of Mortality. At
the same time, Thomas Sydenham was moving clinical thought away from the
classical notion of sickness as the expression of humoral imbalance and toward
that of disease entities. Bernardino Ramazzini in Italy, also in descriptive
mode, arrayed a large number of occupational exposures with connected
pathologies as well as examining a number of epidemics.

No paradigm shift obliterates all other paradigms. Later, in the 18th century,
sharp induction from case series led Percival Pott to the sooty origin of the

scrotal cancer of chimney sweeps and George Baker to the lead colic of cider drinkers. A revolutionary shift did follow early in the early 19th century when the Sanitary Movement adopted the Miasma Theory. This theory postulated a largely environmental source for ill-health in foul emanations from pollution environments.

The laboratory-based Germ Theory supplanted Miasma in the last quarter of the 19th century. It is still manifest in the writings of some laboratory-bound microbiologists and readers of this book will doubtless find it familiar. Among epidemiologists, however, for the past half-century a theory of multiple causes, in recent years exemplified by the metaphor of the Black Box, has dominated the field.

Foreseeing the current paradigm threatened by increasing sterility, Ezra Susser and I have argued that epidemiology is in need of a new paradigm. We argue further that epidemiology has choices to make which can help determine the shape its future takes. Our choice and advocacy is for a multilevel eco-epidemiology, an epidemiology that learns how to range between molecule and macro-environment.

There are of course other choices. I have already referred to one widely canvassed in the UK as a causal theory for chronic disease, namely, David Barker's hypothesis of disordered developmental programming during the fetal period. The hypothesis has been extended, in the light of studies by his group, to encompass infancy.

Charles Stockard in the USA proposed a critical period hypothesis in 1921. When such a critical juncture exists in early development, the appropriate steps must be negotiated if the consequences of delayed development are not to be irreversible. Although similar notions were implicitly entertained by workers before and since, the hypothesis has seldom been addressed in a formal sense outside biology. R. A. McCance and Elsie Widdowson did so in studies of early nutrition—mostly in pigs—in the 1950s, and a decade later, so also did John Dobbing and Myron Winick. Zena Stein and I soon after followed their lead in epidemiological studies of prenatal nutrition, both in Harlem in New York City and in work on the Dutch Famine of 1944/5. But in epidemiology no-one has taken up the general idea with the force and persistence of David Barker.

His group has produced a multitude of studies and a greater multitude of publications. When a respected journal goes on editorial record that this large body of works amounts to a paradigm change, one must call, however mildly, for critical judgment that will ensure balance.

This book does just that. It is indeed a considerable achievement for a multi-author work to sustain, in a conspectus of so many chapters, balanced judgment and interest. Instead of a single critical period hypothesis or fetal programming, the authors adhere to the perspective of cumulative developmental stresses throughout the life course.

The critical period hypothesis can reasonably be equated with the Barker idea of early programming. The hypothesis certainly holds for such unmistakable prenatal insults as rubella, iodine, or folate deficiency that produce well-defined developmental defects. Quite likely it holds for at least a proportion of other less sharply defined chronic disorders such as obesity, schizophrenia, and perhaps breast cancer.

But it cannot by itself account for much of many adult disorders and, even less, for cardiovascular disease. Too much can already be attributed to other factors that accumulate over the life course such as smoking and diet. At best, if not unimportantly, programming could create predispositions and vulnerability to life course experience.

For the common run of chronic diseases the contribution of such early experience, if any, must surely be complementary. We are back, then, with the comfortable, well-tried, and productive formulations that can subsume multiple causes and even, without undue stretch, multilayered relations.

One can commend this book, with its guiding idea of cumulative influences over the life course, as providing the solid and sensible anchor one expects from British epidemiology in approaching the problems of chronic disease in adults.

Preface

In the last forty years adult chronic disease has been the main public health problem of industrialized countries. The aetiological model throughout this period has emphasized adult risk factors, particularly aspects of lifestyle, such as smoking, diet, and lack of physical exercise. In recent years more attention has been paid to possible risk factors in childhood and exciting new research has demonstrated a higher risk of cardiovascular disease, diabetes and chronic bronchitis among those born or brought up in poor childhood circumstances or who experienced poor growth in infancy or utero. The main challenge to the adult life-style model stems from extensive research undertaken from the mid 1980s into the fetal and infant origins of adult disease by David Barker and his research team at the Medical Research Council Environmental Epidemiology Unit in Southampton England. They argue that environmental factors 'programme' particular body systems during critical periods of growth, in utero and infancy, with long term direct consequences for adult chronic disease.

The 'Barker hypothesis' acted as a stimulus for an interdisciplinary group of researchers, mainly based in London, to form a discussion group. This book has evolved as a joint venture among the members of this group who share a common 'life course' approach to chronic disease aetiology. Such an approach studies individual experience from conception to death and does not draw false dichotomies between adult lifestyle and early life influences, or between biological and social risk processes.

The contributors to this book offer a comprehensive and balanced review of recent epidemiological, biological and sociological evidence relating to influences on disease risk in both early and later life. In this one volume the findings of numerous studies which are scattered throughout the scientific press are pulled together. Whilst each chapter reflects the views of individual authors, shared aims and a common framework have provided a more consistent approach than is usually found in such a broad collection of papers.

The contributors ask to what extent early life experiences explain variations in the disease risk of individuals and populations. They discuss the interpretation of the evidence, such as whether early influences act on adult health through independent, synergistic or intermediary mechanisms. Methodological problems, inherent in the study of disease over a long time scale, are raised. The public health implications are discussed, in particular the benefits and risks associated with interventions to improve fetal growth. The book focuses on cardiovascular disease, cancer, diabetes and hypertension; it does not cover all possible diseases which may originate in early life such as schizophrenia, or motor neurone disease. However, both the conceptual and methodological ideas which are described will be sufficiently broad to encompass more than the specific disease entities that are discussed.

The publication of this book is timely as there has been an explosion of publications in the last few years and interest in the research continues to grow rapidly in Britain, Scandinavia, the US and many other countries. This review will make this exciting and varied scientific work more accessible. It will be an invaluable resource for epidemiologists, social scientists, clinicians and public health physicians, and of interest to other medical researchers, policy makers, students and the interested lay reader. It assumes no prior epidemiological knowledge, although some basic understanding of human biology is expected.

As editors, this book has posed an exciting challenge in exchanging intellectual ideas and synthesizing varied opinions. We have learnt an enormous amount in the process of putting the book together. In the last few months it has taken over our lives. We would therefore like to thank our contributors, colleagues and families who have been so supportive of this project. Special thanks are extended to Jeannette Ben-Shlomo, John Carrier, David Green, Peter Kuh and Michael Wadsworth.

London and Bristol   D.K.
March 1997   Y.B.S.

Acknowledgements

Many people have contributed to the production of this book. In particular we would like to thank Professor Michael Wadsworth, who kindly provided information on adult body weight and blood pressure from the MRC National Survey of Health and Development (for table 6.1), Danny Dorling of the Department of Geography, University of Bristol for helping to convert the historical geographical area units into the appropriate contemporary Regional Health Authorities (for table 10.1); Jeremy Schuman of the Office for National Statistics for providing additional unpublished data on mean birth weights from 1986 (for figure 10.2); and Fiona Lampe and Peter Whincup for providing data on the British Regional Heart Study (for table 12.3). Chris Power is supported as a Weston Fellow with the Canadian Institute of Advanced Research. Yoav Ben-Shlomo was a Wellcome Fellow in Clinical Epidemiology when he developed his initial interest in life course epidemiology. Fiona Davison and Anne Rennie provided essential secretarial help, and the staff of the Oxford University Press gave invaluable guidance and support.

The authors would like to thank the following for permission to reproduce published material: Figures 2.1 and 2.2 are reprinted from Kuh, D. and Davey Smith, G., When is mortality risk determined? Historical insights into a current debate, *Social History of Medicine* 1993;**6**:101–23, by kind permission of Oxford University Press; table 7.2 is adapted from Luke, B., Nutritional influences on fetal growth, *Clinical Obstetrics and Gynecology* 1994;**36**:538–49 by kind permission of the author; figure 9.3 is reproduced from Charlton, J., Murphy, M., eds, *The health of adult Britain 1841–1994* (1997) © Crown Copyright 1997, with kind permission of the Controller of HMSO and of the Office for National Statistics.

Finally, we would like to thank Professor David Barker and Professor Jerry Morris for kindly agreeing to be interviewed.

For Allan Frank Lewin

Contents

Contributors

Dr Mel Bartley Principal Research Fellow, Department of Epidemiology and Public Health, University College London Medical School, London.

Dr Yoav Ben-Shlomo Senior Lecturer in Clinical Epidemiology, Department of Social Medicine, University of Bristol.

Dr David Blane Senior Lecturer in Medical Sociology, Academic Department of Psychiatry, Charing Cross and Westminster Medical School, London.

Dr Derek Cook Reader in Epidemiology, St. George's Hospital Medical School, London.

Prof George Davey Smith Professor of Clinical Epidemiology, Department of Social Medicine, University of Bristol.

Dr Jonathan Elford Senior Lecturer in Epidemiology, Department of Primary Care and Population Sciences, Royal Free Hospital School of Medicine, London.

Dr. K. S. Joseph Epidemiologist, Bureau of Reproductive and Child Health, Laboratory Center for Disease Control, Ottawa, Ontario, Canada.

Prof. Michael S. Kramer Professor, Department of Epidemiology and Biostatistics and the Department of Pediatrics, McGill University Faculty of Medicine, Montreal, Quebec, Canada.

Dr Diana Kuh Senior Research Scientist, Medical Research Council National Survey of Health and Development, Department of Epidemiology and Public Health, University College London Medical School, London.

Dr David Leon Senior Lecturer in Epidemiology, Department of Epidemiology and Population Sciences, London School of Hygiene and Tropical Medicine, London.

Dr Paul McKeigue Senior Lecturer in Epidemiology, Department of Epidemiology and Population Sciences, London School of Hygiene and Tropical Medicine, London

Dr Ivan Perry Senior Lecturer in Epidemiology, Department of Epidemiology and Public Health, Imperial College School of Medicine at St. Mary's, London.

Dr Chris Power Reader in Epidemiology and Public Health, Institute of Child Health, University College London Medical School, London.

Dr David Strachan Reader in Epidemiology, Department of Public Health Sciences, St George's Hospital Medical School, London.

Prof Mervyn Susser Emeritus Professor of Epidemiology and Director of the Sergievsky Centre, Columbia University, New York.

Dr Peter Whincup Senior Lecturer in Clinical Epidemiology, Department of Primary Care and Population Sciences, Royal Free Hospital School of Medicine, London .

A Background

1 Introduction: a life course approach to the aetiology of adult chronic disease

Diana Kuh and Yoav Ben-Shlomo

The prevailing aetiological model for adult disease which emphasizes adult risk factors, particularly aspects of adult life style, has been challenged in recent years by research that has shown that poor growth and development and adverse early environmental conditions are associated with a raised risk of adult chronic disease. One early life model hypothesizes that adult chronic disease and many of its adult risk factors are biologically 'programmed' during gestation or early infancy. An alternative model hypothesizes that adult chronic disease reflects cumulative differential lifetime exposure to damaging physical and social environments. The contributors to this book take a broad life course approach, reviewing the epidemiological, social and biological evidence to see which experiences at different stages of the life course may contribute to the development of chronic disease and other aspects of adult health.

1.1 Adult life style and chronic disease

In the last 40 years adult chronic disease has been the main public health problem of industrialized countries. Cardiovascular disease, cancers and respiratory disease have become the most common causes of death, accounting for about three-quarters of all deaths between 30–69 years in the developed world.[1] Despite the secular increases in life expectancy, findings from Britain and the US suggest that increases in 'disability free' life expectancy lag behind,[2–4] and there is little evidence that the onset of degenerative disease has been delayed.[5,6]

The prevailing aetiological model for adult chronic disease emphasizes adult risk factors. Epidemiological research has identified both a number of bodily attributes which predispose individuals to specific chronic diseases, and various personal behaviours, associated with adult life style, which affect underlying

3

biological processes. For example, cigarette smoking is the classic risk factor for lung cancer and chronic bronchitis and contributes to the risk of coronary heart disease along with the other conventional risk factors of high blood pressure, raised cholesterol, diabetes, obesity, and lack of exercise. This evidence has been used to support government health education strategies which encourage adults to adopt a healthier life style.

Classic risk factors are limited in predicting individual risk and only partially explain the striking and well documented social and geographical inequalities in the distribution of chronic disease. This has stimulated further research into genetic markers, other adult risk factors to do with the psychosocial environment, more detailed assessment of adult dietary intake, and possible risk factors in childhood.[7]

1.2 The importance of early life for adult chronic disease

Initially interest in childhood was stimulated by research findings, discussed in later chapters, which suggest that the process of atherosclerosis begins in childhood. For example, the arteries of young children contain fatty streaks. Blood pressure and cholesterol levels in individuals 'track' from childhood to early adult life. Overweight children are at greater risk of becoming overweight adults. Lifelong smoking, dietary and exercise habits are acquired in childhood and adolescence. The life style model, which arose from the study of those in midlife, was gradually extended beyond adulthood as it was increasingly recognised that the establishment of healthy life styles, in terms of the classic risk factors, had to begin in childhood.

A second line of research emphasizes the importance of deprivation rather than affluence in childhood for adult chronic disease and challenges the life style model. This research has investigated environmental conditions and experiences during adolescence, childhood, infancy, and prenatal life, associated with poverty and poor early growth, which may make individuals more susceptible to developing adult chronic disease, either independently or in combination with adult risk factors. In the first instance findings of ecological studies found strong correlations between rates of past infant mortality and present adult mortality from various chronic diseases within the same geographical areas. More extensive studies of this type revealed that mortality rates from coronary heart disease, stroke, obstructive lung disease and lung cancer were differentially correlated with neonatal mortality, postneonatal mortality, mortality from respiratory and enteric disease, maternal mortality, and mean height.

The range of early life factors associated with later adult risk factors or disease in individual studies using prospective or retrospective data has been diverse. It includes various characteristics of the family of origin (such as social class, family size, paternal unemployment, sibling mortality), aspects of maternal characteristics before and during pregnancy (such as height, weight, anaemia, blood pressure, parity), various measures of fetal and infant body size (such as weight at birth or at 1 year, low birth weight relative to placental weight, thinness at birth, or shortness at birth with subsequent failure of infant growth), childhood infectious disease (such as respiratory infections, pneumonia, measles, and whooping cough), height, and educational attainment. The range of adult outcomes associated with these early life markers are equally diverse. They include cardiovascular disease and its risk factors (blood pressure, glucose tolerance, cholesterol and apolipoprotein B, fibrinogen and factor VII, body mass), chronic bronchitis, thyroid function, allergy, stomach cancer, and even suicide.

How are we to interpret the plethora of associations? The statistical associations, in themselves, do not necessarily imply that the underlying environmental causes had their effect in early life. Instead the observed relationships may reflect the effect of lifetime exposure to the underlying causal factor, or simply exposure in adult life. Alternatively, if the early life factors are markers of causal processes operating at this stage of life, what might these be, and what are their biological or social significance relative to causal processes in later life?

1.2.1 Programming during critical periods of development

On the basis of a remarkable series of historical cohort studies[8] and drawing on evidence from animal studies, David Barker and his colleagues at the Medical Research Council (MRC) Environmental Epidemiology Unit at Southampton University have argued strongly that adult chronic disease is biologically programmed in utero or early infancy. The term 'programming' is used to describe the process whereby a stimulus or insult (for example, due to undernutrition, hormones, antigens, drugs, or sensory stimuli) during critical periods of development has lasting or lifelong effects on the structure or function of organs, tissues and body systems.[9,10] Barker has generated a number of hypotheses to explain how undernutrition during different trimesters of pregnancy programmes an individual's adult risk of coronary heart disease, stroke, non-insulin dependent diabetes, and chronic bronchitis. For example, in the case of coronary heart disease it is hypothesized that fetal undernutrition during middle or late gestation, which leads to disproportionate fetal growth, raises the risk of later disease by the programming of blood pressure, cholesterol metabolism, blood coagulation, and hormonal settings.[11]

Barker argues that the current model of adult degenerative disease based on an interaction between genes and an adverse environment in adult life needs to be replaced by a new model, the central feature of which is the concept of environmental programming in fetal and infant life.[12] Since 1986 his MRC unit has published over 200 articles in support of this hypothesis. Such a challenging idea has received both an enthusiastic as well as a skeptical response. In 1993/ 94 the MRC established a major scientific initiative into the fetal and infant origins of adult disease. Just before this an editorial in the *British Medical Journal* suggested that the shift from the 'life style' to the 'early life experience' paradigm was a major scientific revolution.[13] A later, more critical, editorial, was more cautious and demanded both rigorous testing of the hypothesis, and deliberate attempts at refutation.[14]

What is clear is that this broad hypothesis of chronic disease causation is of relevance for a number of research disciplines. In the biological and medical sciences it raises interesting questions about the possible underlying long term biological risk processes. Do exposures in later life simply add additional risk or do they interact with the exposure that occurred during a critical period? To what extent is programming reversible? For example, the failure to develop an anatomical attribute during embryogensis may result in permanent disability. However, the function of certain organs may not just depend on their anatomical structure but may also be sensitive to up- or down-regulation by later exposures. The hypothesis also challenges social scientists to study the extrinsic social risk processes during life which may operate independently or in conjunction with these biological processes.

1.2.2 Accumulation of risk through the life course

The life course approach offers an alternative way of linking early life factors to adult disease. It suggests that throughout the life course exposures or insults gradually accumulate through episodes of illness, adverse environmental conditions and behaviours increasing the risk of chronic disease and mortality.[15-17] Accumulation of risk is different from programming in that it does not require (nor does it preclude) the notion of a critical period. This approach explicitly places more emphasis on a greater range of biological and social experiences in childhood, adolescence, and early adulthood than either the life style or programming models. According to a recent British government report 'it is likely that cumulative differential lifetime exposure to health damaging or health promoting environments is the main explanation for observed variations in health and life expectancy'(p.18).[18]

The study of how risk factors throughout the life course combine to influence adult disease risk is an integral part of this approach. For example, low birth weight is associated with high blood pressure and insulin resistance later in life and recent observations (discussed in Chapters 4 and 6) suggest that this relationship is particularly strong for men and women who are overweight.

Biological and social risk factors at each life stage may be linked to form pathways between early life experiences and adult disease.[17,19] The concept of a 'chain of risk' describes how certain experiences in early life increase the likelihood of future events which in turn lead to a change in the risk of adult disease. Chains can be advantageous or detrimental in their effects.

A life course approach has been favoured in research on psychosocial development. Chains of adversity have been studied extensively by a number of behavioural scientists interested in the psychosocial pathways between childhood and adult life.[20,21] For example, one study of young women showed how parenting breakdown in one generation increased the risk of parenting breakdown in the next.[22] Psychosocial problems in the parents were associated with parenting difficulties and a lack of social support, which in turn led to the daughters being admitted to residential care. An institutional upbringing reduced the girls' expectations of control over their lives. The stressful circumstances experienced on leaving care meant that many married hastily to deviant and disadvantaged men who were unable to offer them support or a rewarding marital relationship. This in turn increased the risks of poor social functioning and parenting breakdown. These scientists are interested in how some experiences in the chain act as protective factors and, by breaking the chain reaction, inhibit continuity. Thus, in the example given above, girls who happened to have more positive school experiences than others showed more planning in their choice of career or marriage and, as a result, married men with whom they were more likely to develop a warm and supportive relationship, which in turn improved their social functioning, increased their parenting skills, and reduced the chance of parenting breakdown. This research not only outlines the pathways between cause and effect, but also has important policy implications for how we may intervene.

The research on chain reactions in psychosocial development has highlighted adolescence and early adulthood as particularly important life stages to negotiate because decisions taken then about education, occupation and marriage may have a considerable impact on an individual's life trajectory. This is of importance in a life course approach to adult chronic disease because different life trajectories are associated with differential disease risks (see Chapter 8).

The study of the effects of exposures throughout life on adult disease risk raises a number of problems of analysis and interpretation which are discussed in later chapters. Most are not unique to studies of the life course but are exacerbated by the length of follow up required. The key epidemiological concepts are defined in the following section to help readers understand the arguments and interpret the evidence for themselves.

1.3 Epidemiological concepts and methodological problems encountered in studying the life course

Longitudinal designs are most appropriate for the study of accumulation of risk particularly where the effects of exposures in later life vary among individuals according to past experience and development. Studies which collect data repeatedly provide the most accurate time sequences of events and intra-individual change over time necessary to test causal hypotheses and to study 'escape' from risk. But longitudinal studies are expensive and do not yield quick returns unless the appropriate prospective data have already been collected. Historical cohort studies, where new data are collected on a population for whom data was collected earlier (perhaps for another purpose), are more cost effective but the detail on early life factors is often restricted to routine data and any information on the intervening years has to be recalled. In any type of study reliance on recall data is not possible for many exposures of interest (for example, where measurements are needed), memory is often unreliable and details of the timing or duration of exposures are limited. Characteristics of the longitudinal studies discussed in later chapters are provided in a table at the end of this chapter.

Losses to follow up are an inevitable feature of longitudinal and historical cohort studies and raise the possibility of selection bias, especially if migrants are not traced or have a higher loss rate. If sufficient data have been collected before loss occurs some account may be taken of the likely effects of this bias.

A long intervening period between the exposure and outcome raises the distinct possibility that any association may be due to confounding by a third factor. For example, low birth weight may be associated with heart disease, because small babies are more likely to smoke as adults. Birth weight, in this case, may be acting as a surrogate marker for smoking behaviour. Multivariate statistical methods enable the adjustment of risk estimates so that the size of any effect is independent of the confounding factor but are limited if the exposure and confounder are very closely correlated[23] or there is a difference in the measurement error ('misclassification')[24] of exposure and confounder.[25] The latter may be particularly likely to occur in studies where early life experiences are collected retrospectively whereas current ones are measured or more detailed, or in longitudinal studies when better measurement techniques are available at the later follow ups. One strategy is to break the confounding by testing the association between exposure and disease in a population where the confounding variable is not related to the exposure.[26]

A variable may also act as an 'effect modifier' altering the relationship between a causal variable and an outcome (for example, adult weight appears to modify the effect of birth weight on blood pressure). In this case the relationship between the causal variable and outcome is not consistent and will vary according to the presence or absence of this third variable. This general process is known as 'interaction' and either 'synergism' if the third variable enhances the effect of the causal variable or 'antagonism' if it diminishes it.[27,28] An effect modifier may either independently act as a causal factor or may have no effect in the absence of other variables.

Studying the relationship between exposure and disease is further complicated because of variation in the time between exposure and initiation of the disease process (induction period), or between disease initiation and detection (latency period).. This variability makes it difficult to detect risk factors, and the strength between an exposure and disease can be diluted or missed if the wrong time frame of exposure is measured.[29] Similarly if an exposure has a long latency period, its public health importance will vary according to when in the lifecourse one is exposed. Hence a 30 year induction is important if an individual is young but may be irrelevant if the individual is in their eighties.

1.4 The aims of this book

Discussion of the aetiological importance of early life for adult chronic disease has focused on the role of programming and the underlying biological risk processes. This book aims to widen this discussion within a broad life course approach which studies individual experience from conception to death and does not draw false dichotomies between adult and early life influences, or between biological and social risk processes. Such an approach explores evidence both for programming during critical periods of growth and development and the cumulative risk attached to a number of different exposures throughout the life course.

The contributors to this book are faced with the challenge of reconceptualizing current empirical evidence within a life course framework. An historical overview in Chapter 2 traces the twentieth century development of the idea that experiences early in life may have long term effects on the development of chronic disease. The next four chapters review the evidence and assess the relative contribution of early life and later life risk factors for cardiovascular disease, breast cancer, diabetes, respiratory disease and high blood pressure. The following two chapters explore possible risk mechanisms: Chapter 7 examines gestational and maternal influences on fetal growth and development; Chapter 8 examines the evidence for social processes acting throughout life which affect adult disease risk by ameliorating or exacerbating biological factors.

The contributors to the fourth section of the book address the question of whether differences in early life experience explain variations in the health of populations, rather than the risk of individuals within a given population. How do they relate to time trends in chronic disease or to what extent to they account for social and geographical variations in disease risk?

Programming presents a direct challenge to the contemporary wisdom of health education strategies which focus on health behaviour and life style, and the final section of the book is concerned with the policy implications of this model. It assesses the evidence from intervention studies which have attempted to improve the nutritional state of young women or alter fetal and infant growth and survival. It asks whether there would be a positive change in the nation's health if current health promotion strategies shifted towards an emphasis on early life risk factors facing the next generation of mothers and babies.

Research findings on the biological and social risk factors which have long term effects on adult disease risk are scattered throughout the scientific press. It is our hope that by making this important and varied scientific work more accessible will encourage the development of a life course approach in epidemiology and, at the same time, prove stimulating to other medical and social scientists, policy makers and interested lay readers.

The key studies which are reviewed in the following chapters are summarized in Table 1.1.

References

Those marked with an asterisk are especially recommended for further reading.

1 Murray CJL, Lopez AD. Global and regional cause-of-death patterns in 1990. In: Murray CJL, Lopez AD, eds. *Global comparative assessments in the health sector. Disease burden, expenditures and intervention packages.* Geneva: World Health Organization, 1994: 21-54

2 Bebbington AC. The expectation of life without disability in England and Wales. *Soc Sci Med* 1988;**27**:321-6.

3 Bebbington AC. The expectation of life without disability in England and Wales. *Popul Trends* 1991;**66**:26-9.

4 Robine JM, Ritchie K. Healthy life expectancy: evaluation of global indicator of change in population health. *Br Med J* 1991;**302**:457-60.

5 Fries JF, Green LW, Levine S. Health promotion and the compression of morbidity. *Lancet* 1989;**333**:481-3.

6 Barrett-Connor E. Are we living longer or dying longer? In: Poulter N, Sever P, Thom S, eds. *Cardiovascular disease: risk factors and intervention.* Oxford: Radcliffe Medical Press, 1993:89-99.

7 Marmot M, Elliot P, eds. *Coronary heart disease epidemiology: from aetiology to public health.* Oxford: Oxford Medical Publications, Oxford University Press, 1992.

8* Barker DJP, ed. *Fetal and infant origins of adult disease*. London: BMJ Publishing Group, 1992.

9 Lucas A. Programming by early nutrition in man. In: Bock GR, Whelan J, eds. *The Childhood Environment and Adult Disease*. Chichester: John Wiley and Sons, 1991:38-55.

10* Barker DJP. Mothers, babies, and disease in later life. London: BMJ Publishing Group, 1994.

11* Barker DJP. Fetal origins of coronary heart disease. *Br Med J* 1995;**311**:171-4.

12 Barker DJP. The fetal and infant origins of adult disease. *Br Med J* 1990;**301**:1111.

13 Robinson RJ. Is the child father of the man? Controversy about the early origins of cardiovascular disease. *Br Med J* 1992;**304**:789-90.

14* Paneth N, Susser M. Early origin of coronary heart disease (the "Barker hypothesis"). *Br Med J* 1995;**310**:411-2.

15* Forsdahl A. Are poor living conditions in childhood and adolescence an important risk factor for arteriosclerotic heart disease? *Br J Prev and Soc Med* 1977;**31**:91-5.

16 Riley JC. *Sickness, Recovery and Death*. Hampshire: MacMillan Press, 1989.

17 Ben-Shlomo Y, Davey Smith G. Deprivation in infancy or adult life: which is more important for mortality risk? *Lancet* 1991;**337**:530-4.

18 Department of Health. *Variations in Health: What Can the Department of Health and the NHS Do?* London: Department of Health, 1995.

19 Wadsworth MEJ. Health inequalities in the life course perspective. *Soc Sci Med* 1997;**44**:859-70.

20* Rutter M. Pathways from childhood to adult life. *J Child Psychol Psychiatry* 1989;**30**:25-51.

21 Robins L, Rutter M. *Straight and devious pathways from childhood to adulthood*. Cambridge: Cambridge University Press, 1990.

22 Quinton D, Rutter M. *Parental breakdown. The making and breaking of intergenerational links*. Aldershot: Gower, 1988.

23 Davey Smith G, Phillips A. Declaring independence: why we should be cautious. *J Epidemiol Community Health* 1990;**44**:257-8.

24 Leon DA. Failed or misleading adjustment for confounding. *Lancet* 1993;**342**:479-81.

25 Phillips AN, Davey Smith G. How independent are "independent" effects? Relative risk estimation when correlated exposures are measured imprecisely. *J Clin Epidemiol* 1991;**44**:1223-31.

26 Davey Smith G. Confounding in epidemiological studies: why 'independent effects' may not be all they seem. *Br Med J* 1992;**305**:757-9.

27 Rothman KJ. Synergy and antagonism in cause-effect relationships. *Am J Epidemiol* 1974;**99**:385-8.

28   Rothman KJ, Greenland S, Walker AM. Concepts of interaction. *Am J Epidemiol* 1980;**112**:467-70.

29   Rothman KJ. Induction and latent periods. *Am J Epidemiol* 1981;**114**: 253-9.

30   Barker DJP, Osmond C, Winter PD, Margetts B, Simmonds SJ. Weight in infancy and death from ischaemic heart disease. *Lancet* 1989;**2**: 577-80.

31   Barker DJP, Osmond C, Simmonds SJ, Wield GA. The relation of small head circumference and thinness at birth to death from cardiovascular disease. *Br Med J* 1993;**306**:422–6.

32   Barker DJP, Bull AR, Osmond C, Simmonds SJ. Fetal and placental size and risk of hypertension in adult life. *Br Med J* 1990;**301**:259-63.

33   Leon DA, Koupilova I, Lithell HO, Berglund L, Mohsen R, Vagero D, Lithell U-B, McKeigue PM. Failure to realise growth potential in utero and adult obesity in relation to blood pressure in 50 year old Swedish men. *Br Med J* 1996;**312**:401-6.

34   The Caerphilly and Speedwell Collaborative Group. Caerphilly and Speedwell collaborative heart disease studies. *J Epidemiol Community Health* 1984;**38**:259-62

35   Shaper AG, Pocock SJ, Walker M, Cohen NM, Wale CJ, Thomson AG. British Regional Heart Study: cardiovascular risk factors in middle aged men in 24 towns. *Br Med J* 1981;**283**:179-86.

36   Whincup PH, Cook DG, Adshead F, Taylor S, Papacosta O, Walker M, Wilson V. Cardiovascular risk factors in British children from towns with widely differing adult cardiovascular mortality. *Br Med J* 1996;**313**: 79-84.

37   Wadsworth MEJ, Kuh DJL. Childhood influences on adult health: a review of recent work in the British 1946 national birth cohort study, the MRC National Survey of Health and Development. *Paediat Perinat Epidemiol* 1997;**11**:2–20.

38   Power C. A review of child health in the 1958 cohort: National Child Development study. *Paediat Perinat Epidemiol* 1992;**6**:91-110.

39   Butler NR, Golding J, Howlett BC (eds) *From birth to five: a study of the health and behaviour of a national birth cohort.* Oxford: Pergamon 1985.

Table 1.1. Characteristics of main studies with data on life course influences on adult disease

Title	Type of study	Index sample	Sample size	Period of birth	Age at last examination[a] or current age[b]
1 Hertfordshire[30]	historical cohort	All births notified in east Hertfordshire	10,141	1911–30	66–85[b]
2 Sheffield[31]	historical cohort	All births notified at Jessop hospital, Sheffield	1,586	1907–24	72–89[b]
3 Preston[32]	historical cohort	All births recorded in Sharoe Green General hospital, Preston	449	1935–44	45–54[b]
4 Uppsala[33]	historical cohort and cross-sectional survey	Men living in Uppsala between 1970–73 and aged 46–53	1,335	1920–24	50–74[b]
5 Caerphilly[34]	prospective cohort	Total population of men aged 45–59 from electoral rolls, Caerphilly, S. Wales	2,442	1921–35	60–75[b]
6 British Regional Heart Study[35]	prospective cohort	Random sample of men aged 40–59 from a general practice register across 24 towns selected on range of water hardness	7,727	1921–40	56–75[b]
7 Ten Towns Study[36]	repeat cross-sectional surveys	Random sample of children from schools based in ten towns selected on basis of high or low adult cardiovascular mortality	3,415	1983–85	10–12[a]
8 MRC National Survey of Health and Development[37]	prospective cohort	Stratified sample of births in one week in March in England, Scotland and Wales	5,362	1946	50[a]
9 National Child Development Study[38]	prospective cohort	All births in one week in March in England, Scotland and Wales	17,733	1958	33[a]
10 Child Health and Education Study[39]	prospective cohort	All births in one week in March in England Scotland and Wales	16,567	1970	16[a]

				Exposures			
					adulthood		
parental	gestational	post-natal	childhood	adolescence	early	middle	late
✓	✓	✓					✓
✓	✓						✓
✓	✓					✓	
	✓					✓	✓
	✓					✓	✓
		✓				✓	✓
✓	✓		✓				
✓	✓	✓	✓	✓	✓	✓	
✓	✓	✓	✓	✓	✓		
✓	✓	✓	✓				

2 The life course and adult chronic disease: an historical perspective with particular reference to coronary heart disease

Diana Kuh and George Davey Smith

In the first half of the twentieth century there was considerable public health and epidemiological interest in the idea that early life experiences influenced adult vitality and mortality risk. This was complementary to ideas that emerged in the biological and psychological sciences at that time. A key feature of the scientific debate was the relative contribution of the early environment as compared with heredity.

During the inter war period the 'epidemics' of coronary heart disease and lung cancer shifted attention to the aetiology of specific chronic diseases. The potential of the environment at different life stages to modify an individual's constitution and disease susceptibility was recognized but interest grew in the possible effects of adult physiological function, habits, and the socioeconomic environment on the development of chronic disease.

In the early postwar period adult risk factors were emphasized because of the natural interests of the cardiologists and physiologists who initiated cardiovascular epidemiology, the use of the prospective cohort to study disease incidence, and the need to develop preventive strategies to a pressing public health problem. The re-emergence of interest in early life factors from the 1970s stemmed first from the need to understand the natural history of these adult risk factors, and secondly, and more importantly, from the inability of the life style model to explain social and geographical variations in chronic disease risk. Epidemiological research is increasingly concerned with the independent and combined effects of early life and later life influences on chronic disease risk.

2.1 Introduction

This chapter traces the twentieth century development of the idea that experiences early in the life course may have long term effects on the development of chronic disease. This may be either because they occur at some critical period of development or because they contribute to a more gradual process of risk accumulation (see chapter 1). Why, in postwar chronic disease epidemiology, were these ideas eclipsed by the adult life style model, and how do they relate to the recent emergence of the environmental programming model in fetal and infant life outlined in Chapter 1?

2.2 Child health, adult vitality and mortality risk: the 'generation effect'

Between 1851 and 1940 there was a dramatic decline in all cause mortality rates of children and young adults under 45 years of age in Britain, mainly due to the decline in mortality from infectious diseases which were common at younger ages. Despite these improvements the widespread concern at the beginning of the twentieth century about a possible deterioration in national fitness which might impede economic or military success focused public health attention on infant mortality which had shown no signs of improvement during the nineteenth century.[1,2] Although bacteriological research dominated public health in the first four decades of this century[3] the idea that early life conditions and experiences affected adult health was a component of the prevailing public health model in Britain and the US.[4] To British public health officials it was evident that fitness and general vitality depended on the development of a stock of good health in early life, itself dependent on adequate care and nutrition in childhood. According to George Newman writing in 1914 when he was Chief Medical Officer to the Board of Education, 'recent progess has shown a) that the health of the adult is dependent upon the health of the child...[and]......b) that the health of the child is dependent upon the health of the infant and its mother.'(p.16).[5]

These ideas and the research studies that were undertaken to support them, discussed in more detail elsewhere,[6-8] lay behind the development of infant and child health services in Britain and the US. These social reforms were seen as misguided by the eugenicists such as Karl Pearson who believed that good health was inherited rather than nurtured by a good environment. He argued that interfering with natural selection by adapting the environment to man would lead to a British race of 'degenerate and feeble stock'(p.29).[9]

Early cohort analysis, applied to the age specific British death rates for the period 1841–1925 revealed the existence of a 'generation effect',[10,11] in that the mortality risk of each successive generation was found to be lower at all ages (see Fig. 2.1). The medical scientists who published the later paper[11] interpreted the generation effect as evidence of the importance of early environmental factors for adult health and used it to refute Pearson's concern about national degeneration. To Kermack and his colleagues their findings suggested that 'the expectation of life was determined by the conditions which existed during a child's earlier years' and that 'a good environment in childhood builds up a stronger constitution and raises the standard of physique'(p.703),[11] and that this had a decisive effect at all later ages. This mention of constitution and physique was part of a wider revival of interest in this subject (see Section 2.4.1)

The generation effect was discussed widely in the 1930s although other medical scientists were more cautious about the overwhelming importance of the childhood years. For example, Major Greenwood, in his valedictory address for Pearson, argued that 'persons over the age of 40 need not abandon hope that social and hygienic betterments introduced after their school days may increase their expectations of life,' (p.706) while in the discussion George Yule commented that the more interesting question was the 'relative influences on the mortality of any age group of a) the conditions to which they had been earlier subjected, especially at the beginning of life and of b) the contemporaneous conditions'.(p.710).[12] The notion that early life factors affected adult health by modifying the constitution and altering vitality clearly underlay the studies of child nutrition[13] and child health[14] in the 1930s, with the emphasis on the accumulation of environmental effects on health throughout childhood. Developmental critical periods were being discussed in psychoanalysis,[15] in behavioural psychology,[16,17] and in the biological sciences,[18-22] although this interest generally focused on very early life, when particular experiences might have long term effects. In the post war period the idea of a critical period became a central concept in research into animal behaviour, growth, and psychosocial development.[23-30] Paediatric epidemiology recognized the importance of the mother's early experience for the health of her offspring[31-33] and some theories of ageing used ideas of insult accumulation or a 'frailty' model.[34-37] In contrast, public health interest in early life determinants of susceptibility to adult disease waned as attention was drawn to the poor health of adults which occurred despite the improvements in child health.

2.3 Growing interest in adult chronic disease

Predictions made on the basis of the 'generation effect' suggested that death rates in middle age would begin to fall sharply as the cohorts who had

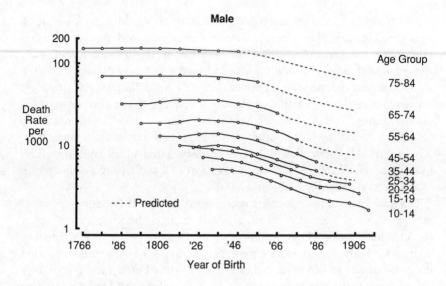

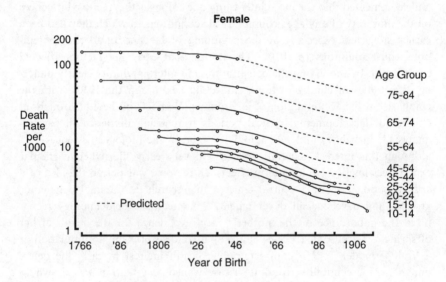

Figure 2.1 Changes in generation mortality (England and Wales).[10] Based on age specific death rates 1841–1925

experienced dramatic improvements in survival during childhood reached this age. These predictions failed to be confirmed (see Fig. 2.2) and concern in Britain and the US at the lack of improvements in middle age life expectancy, raised during the 1920s and 1930s,[38,39] became a major focus of social medicine and public health.

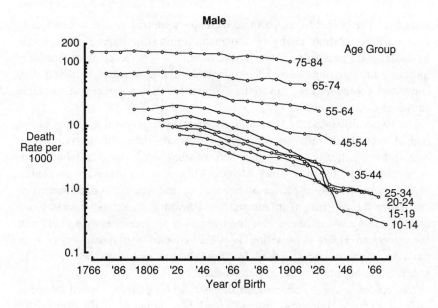

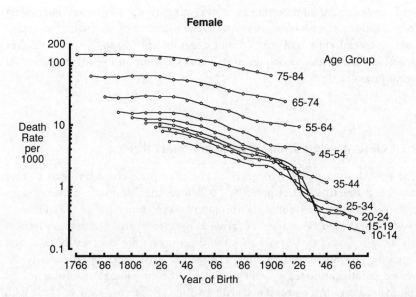

Figure 2.2 Changes in generation mortality (England and Wales).[195] Based on age specific death rates 1841–1990

Increases in the numbers of deaths attributed to heart disease and cancer were observed. Although some of this increase was the inevitable result of an ageing population, this could not explain the upward trends in age-specific rates.[40–50] The degree to which these increases were real or due to changes in cause-of-death coding, changing diagnostic fashions or improved diagnostic methods, was, and still is, much discussed.[51–57] The reversal of declining mortality rates among the middle aged which occured between 1920 and 1940 convinced contemporary[58] and later[59] observers that real increases in some causes of death did occur.

For those influenced by Pearson's arguments, the worsening trends in the middle aged death rates were a sign of reduced vitality of the population caused by genetically weaker members of the population surviving child-hood. Newman, by then Chief Medical Officer at the Ministry of Health denied there was any evidence of national deterioration[56] and continued to emphasize the key role of infant and child health. In contrast the establishment of the American Society for the Control of Cancer as early as 1913 and the American Heart Association in 1922 reflected widespread concern in the US[39] with the threat posed by these diseases and calls for preventive programmes of 'adult hygiene' were voiced.[60]

The 'epidemics' of coronary heart disease and lung cancer shifted attention away from acute infectious disease[61] and gave impetus to the concept of host, environment and agent, as it was already apparent that interacting factors influenced chronic disease risk. Demonstration of differential mortality risks by social class and sex[62,63] and geographical regions[64] suggested that potentially modifiable environmental factors were responsible for the increased death rates.[39]

2.3.1 Clinical recognition of coronary heart disease

The early history of the emergence of the concept of coronary heart disease has been described elsewhere.[56,65–69] Before the twentieth century myo-cardial infarction and coronary thrombosis were generally seen as terminal events[68] and reports of their occurrence were rare. In 1912 James Herrick, a Chicago physician, showed that the disease was not necessarily fatal and could be diagnosed during life.[70] Diagnosis was aided by the newly in-vented electrocardiograph which allowed the physiological properties of the living heart to be correlated with various symptoms, such as chest pain and breathlessness, and, subsequently, with underlying organic disorder. Clinicians became interested in coronary thrombosis as a clinical entity after Herrick's second paper in 1918[71] which linked his clinical information with electrocardiogram evidence from experimental canine and human subjects. Clinical awareness of coronary thrombosis occurred later in Britain[72–74] but in both places its emergence helped to define the territory of a new speciality of cardiology.[69]

2.4 Clues to the aetiology of coronary heart disease and atherosclerosis

Paul Dudley White and Samuel Levine, two of the first US cardiologists, were interested in the aetiology and prevention of heart disease in general,[75,76] and of coronary thrombosis in particular.[77] Influenced by Sir James Mackenzie and Sir Thomas Lewis, two of the earliest British physicians to specialise in the study of the heart and blood vessels, White and Levine used their detailed patient records as a basis for some of the first clinical studies of coronary thrombosis to investigate aetiological factors. In 1929 Levine published a detailed review based on his clinical records of 145 patients with the disease who subsequently died and were autopsied.[77] His findings indicated that previously existing hypertension was 'probably the most common single aetiological factor in the development of coronary thrombosis'(p.10).[77] Hypertension was a natural candidate for investigation because it was already recognised as a marker of underlying arterial or renal disease. Levine also observed a greater frequency of coronary thrombosis among men, those of muscular build, and those with a history of diabetes but not infectious disease (discussed in relation to other research below). In 1937 Levine, Glendy and White published an early case control study comparing the characteristics of 100 coronary heart disease patients with a rather odd control group of 300 healthy men aged 80 years or older.[78] Levine's earlier observations were confirmed, and, additionally, smoking, lack of exercise, and nervous strain distinguished the cases from the controls. With other colleagues White went on to conduct a series of studies of hypertension among the armed services.[79–83] At the same time life insurance data were showing that even moderate elevations of blood pressure raised disease risk.

The possible effects of adult habits and behaviour on adult mortality risk and chronic disease were already under scrutiny. Research suggested that the physical labour of working men shortened life expectancy[84] and increased the risk of coronary thrombosis[77] and arteriosclerosis[85] through blood pressure elevation, although the case control study just discussed suggested physical activity might have a protective effect.[78] Tobacco and alcohol consumption also shortened life expectancy[86,87] and had adverse effects on physiological function in ways that might cause long term damage to the heart or its arteries,[88,89] but the findings of the first few clinical studies of coronary patients were contradictory.[78,90,91] Many were unconvinced of the harmful effects of tobacco[47,92] or alcohol, and the research debate was clouded with moral overtones.[88,93]

Attention also turned to diet. A review of chemical, experimental and pathologic studies of atherosclerosis concluded that 'the pathogenesis of atherosclerosis of the aorta is principally dependent on age, cholesterol metabolism and blood pressure'(p.684).[94] This consideration of the possible role of cholesterol metabolism in humans built on the knowledge gained from animal experiments regarding diet and atherosclerosis which had been ongoing from the turn of the century.[68] Rosenthal reported that evidence from 28 studies of the relationship of diet and blood pressure to atherosclerosis undertaken all over the world among different ethnic and racial groups showed that 'in no race for which a high cholesterol intake (in the form of eggs, butter and milk) and fat intake are recorded is atherosclerosis absent'(p.493-494).[94] Early clinical investigations showed that those with diseases associated with serious lipid disorders, such as diabetes and hypothyroidism, had a higher risk of atherosclerosis and coronary thrombosis.[95,96]

Those involved in the development of social medicine such as John Ryle were particularly interested in aspects of the social and economic environment associated with chronic disease.[97] Some blamed the stress of living and working in the modern era for the rising rates of heart disease.[39,98] Generally attention focused on the contemporary environment although several observers who speculated that the considerable hardships suffered by recruits during the first world war might have caused the subsequent increase in heart disease were more concerned with the life course.[99,100]

2.4.1 Constitution and disease

The interwar period saw a revival of interest in the relationship between an individual's constitution and their risk of disease.[19,101–105] The notion of constitution was accorded many different meanings but, in essence, it referred to the total nature of the organism and, in particular, to those intrinsic characteristics which determined an individual's reaction, successful or unsuccessful, to the stress of the environment. Some, like Pearson, maintained that a person's constitution was dependent solely on genetic factors.[104] Others took what we would now describe as a life course approach.[101,105] For example, George Draper divided the life span into five great epochs: fetal life, infancy, childhood, the central span of adult life (marked by the two main dividing points, puberty and the climacteric), and the final stage of life. 'It is probable', speculated Draper, 'that the results of an individual's reaction to environment in one phase of growth has an important bearing on the next. This is especially true of the first, second and third stages during which the skeleton is forming and solidifying in its fixed condition.'(p.27)

Raymond Pearl, referring to the work of the early embryologists such as Charles Stockard,[21] saw constitution as the outcome of an interaction between an individual's genetic make up and environmental forces acting 'during development primarily, but also in some degree throughout the duration of the life of the individual'(p.36). Thus the constitution of the individual at any given moment is in part the resultant of his past history—the diseases he has had, the vicissitudes of embryonic development through which he has passed, and so on'(p.34).[105] The idea that disease episodes could have long term effects was not new; for example, the long term heart sequelae of rheumatic fever were recognised[75,106] and there was also interest in whether other infectious diseases predisposed sufferers to the subsequent development of arteriosclerosis and cancer.[107–109] However, the early clinical studies found that coronary heart disease patients reported fewer of the common infectious diseases.[77,78]

By observing and measuring anatomical, physiological, biochemical, psychological and emotional characteristics, researchers sought to distinguish constitutional types who were more or less predisposed to certain diseases. A number investigated the relationship between human form and human nature. Studies took detailed measurements of body build in order to classify the somatological variations into broad categories and to examine their relationship with different disease types.[101,104,110-114] The early clinical studies showed that muscular mesomorphs were more prone to coronary heart disease.[77,78] The relationship of various chronic diseases to overweight and short stature was also being revealed by studies of life insurance data.[115–118] Pearl and Ciocco, in a study of somatological differences associated with heart disease,[110] published this photograph in 1934 to illustrate the differences between the cardiac and the non cardiac individual. In fact, this study found that the most significant differences were the greater body weight and functional deficiency of the chest in the cardiac group compared with the non cardiac group and the authors concluded these were 'not innate constitutional differences but rather due to accumulation of body fat from relative over-eating and lack of physical exercise'(p.711).[110]

2.5 Chronic disease epidemiology in the early post war period: the rise of adult life style

Despite the advances made by almost every method of medical research, Paul Dudley White was convinced that the identification of the causes of heart disease would be advanced by population studies, both between and within countries, and by follow up studies of healthy persons as well as those with heart disease. In the Biggs lecture to the New York Academy of Science in 1940 he argued:

'Nature has for centuries been conducting gigantic experiments as to the effect of climate, of type of work, of diet, and of local or world-wide diseases on men, women, and children of different races, are spread out before our very eyes for us to record and analyze.... We need a large, well organized study that can in a several year program collect information, not just from hospital clinics or private practice, but from entire communities that will really show how common are hypertension and rheumatic valvular disease and syphilitic aortitis and coronary heart disease in relation to climate and mode of life.

Several well and similarly trained groups armed with good clinical observers, stethoscopes, sphgmomanometers, electrocardiographs, x-ray apparatus, and autopsy technic could in a few years accomplish more than the next century of desultory work, and cost less than a single air raid over a city at war.'(p.436).[119]

Early cardiologists like White sowed the seeds of a new epidemiological approach to the study of heart disease which used the new cardiac technology and biochemical tests of the laboratory to measure the prevalence, incidence and causes of heart disease in the general population. Although the Second World War delayed the putting into practice of this idea, the social changes it brought about enabled the organisation and funding of such studies in the post war era.

After the Second World War adult chronic diseases became a major public health concern because of the ageing of the population, the general public

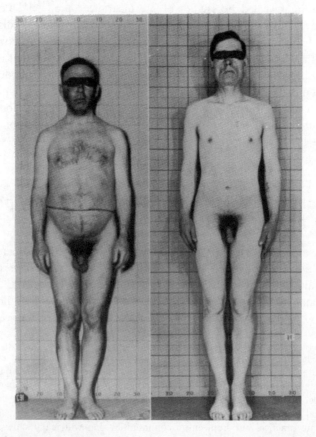

Figure 2.3 Front view of approximately 'average' cardiac individual (on the left) and of approximately 'average' non-cardiac individual (on the right)[110]

insistence that efforts should made to prevent all forms of illness and disability and the fact that mortality rates from cancer and coronary heart disease rose rapidly after the war, particularly among men during the most productive stage of their working life.[45,120] They were now seen as a preventable problem and there was widespread belief in the power of medical research to deal as successfully with the new diseases of affluence as it had done with the infectious diseases. The decline in the latter and the obvious improvement in child health also encouraged more emphasis to be placed on adult chronic disease.

The international and national institutions which were put into place after the war served an important function in the organisation and funding of large epidemiological studies. The creation of the World Health Organization in 1948 marked a new era in international cooperation and made worldwide research collaboration more possible. In the US, the reorganisation of the National Institutes of Health (NIH)[121] and of public voluntary health organisations, such as the American Heart Association,[122] encouraged greater emphasis on chronic disease and large scale funding of preventive medical research. In Britain, investment in this type of research was more modest, but a number of important epidemiological studies were funded by the Medical Research Council (MRC). Among them was Richard Doll and Bradford Hill's prospective study of 40 000 doctors,[123–125] which showed that smoking was a risk factor for lung cancer, coronary heart disease and chronic bronchitis. This study gave great impetus both to the prospective study as a powerful epidemiological tool and to the possibility that ways of life, modifiable by changes in personal behaviour, might be behind the poor health of middle aged men and women.

2.5.1 British cardiovascular epidemiology

After the war the MRC funded a new unit of Social Medicine with Jerry Morris as its director. His analysis of a long series of postmortem records from the London hospital revealed no increase in coronary atheroma over the previous 40 years, while there had been an apparent increase in coronary thrombosis.[46,58] This caused him to question the traditional view that atheroma underlay thrombosis and coronary occlusion and directed his attention to the thrombotic processes which precipitated the disease. As a strong supporter of social medicine he was particularly interested in the social and economic factors that might have caused the rise in disease, and less interested in the more proximal factors which he called the 'pathological precursors', such as cholesterol and blood pressure. The occupational studies by Morris and his colleagues confirmed that coronary heart disease was on the increase and, contrary to the findings of earlier studies, showed that men in jobs which demanded more physical activity (bus conductors and postmen) had a lower incidence of coronary heart disease and a lower early case-fatality than those in less active occupations (bus drivers and civil servants in sedentary grades).[126-128] At the same time other British investigators expanded their community surveys of respiratory disease to include studies of coronary heart disease and from the late 1960s the MRC and other bodies provided more extensive funding of prospective cohorts.[30,129-133]

2.5.2 US cardiovascular epidemiology

In contrast to the British experience, the clinicians and laboratory scientists who initiated American cardiovascular epidemiology were more interested in the pathological precursors to coronary thrombosis rather than the social and occupational factors that might underlie them. This was reflected in a strong attachment to the lipid theory of coronary heart disease, extensively reviewed in the 1950s[95,134] and systematically developed by Ancel Keys, director of the Laboratory of Physiological Hygiene at the University of Minnesota, in the postwar period.[135,136]

Immediately after the war White and his medical colleagues began a new case control study of young coronary heart patients which included a full appraisal of physique (thus maintaining their earlier interest in constitution) but also examined the newer hormonal and biochemical aspects of coronary heart disease.[48,137] Keys initiated a longitudinal study of 279 healthy professional men.[138,139]

Keys, despite his background as an experimental physiologist, shared White's interest in population studies.[140] With the support of White and a grant from NIH, he became principal investigator on the Seven Countries study, coordinating parallel cohort studies on men aged 40–59 years of age in countries with different diet or reputed incidence of heart disease. In most countries these cohorts were followed up for 30 years.[141]

The first major American prospective study of heart disease, also funded by NIH, was set up in 1948, in Framingham, Massachusetts. In his role as adviser to the National Heart Institute, White's endorsement of this study was of great importance.[142] The medical profession, including Levine and three other cardiologists, dominated the advisory committee and doubtless were influential in identifying the main hypotheses for study. Naturally their interest was in testing the pathological precursors of coronary heart disease, namely hypertension and elevated cholesterol. Drawing on the aetiological clues from the interwar studies[142] the importance of various diseases (such as diabetes and hypothyroidism), overweight, a number of personal habits (dietary intake, alcohol consumption, smoking, and physical activity), and physique were also considered. Other smaller cohort studies in Albany,[143] Los Angeles[144] and Chicago[145] followed behind the Framingham study, mostly funded by NIH, often in collaboration with state health departments.

The historical details of the Seven Countries Study and the Framingham Study, their important role in the development of postwar epidemiology and in dispelling earlier clinical misconceptions, have been discussed elsewhere.[146–151] Mervyn Susser described the Framingham Study as one of the 'intellectual levers' of modern epidemiology, the other being Doll and Hill's prospective study.[146] The point that concerns us here is that, despite initial differences in approach among British and US researchers, a general consensus gradually emerged about the classic risk factors connected with adult life style which raised individual risk, and in some cases population risk, of the most common adult chronic diseases.[152]

2.6 Early life factors and chronic disease epidemiology in the post war period

In the first 25 years after the war little attention was given to early life factors or to a consideration of the life course in the aetiology of coronary heart disease. Morris and his colleagues did consider the possibility that constitutional differences might explain the excess coronary heart disease rates in bus drivers compared with conductors.[153] Similarly he noted that new cohorts suffering more from coronary heart disease might have differed from their predecessors at an even earlier stage of the life course when he commented in his 1951 paper that it 'may be that those now living to middle age are qualitatively different; they have survived, or been preserved through, hazards that would previously have been mortal. Consequently they may be in some way constitutionally more liable than their coevals of forty years ago to succumb to diseases that are prevalent, including coronary heart-disease.'(p.72).[46] A decade later Geoffrey Rose echoed the same theme after a small study of familial patterns in ischaemic heart disease revealed that those who in adult life suffered from ischaemic heart disease came from families who had experienced excess mortality, particularly in infancy. One interpretation discussed by Rose was that these individuals came from 'a constitutionally weaker stock, more liable to succumb to a variety of diseases.'(p.80).[154] These ideas were not taken up at the time. According to Morris,[46] this was because of methodological problems inherent in life course research but other factors also inhibited investigation of a possible link between childhood experience and adult disease. In Britain a number of organisational and administrative changes in state health and welfare services, discussed in more detail elsewhere,[6] broke the prewar public health connection between child and adult health. The generation effect had failed to materialize and coronary heart disease appeared more prevalent at the time among the upper social groups whose early experiences were likely to have been more favourable than those of their lower social class peers. Lower child mortality had been accompanied by evidence of better child health and reductions in social inequalities, of which Morris and others were well aware,[56,155] and did not suggest that the origins of adult disease lay in early life.

In the first era of American prospective studies no attention was paid to childhood risk factors, for similar reasons. Although a full appraisal of physique was carried out on most members of the Framingham study few interesting results emerged[156] and it was adult body weight, rather than the more long term aspects of body build, that later became a classic risk factor. The clinicians' and physiologists' interests lay more in proximal rather than distal risk factors and there were no indications from the early clinical studies that those who suffered poor growth or infections in childhood were more likely to have coronary thrombosis. Indeed, one study had suggested that young men destined to die from coronary heart disease had, compared with their controls, been physically early developers and had mothers who had been in better condition during pregnancy.[157]

On a practical level individual prospective studies could not be applied to the whole life course without an unacceptable time lag, even the adult studies had to plan a long follow up to get sufficient cases for analysis. Not until the classic risk factors were established and the question of their natural history was raised did researchers begin to look back to the childhood years.

2.6.1 The growing importance of early life factors

In the intervention studies that began in the late 1960s it was clear that adults were finding it difficult to change their life styles, and consideration was given to the establishment of adult life styles in childhood.[158–161] Longitudinal research revealed that blood pressure and serum cholesterol 'tracked' through childhood and adolescence, in that children maintained their percentile position in the distribution. (see, for example, references[162–166])

Increasing attention was paid to atherosclerosis in young people after it was found that over three-quarters of young soldiers killed in the Korean war had gross evidence of coronary disease.[167] Fatty streaks were present in the aortas of 3 year olds[168] and appeared in the coronary arteries in the second decade of life[169] and in a later study these were found to relate to measures of cholesterol taken before death.[170] Atherosclerosis from a paediatric perspective[171] meant the encouragement of healthy lifestyles in childhood, such as lower fat consumption, which might directly inhibit early atherosclerosis and, to the extent that behaviours were maintained throughout life (see reference[6] and Chapter 8) indirectly reduce adult risk by improving adult risk factor profile. In more directly pathological terms, Osborn[172] argued that artifical infant feeding led to arterial damage, but these ideas were not taken up at the time.[8]

The inability of the life style model to explain social and geographical variations in chronic disease risk also encouraged others to consider the possible effects of early deprivation on adult disease. Since the late 1970s and 1980s there has been a growing body of evidence, discussed in later chapters, to suggest that poor living conditions in early life, and more specifically, poor growth, undernutrition and infectious disease, increase the risk of adult cardiovascular and respiratory diseases. This work has originated mainly from David Barker and his research team at the MRC Environmental Epidemiology Unit (reviewed in references[27,173-176]), but also from the Norwegian researcher Anders Forsdahl,[177-179] the maturing British cohorts[180-184] and studies of adult height and chronic disease.[185-189]

In interpreting his findings, Forsdahl suggested that 'various types of injury to health may add up so as to cause an increased risk of early ageing and death'(p.95),[177] thereby emphasizing the accumulation of risk over the life course. In contrast, Barker's model of biological programming in utero and infancy (see Chapters 1 and 7) is a development of the longstanding concept of critical periods in the biological sciences. In emphasising the role of fetal undernutrition and studying body proportions[175] he draws on the findings of earlier postwar research on nutrition and growth which had been previously neglected by those studying chronic adult disease.[29,30] Others, drawing on similar material,[190] emphasize the role of childhood nutrition.[191]

2.7 Conclusions: a modern revivial of constitution?

In the first half of this century the importance of the life course in health and disease was generally recognised through the notion of constitution; controversy centred on the relative influence of nurture and nature. Pearson attributed long term constitutional vulnerability to hereditary factors because social reforms *prevented* the weak from dying in infancy, whereas others attributed such vulnerability to both genetic and environmental factors. In the modern revival of interest in constitution it is the early environmental conditions that are seen to determine constitutional susceptibility to adult disease. Forsdahl argued that 'whereas the weaker of the cohort die in infancy, the fit survive and carry with them a life-long vulnerability'(p.95).[177] He refers to poor living conditions in early years followed by later affluence;[177] for Barker the most important environmental factor is undernutrition in pregnancy.[27]

One key question in the current debate is how the early environment affects later disease risk. This chapter has shown that both the idea of accumulation of risk over the life course and the concept of developmental critical periods have been discussed in the scientific literature throughout this century. The novel development in the current debate has been Barker's biological programming hypothesis which links differential development during critical periods to adult chronic disease risk. The other question concerns the relative influence on disease and mortality risk of conditions in early and later life,[192] and the extent to which these are independent or interactive effects.[193,194] As we have seen this question was posed by Yule in 1936 but was not taken up in the early postwar period when cardiologists and physiologists instigated prospective cohort studies of those in middle age and emphasized the role of adult life style. The recent interest by chronic disease epidemiologists in early life factors and the combined effects of exposures at different stages of the life course has been stimulated by the empirical evidence from imaginative historical cohort studies which have followed up adults on whom there is early life data from official records or previous surveys, and from maturing longitudinal studies. The next chapters review this evidence with respect to a number of adult chronic diseases.

References

Those marked with an asterisk are especially recommended for further reading.

1   Great Britain Parliamentary Papers. *Report of the Inter-departmental Committee on Physical Deterioration. Vol I: Report and Appendix Cmnd. 2175; Vol II: List of Witnesses and Minutes of Evidence, Cmnd. 2210; Vol III: Appendix and General Index, Cmnd. 2186.* London: HMSO, 1904.

2   Newman G. *Infant mortality. A social problem.* London: Methuen, 1906.

3   Rosen G. *A history of public health.* New York: MD Publications, 1958.

4   Fisher I. *Report on National Vitality, its Wastes and Conservation.* Washington Government Printing Office: National Conservation Commission. Bulletin 30 of the Committee of One Hundred, 1909.

5   Great Britain. *Annual Report for 1913 of Chief Medical Officer of the Board of Education, Cd 7330.* London: HMSO 1914.

6   Kuh DJL. *Assessing the influence of early life on adult health.* PhD thesis. London University, 1993.

7*   Kuh D, Davey Smith G. When is mortality risk determined? Historical insights into a current debate. *Social History of Medicine* 1993;**6**: 101–23.

8   Davey Smith G, Kuh D. Does early nutrition affect later health? Views from the 1930s and 1980s. In: Smith D, ed. *The history of nutrition in Britain in the twentieth century: science, scientists and politics.* London: Routledge, 1997:214–37.

9   Pearson K. *Darwinism, medical progress and eugenics. The Cavendish Lecture.* London: Eugenics Laboratory Lecture Series IX, 1912.

10   Derrick VPA. Observations on (1) errors of age on the population stat-
     istics of England and Wales and (2) the changes in mortality indicated
     by the national records. *J Instit Actuaries* 1927;**58**:117–59.

11* Kermack WO, McKendrick AG, McKinlay PL. Death rates in Great
     Britain and Sweden: Some general regularities and their significance.
     *Lancet 1934;***226**:698–703.

12   Greenwood M. English death-rates, past, present and future. A vale-
     dictory address. *J R Stat Soc* 1936;**99**:674–713.

13   Boyd Orr J. *Food, health and income*. London, 2nd edition Macmillan,
     1937.

14   M'Gonigle GCM, Kirby J. *Poverty and Public Health*. London:
     V Gollancz, 1936.

15   Freud S. The claims of psycho-analysis to scientific interest: the interest
     of psycho-analysis from a developmental point of view (1913). In:
     Strachey J, ed. *The complete psychological works of Sigmund Freud,
     Vol XIII*. London: Hogarth Press, 1955:182–4.

16   Watson JB. *Psychological care of infant and child*. New York: Norton,
     1928.

17   Watson JB. *Behaviourism*. Chicago: University of Chicago Press. Revised
     edition 1930.

18   Stockard CR. Developmental rate and structural expression: an
     experimental study of twins, "double monsters" and single deformities
     and their interaction among embryonic organs during their origins and
     development. *Am J Anat* 1921;**28**:115–225.

19   Stockard CR. Constitution and type in relation to disease. In: *De Lamar
     Lectures 1925–1926*. The Johns Hopkins University School of Hygiene
     and Public Health. Baltimore: The Williams and Wilkins Co., 1927:
     154–68.

20   Stockard CR. *Hormones and structural development. The Beaumont
     Foundation Lecture. Series number six*. Detroit, Michigan: Wayne County
     Medical Society, 1927.

21   Stockard CR. *The physical basis of personality*. London: George Allen &
     Unwin Ltd, 1931.

22   Speman H. *Embryonic development and induction*. New Haven: Yale
     University Press, 1938.

23   Bowlby J. *Maternal care and mental health*. World Health Organisation
     Monograph Series no.2. Geneva: World Health Organisation, 1951.

24   Bowlby J. *Child care and the growth of love*. Harmondsworth: Penguin,
     1953.

25   Beach FA, Jaynes JA. Effects of early experience upon the behavior of
     animals. *Psychol Bull* 1954;**51**:239–63.

26   Henderson ND. Effects of early experience upon the behavior of animals:
     the second twenty five years of research. In: Simmel EC, Baker G, eds.

Early experiences and early behavior. Implications for social development. New York: Academic Press, 1980:45–77.

27* McCance RA, Widdowson EM. The determinants of growth and form. *Proc R Soc Lond* 1974;**185**:1–17.

28 Clarke AM, Clarke ADB. The formative years? In: Clarke AM, Clarke ADB, eds. *Early experience: myth and evidence.* New York: The Free Press, 1976:3–24.

29 McCance RA. Food, growth, and time. *Lancet* 1962;**ii**:621–6 & 671–5.

30 Barker DJP. *Mothers, babies, and disease in later life.* London: BMJ Publishing Group, 1994.

31 Drillien CM. The social and economic factors affecting the incidence of premature birth. *J Obstet Gynaecol Br Emp* 1957;**64**:161–84.

32 Baird D. Epidemiology of congenital malformations of the central nervous system in (a) Aberdeen and (b) Scotland. *J Biosoc Sci* 1974;**6**:113–37.

33 Lumey LH, Van Poppel FWA. The Dutch famine of 1944–5: mortality and morbidity in past and present generations. *Social History of Medicine* 1994;229–46.

34 Jones HB. A special consideration of the ageing process, disease, and life expectancy. In: Lawrence JH, Tobias CA, eds. *Adv Biolog Med Phys* 1956;**4**:281–337.

35 Jones HB. The relation of human health to age, place, and time. In: Birren JE, ed. *Handbook of aging and the individual.* Chicago: University of Chicago Press, 1959:336–63.

36 Riley JC. *Sickness, recovery and death.* Hampshire: MacMillan Press, 1989.

37 Alter G, Riley JC. Frailty, sickness, and death: models of morbidity and mortality in historical populations. *Popul Stud* 1989;**43**:25–45.

38 Ministry of Health. *Report of the Chief Medical Officer for 1921.* London: HMSO, 1921.

39* Sydenstricker E. *Health and environment.* New York and London: McGraw-Hill Book Campany, Inc., 1933.

40 Registrar General. *Eightieth Annual Report (1917).* London: HMSO, 1919.

41 Wiehl DG. Some recent changes in the mortality among adults. *J Prev Med* 1930;**4**:215–37.

42 Dublin LI, Armstrong DB. *Favorable aspects of heart disease with special reference to the health officer.* New York: Metropolitan Life Insurance Company, 1933.

43 Greenwood M. *Epidemics and crowd diseases. An introduction to the study of epidemiology.* New York: The MacMillan Company, 1935.

44 Woolsey TD, Moriyama IM. Statistical studies of heart disease. II. Important factors in heart disease mortality trends. *Public Health Rep* 1948;**63**:1247–73.

45   Moriyama IM, Woolsey TD. Statistical studies of heart disease. *Public Health Rep* 1951;**66**:355–68.

46*   Morris JN. Recent history of coronary heart disease. *Lancet* 1951;**1–7**: 69–73.

47   Ryle JA, Russell WT. The natural history of coronary disease. *Br Heart J* 1949;**XI**:370–89.

48*   Gertler MM, White PD. *Coronary heart disease in young adults.* Cambridge, Mass: Harvard University Press, 1954.

49   Acheson RM. The etiology of coronary heart disease: a review from the epidemiological standpoint. Yale J Biol Med 1962;**35**:143–70.

50   Case RAM. Cohort analysis of cancer mortality in England and Wales, 1911-1954 by site and sex. *Br J Prev Soc Med* 1956;**10**:172–99.

51   Bolduan CF, Bolduan NW. Is the "appalling increase" in heart disease real? *J Prev Med* 1932;**6**:321–33.

52   Levy RL, Bruenn HG, Kurtz D. Facts on disease of the coronary arteries, based on a survey of the clinical and pathologic records of 762 cases. *Am J Med Sci* 1934;**187**:376–90.

53   Lew AE. Some implications of mortality statistics relating to coronary artery disease. *J Chron Dis* 1957;**6**:192–209.

54   Campbell M. Death rate from diseases of the heart: 1876 to 1959. *Br Med J* 1963;**2**:528–35.

55   Robb-Smith AHT. *The enigma of coronary heart disease.* Chicago: Year Book Medical Publishers, 1967.

56*   Bartley M. Coronary heart disease and the public health 1850-1983. *Sociol Health Illness* 1985;**7**:289–313.

57   Stehbens WE. An appraisal of the epidemic rise of coronary heart disease and its decline. *Lancet* 1987;**I**[1]:606–10.

58   Morris JN. Epidemiology and cardiovascular disease of middle age: part I. *Mod Concepts Cardiovasc Dis* 1960;**29**:625–32.

59   Davey Smith G, Marmot M. Trends in mortality in Britain 1920-1986. *Ann Nutr Med* 1991;**35 (Suppl 1)**:53–63.

60   Bigelow GH, Lombard HL. *Cancer and other chronic diseases in Massachusetts.* Cambridge: The River Side Press, 1933.

61   Gordon JE. Epidemiology—old and new. *J Mich St Med Soc* 1950;**49**: 194–9.

62   Stevenson THC. The social distribution of mortality from different causes in England and Wales 1910–12. *Biometrika* 1923;**15**:382–400.

63   Stocks P. The effects of occupation and its accompanying environment on mortality. *J R Stat Soc* 1938;**101**: 690–7.

64   Askanazy M (ed). *Deuxieme conference internationale de pathologie geographique.* Utrecht: A Oostoek, 1934.

65   Leibowitz JO. *The history of coronary heart disease.* London: Wellcome Institute of the History of Medicine, 1970.

66 Proudfit WL. Origin of concept of ischaemic heart disease. *Br Heart J* 1983;**50**:209–12.

67 Michaels L. Aetiology of coronary artery disease: an historical approach. *Br Heart J* 1966;**28**:258–64.

68* Acierno LJ. *The history of cardiology*. London: Parthenon, 1994.

69* Lawrence C. "Definite and Material": Coronary thrombosis and cardiologists in the 1920s. In: Rosenberg CE, Golden J, eds. *Framing disease*. New Brunswick, New Jersey: Rutgers University Press, 1992.

70 Herrick JB. Clinical features of sudden obstruction of the coronary arteries. *JAMA* 1912;**59**:2015–20.

71 Herrick JB, Nuzum FR. Angina pectoris, clinical experience with two hundred cases. *JAMA* 1918;**70**:67–70.

72 McNee JW. The clinical syndrome of thrombosis of the coronary arteries. *Q J Med* 1925;**19**:44–53.

73 Gibson AG. The clinical aspects of ischaemic necrosis of the heart muscle. *Lancet* 1925;**ii**:1270–75.

74 Parkinson J, Bedford DE. Cardiac infarction and coronary thrombosis. *Lancet* 1928;**i**:4–11.

75 White PD. *Heart disease*. New York: Macmillan Co., 1931.

76 White PD, Parton M. *My life and medicine*. Boston: Gambit, 1971.

77* Levine SA, Brown CL. Coronary thrombosis: its various clinical features. *Medicine* 1929;**8**:245–418.

78* Glendy RE, Levine SA, White PD. Coronary disease in youth. *JAMA* 1937;**109**:1775–81.

79 Hillman CC, Levy RC, Stroud WD, White PD. Studies of blood pressure in army officers. *JAMA* 1944;**125**:699–701.

80 Levy RL, Hillman CC, Stroud WD, White DD. Transient hypertension. Its significance in terms of later development of sustained hypertension and cardiovascular-renal diseases. *JAMA* 1944;**126**:829–33.

81 Levy RL, White PD, Stroud WD, Hillman CC. Transient hypertension. The relative prognostic importance of various systolic and diastolic levels. *JAMA* 1945;**126**:1059–61.

82 Levy RL, White PD, Stroud WD, Hillman CC. Transient tachycardia prognostic significance alone and in association with transient hypertension. *JAMA* 1945;**129**:585–8.

83 Levy RL, White PD, Stroud WD, Hillman CC. Sustained hypertension, predisposing factors and causes of disability and death. *JAMA* 1947; **135**:77–80.

84 Pearl R. *Studies in human biology*. Baltimore: Williams and Wilkins, 1924.

85* Hueper F. Arteriosclerosis. *Arch Path* 1945;**39**:187–216.

86 Pearl R. *Alcohol and longevity*. New York: Knopf, 1926.

87 Pearl R. Tobacco smoking and longevity. *Science*1938;**87**:216–7.

88 Burnham JC. American physicians and tobacco use: two surgeon generals, 1929 and 1964. *Bull Hist Med* 1989;**63**:1–31.

89 Grollman A. The action of alcohol, caffeine, and tobacco, on the cardiac output (and its related functions) of normal man. *J Pharmacol Exp Ther* 1930;**39**:313–27.

90 White D, Sharber T. Tobacco, alcohol and angina pectoris. *JAMA* 1934;**102**:655–7.

91 English JP, Willius FA, Berkson J. Tobacco and coronary disease. *JAMA* 1940;**115**:1327–8.

92 Cassidy Sir,M. Coronary heart disease: the Harveian Oration of 1946. *Lancet* 1946;**ii**:587–90.

93 Weeks CC. *Alcohol and human life*. London: Lewis & Co, 1938.

94* Rosenthal SR. Studies in atherosclerosis: chemical, experimental and morphologic. *Arch Pathol* 1934;**18**:473–506, 660–98, 827–42.

95 Katz LN, Stamler J. *Experimental atherosclerosis*. Illinois: Charles C Thomas, 1953.

96* Hueper F. Arteriosclerosis. *Arch Pathol* 1945;**38**:162–81.

97 Ryle JA. *Changing disciplines*. London: Oxford University Press, 1948.

98 Stewart I. Coronary disease and modern stress. *Lancet* 1950;**ii:867–70.**

99 Registrar General. *Statistical review of England and Wales for the years 1938 and 1939. New Annual Series Nos.18 and 19*. London: HMSO, 1947.

100 Stocks P. The mortality of men between the ages of 50 and 65. *Lancet* 1943;**i**:543–9.

101* Draper G. *Human constitution: a consideration of its relationship to disease*. Philadelphia and London: Saunders, 1924.

102 Petersen WF. Constitution and disease. *Physiol Rev* 1932;**12**: 283-308.

103 Ciocco A. The historical background of the modern study of constitution. *Bull Hist Med* 1936;**4**:23-38.

104 Bauer J. *Constitution and disease*. New York: Grune and Stratton, 1943.

105 Pearl R. *Constitution and disease*. London: Kegan Paul, Trench, Trubner & Co Ltd, 1933.

106 Wilson MG, Lubschez R. Longevity in rheumatic fever. *JAMA* 1948;**138**:794–8.

107 Thayer WS. On the late effects of typhoid fever in the heart and vessels. *Am J Med Sci* 1904;**127**:391–415.

108 Ophuls W. Arteriosclerosis, cardiovascular disease: their relation to infectious diseases. *Medical Sciences* 1921;**1**:5–102. Stanford: Stanford University Publications.

109 Cherry T. Cancer and acquired resistance to tuberculosis. *Med J Aust* 1924;**2**:372–8.

110 Pearl R, Ciocco A. Studies in constitution II. Somatological differences associated with disease of the heart in white males. *Hum Biol* 1934;**6**: 650–713.

111 Reed LJ, Love AG. Biometric studies on U.S. army officers—somato-logical norms in disease. *Hum Biol* 1993;**V**:61–93.

112 Pearl R. An index of body build. *Am J Phys Anthropol* 1940;**26**:315–48.

113 Sheldon WH, Stevens SS, Tucker WB. *The varieties of human physique.* New York: Harper and Bros, 1940.

114 Draper G, Dupertuis CW, Caughey JL. *Human constitution in clinical medicine.* New York: Paul B Hoeber Inc., 1944.

115 Du Bray ES. Comments on body weight in relation to health and disease. *Am J Med Sci* 1925;**170**:564–75.

116 Dublin LI. The influence of weight on certain causes. *Hum Biol* 1930; **II**:159–83.

117 Dublin LI, Marks HH. The weight standard and mortality of very tall men. *Proc Assoc Life Insurance Directors America* 1937;**23**:153–81.

118 Dublin LI, Marks HH. Mortality of women according to build—experience in substandard issues. *Proc Assoc Life Insurance Directors America* 1938;**22**:203–36.

119* White PD. Heart disease, a world problem. *Bull N Y Acad Med* 1940; **16**:431–43.

120 Kaiser RF. Why cancer "control"? *Public Health Rep* 1950;**65**:1203–8.

121 Williams RC. *The United States Public Health Service 1798–1950.* Washington D.C.: Commissioned Officers Association of the United States Public Health Service, 1951.

122 Blackburn H, Epstein FH. History of the Council on Epidemiology and Prevention, American Heart Association. *Circulation* 1995;**91**: 1253–62.

123 Doll R, Hill AB. Mortality in relation to smoking: 10 years of obser-vations on male British doctors. *Br Med J* 1964;**1**:1399–460.

124 Doll R, Peto R. Mortality in relation to smoking: 20 years' observations on male British doctors. *Br Med J* 1976;**2**:1525–36.

125 Doll R, Peto R, Wheatley K, Gray R, Sutherland I. Mortality in relation to smoking: 40 years' observations on male British doctors. *Br Med J* 1994;**309**:901–11.

126 Morris JN, Heady JA, Barley RG. Coronary heart disease in medical practitioners. *Br Med J* 1952;**1**:503–20.

127 Morris JN, Heady HA, Raffle PAB, Roberts CG, Parks JW. Coronary heart-disease and physical activity of work. *Lancet* 1953;**ii**:1052–7, 1111–20.

128 Morris JN, Kagan A, Pattison DC, Gardner MJ, Raffle PAB. Incidence and prediction of ischemic heart disease in London busmen. *Lancet* 1966;**ii**:553–9.

129 Reid DD, Brett GZ, Hamilton PJS, Keen H, Jarrett RJ, Rose G. Cardiorespiratory disease and diabetes among middle-aged male civil servants. *Lancet* 1974;**i**:469–73.

130 Shaper AG, Pocock SJ, Walker M, Cohen NM, Wale CJ, Thomson AG. British Regional Heart Study: Cardiovascular risk factors in middle-aged men in 24 towns. *Br Med J* 1981;**283**:179–86.

131 Meade TW, North WRS, Chakrabarti R, Stirling Y, Haines AP, Thompson SG, Brozovic M. Haemostatic function and cardiovascular death: early results of a perspective study. *Lancet* 1980;**i**: 1050–54.

132 Thomas AJ, Cochrane AL, Higgins ITT. The measurement of the prevalence of ischaemic heart-disease. *Lancet* 1958;**ii**:540–4.

133 Higgins ITT, Cochrane AL, Thomas AJ. Epidemiological studies of coronary disease. *Br J Prev Soc Med* 1963;**17**:153–65.

134 Katz LN, Stamler J, Pick R. *Nutrition and atherosclerosis*. London: Henry Kimpton, 1959.

135 Keys A. Atherosclerosis: a problem in newer public health. *J Mt Sinai Hosp* 1953;**20**:118–39.

136 Keys A. Prediction and possible prevention of coronary disease. *Am J Public Health* 1953;**43**:1399–407.

137 Gertler MD, Garn SM, White PD. Young candidates for coronary heart disease. *JAMA* 1951;**147**:621–5.

138 Keys A, Longstreet Taylor H, Blackburn H, Brozek J, Anderson JT, Simonson E. Coronary heart disease among Minnesota business and professional men followed fifteen years. *Circulation* 1963;**28**:381–95.

139 Keys A, Taylor HL, Blackburn H, Borzek J, Anderson JT, Simonson E. Mortality and coronary heart disease among men studied for 23 years. *Arch Intern Med* 1971;**128**:201–14.

140 Keys A. Nutrition in relation to the etiology and the course of degenerative diseases. *J Am Diet Assoc* 1948;**24**:281–5.

141* Keys A. *Seven Countries: A multivariate analysis of death and coronary heart disease*. London: Harvard University Press, 1980.

142* Dawber TR. *The Framingham Study. The epidemiology of atherosclerotic disease*. London: Harvard University Press, 1980.

143 Doyle JT, Heslin AS, Hilleboe HE, Formel PF, Korns RF. A prospective study of degenerative cardiovascular disease in Albany: report of three years' experience—1. Ischemic heart disease. In: Measuring the risk of coronary heart disease in adult population groups. *Am J Public Health* 1957; **(Suppl, April)**:25–32.

144 Chapman JM, Goerke LS, Dixon W, Loveland DB, Phillips E. The clinical status of a population group in Los Angeles under observation for two to three years. In: Measuring the risk of coronary heart disease in adult population groups. *Am J Public Health* 1957; **(Suppl, April)**: 33–42.

145 Stamler J, Lindberg HA, Berkson DM, Shaffer A, Miller W, Poindexter A, Colwell M, Hall Y. Prevalence and incidence of coronary heart disease

in strata of the labor force of a Chicago industrial corporation. *J Chron Dis* 1960;**11**:405–20.

146* Susser M. Epidemiology in the United States after World War II: the evaluation of technique. *Epidemiol Rev* 1985;**7**:147–77.

147 Blackburn H. *On the trail of heart attacks in seven countries*. Minnesota: University of Minnesota, 1995.

148* Kromhout D, Menotti A, Blackburn H. *The Seven Countries Study: a scientific adventure in cardiovascular epidemiology*. Utrecht: Brouwer Offset, 1994.

149 Epstein FH. Cardiovascular disease epidemiology. A journey from the past into the future. *Circulation* 1996;**93**:1755–64.

150 Kannel WB. Clinical misconceptions dispelled by epidemiological research. *Circulation* 1995;**92**:3350–60.

151 Kuh DJL, Davey Smith G. The origins of cardiovascular epidemiology (abstract). *J Epidemiol Community Health* 1996;**50**:584.

152 Kannel WB. An overview of the risk factors for cardiovascular disease. Reprinted in: Buck C, Llopis A, Najera E, Terris M, eds. *The challenge of epidemiology. Issues and selected readings*. Pan American Health Organization. Scientific Publication No. 505. Washington: World Health Organization, 1988:699–718.

153 Morris JN, Heady JA, Raffle PAB. Physique of London busmen. *Lancet* 1956;**ii**:569-70.

154 Rose G. Familial patterns in ischaemic heart disease. *Br J Prev Soc Med* 1964;**18**:75–80.

155 Anon. Health and social class. *Lancet* 1959;**i**:303–5.

156 Damon A, Damon ST, Harpending HC, Kannel WB. Predicting coronary heart disease from body measurements of Framingham males. *J Chron Dis* 1969;**21**:781–802.

157 Yater WM, Traum AH, Spring S, Brown WG, Fitzgerald RP, Geisler MA, Wilcox BB. Coronary artery disease in men eighteen to thirty-nine years of age. *Am Heart J* 1948;**36**:334–722.

158 Falkner F. *Prevention in childhood of health problems in adult life*. Geneva: WHO, 1980.

159 United States Department of Health and Human Services. *Healthy People. Surgeon-General's Report on health promotion and disease prevention*. Washington DC: US Government Printing Office, 1979.

160 Coronary Prevention Group. *Children at risk: should the prevention of coronary heart disease begin in childhood?* London: Coronary Heart Prevention Group, 1989.

161 World Health Organisation. *Prevention in childhood and youth of adult cardiovascular diseases: Time for Action*. Geneva: WHO Technical Report Series 792, 1990.

162 Lauer RM, Clarke WR, Rames LK. Blood pressure and its significance in childhood. *Postgrad Med J* 1978;**54**:206–10.

163 Strasser T. Prevention in childhood of major cardiovascular diseases of adults. In: Falkner F, ed. *Prevention in childhood of health problems in adult life.* Geneva: WHO, 1980.

164 de Swiet M. The epidemiology of hypertension in children. *Br Med Bull* 1986;**42**:172–5.

165 Cresanta JL, Borke GL. Determinants of blood pressure levels in children and adolescents. In: Berenson GS, ed. *Causation of cardiovascular risk factors in children.* New York: Raven Press, 1986:157–89.

166 Webber LS, Freedman DS, Cresanta JL. Tracking of cardiovascular disease risk factor variables in school-age children. In: Berenson GS, ed. *Causation of cardiovascular risk factors in children.* New York: Raven Press, 1986:42–64.

167 Enos WF, Holmes RH, Beyer J. Coronary disease among United States soldiers killed in action in Korea. *JAMA* 1953;**152**:1090–3.

168 Holman KL, McGill HC, Strong JP, Geer JC. The natural history of atherosclerosis: the early aortic lesions as seen in New Orleans in the middle of the 20th century. *Am J Pathol* 1958;**35**:209–35.

169 Strong JP, McGill HC. The natural history of coronary atherosclerosis. *Am J Pathol* 1962;**40**:37-49.

170 Newman WP, Freedman DS, Voors AW, Gard PD, Srinivasan SR, Cresanta JL, Williams GD, Webber LS, Berenson GS. Relation of serum lipoprotein levels and systolic blood pressure to early atherosclerosis. *N Engl J Med* 1986;**314**:138-44.

171 Subbiah R. *Atherosclerosis: a pediatric perspective.* Florida: CRC Press Inc, 1989.

172 Osborn GR. Stages in development of coronary disease observed from 1,500 young subjects. Relationship of hypotension and infant feeding to aetiology. *Colloques Internationaux du Centre National de la Recherche Scientifique* 1967;**169**:93–139.

173 Barker DJP. *Fetal and infant origins of adult disease.* London: BMJ Publishing Group, 1992.

174 Barker DJP. The Wellcome Foundation lecture, 1994. The fetal origins of adult disease. *Proc R Soc Lond* 1995;**262**:37–43.

175 Barker DJP. Fetal origins of coronary heart disease. *Br Med J* 1995; **311**:171–4.

176 Barker DJP. The intrauterine origins of cardiovascular and obstructive lung disease in adult life. The Marc Daniels Lecture 1990. *J R Coll Physicians Lond* 1991;**25**:129–33.

177 Forsdahl A. Are poor living conditions in childhood and adolescence an important risk factor for arteriosclerotic heart disease? *Br J Prev Soc Med* 1977;**31**:91–5.

178 Forsdahl A. Living conditions in childhood and subsequent development of risk factors for arteriosclerotic heart disease. *J Epidemiol Community Health* 1978;**32**:34–7.

179 Arnesen E, Forsdahl A. The Tromso heart study: coronary risk factors and their association with living conditions during childhood. *J Epidemiol Community Health* 1985;**39**:210–4.

180 Colley JRT, Douglas JWB, Reid DD. Respiratory disease in young adults; influence of early childhood lower respiratory tract illness, social class, air pollution, and smoking. *Br Med J* 1973;**2**:195–8.

181 Kiernan KE, Colley JRT, Douglas JWB, Reid DD. Chronic cough in young adults in relation to smoking habits, childhood environment and chest illness. *Respiration* 1976;**33**:236–44.

182 Britten N, Davies JMC, Colley JRT. Early respiratory experience and subsequent cough and peak expiratory flow rate in 36 year old men and women. *Br Med J* 1987;**294**:1317–20.

183 Strachan DP, Anderson HR, Bland JM, Peckham C. Asthma as a link between chest illness in childhood and chronic cough and phlegm in young adults. *Br Med J* 1988;**296**:890–3.

184 Wadsworth MEJ, Cripps HA, Midwinter RA, Colley JRT. Blood pressure at age 36 years and social and familial factors, cigarette smoking and body mass in a national birth cohort. *Br Med J* 1985;**291**: 1534–8.

185 Notkola V, Punsar S, Karvonen MJ, Haapokoski J. Socio-economic conditions in childhood and mortality and morbidity caused by coronary heart disease in adulthood in rural Finland. *Soc Sci Med* 1985;**21**:517–23.

186 Marmot MG, Rose GA, Shipley MJ, Hamilton PJS. Employment grade and coronary heart disease in British civil servants. *J Epidemiol Community Health* 1978;**32**:244–9.

187 Waaler HTH. Height, weight and mortality. The Norwegian experience. *Acta Med Scand* 1984; **(Suppl 679)**:1–56.

188 Yarnell JWG, Limb ES, Layzell JM, Baker IA. Height: a risk marker for ischaemic heart disease: prospective results from the Caerphilly and Speedwell heart disease studies. *Eur Heart J* 1992;**13**:1602–5.

189 Leon D, Davey Smith G, Shipley M, Strachan D. Height and mortality in London: early life influences, socio-economic confounding or shrinkage? *J Epidemiol Community Health* 1995;**49**:5–9.

190 Leitch I. Growth and health. *Br J Nutr* 1951;**5**:142–51.

191 Gunnell DJ, Davey Smith G, Frankel SJ, Nanchqhal K, Braddon FEM, Peters TJ. Childhood leg length and adult mortality—follow up of the Carnegie survey of diet and growth in pre-war Britain (abstract). *J Epidemiol Community Health* 1996;**50**:580–1.

192 Ben-Shlomo Y, Davey Smith G. Deprivation in infancy or adult life: which is more important for mortality risk? *Lancet* 1991;**337**:530–4.

193 Leon DA, Koupilova I, O Lithell H, Berglund L, Mohsen R, Vagero D, Lithell U-B, McKeigue PM. Failure to realise growth potential in utero and adult obesity in relation to blood pressure in 50 year old Swedish men. *Br Med J* 1996;**312**:401–6.

194 O Lithell H, McKeigue PM, Berglund L, Mohsen R, Lithell U-B, Leon DA. Relation of size at birth to non-insulin dependent diabetes and insulin concentrations in men aged 50–60 years. *Br Med J* 1996;**312**: 406–10.

195 Office of Population Censuses and Surveys Mortality statistics 1841–1990. Serial Tables DH1 No.25. London: HMSO, 1992.

B Development of disease risk throughout life

3 Preadult influences on cardiovascular disease and cancer

David Leon and Yoav Ben-Shlomo

Recent evidence suggests that factors acting across the life course, rather than just adulthood, are important in determining the risk of cardiovascular disease and cancer. Consistent evidence, from different settings, demonstrates an inverse association between birthweight and risk of coronary heart disease, fetal growth retardation being associated with an increased risk. These relationships do not appear to be explained by confounding factors such as socioeconomic status, or other risk factors. Specific patterns of growth retardation, rather than birthweight *per se*, may be particularly important and explain the paradoxical observation that twin births, despite being lighter, do not show an increased risk. Weight at 1 year, exposure to enteric infections, and growth in childhood may also independently increase disease risk, through possibly different mechanisms. Natural history studies of children also demonstrate how adult risk factors track from an early age and predict early markers of atherosclerosis. Breast cancer is similarly associated with age at first birth, height, age at menarche, and possibly birthweight and pre-eclampsia. The latter findings are, however, inconsistent and based on proxy measures of ooestrogen exposure in utero. This has been hypothesised to alter the number or susceptibility of stem cells that may undergo future malignant change.

Fetal development is obviously a period when the in utero milieu can programme the structure and function of many organ systems. Whether such changes are permanent or reversible remains less clear but there is already evidence that early exposures can interact with exposures in adulthood. Future public health policy will need to consider the implications of a life course approach for disease prevention.

3.1 Introduction

Cardiovascular disease and cancers account for the majority of deaths in the developed world. In 1990, coronary heart disease (CHD), cerebrovascular disease and malignant neoplasms accounted for 60% and 64% of deaths amongst men and women respectively aged 30 years or older.[1] These diseases are rare until middle age and over half of deaths occur over the age of 70 years. Until recently,[2] most of our knowledge concerning aetiological risk factors focused on factors acting in adult life such as diet, smoking, physical activity, hypertension and adult obesity.[3] Little evidence existed concerning the role of factors in childhood or even earlier. This Chapter sets out to review current ideas concerning the potential role of preadult influences and to discuss the various models and mechanisms that might explain how circumstances in the first two decades of life may influence occurrence of CHD, stroke and cancer in middle or old age.

3.1.1 Evidence concerning the importance of early life influences

Much of our reliable knowledge about the aetiology and natural history of cardiovascular disease and cancer has come from prospective cohort studies. Early cohort studies recruited people already in adult life, many being restricted to people in middle age or older. Cohorts studies are expensive and time consuming and therefore recruiting older subjects increases efficiency as within a given follow up period there will be more events to analyse. (see also Chapter 2, Section 2.5) They provided little, if any, information about the influence of factors in childhood on the incidence of cardiovascular events and cancer. Instead, a wide variety of other sources indicated the potential role of childhood and early life factors (see Table 3.1). Until recently, most of this evidence has been relatively weak and indirect, using either ecological or proxy measures, such as height. However, both prospective[4] and historical cohort studies,[5] have now provided far more rigorous evidence to test associations between circumstances and outcomes many decades apart.

3.2 Cardiovascular disease

3.2.1 Geographical studies

Descriptive studies have demonstrated marked geographical differences in mortality and morbidity from CHD, both within and between countries (see Chapter 10, Section 10.2 for a more detailed discussion). Attempts to consider preadult influences have noted strong positive correlations between infant mortality in the past and subsequent adult mortality from heart disease.[6–8] Areas with high infant mortality rates experienced higher rates of CHD, over half a century later. These associations did not appear to be related to a specific cause of infant mortality, and were found with both neonatal and postneonatal mortality.[8] As well as infant mortality, areas with lower mean adult or child height have been noted to show higher rates of coronary heart disease.[9–11]

Various interpretations have been made of these findings. Forsdahl[6] suggested an interaction between poverty in adolescence followed by later affluence, whilst Barker and colleagues have postulated the importance of poor intrauterine development and the immediate neonatal period.[8] Others have suggested that this reflects continued deprivation acting across the life course from birth to adulthood rather than a specific influence of early life events.[12]

3.2.2 Social and geographic mobility

Adults often end up living in a place that is either geographically or socio-economically removed from their family of origin. This mobility has been exploited in a number of studies to investigate the relative contribution of circumstances in childhood and adult life on disease risk. The logic of these studies is that place of residence or socioeconomic position are proxy measures for pertinent environmental exposures at different points in time.

In a study of men and women whose childhood place of residence in England and Wales differed from that in adult life, mortality rates from CHD were found to be independently related to place of residence at both points in the life course.[13] This was interpreted as suggesting that childhood and adult risk factors were involved in determining risk of death from CHD. However, an analysis from the British Regional Heart Study[14] of CHD risk in relation to migration between place of birth and place of examination in middle age found that place of birth had little independent effect on risk, although its conclusions were based on few CHD events.

Early studies of social mobility and CHD focused on the stress of upward or downward mobility leading to an increased risk of disease[15,16] (see also Chapter 11, Section 11.2). These studies suggested an independent effect of paternal socioeconomic status after controlling for adult socioeconomic status and a range of cardiovascular risk factors. A case control study in Wales, similarly found that father's social class was an independent risk factor for myocardial infarction, but found no adverse effects of upward mobility *per se*[17], as predicted by the Forsdahl hypothesis.[6]

Socioeconomic conditions in childhood in Finland were also found to be related to risk of CHD in men, independent of socioeconomic position in adulthood, smoking, and serum cholesterol.[18] Two different analyses of another Finnish data set reached opposite conclusions on this question.[19,20]

Table 3.1 Evidence for pre-adult influences on adult disease

Type or source of information on early life	How information is used to infer pre-adult influences on adult disease risk	Examples	Strengths and limitations
Recalled events or behaviour	Information on events or behaviour in pre-adult life obtained from adults in case-control or cohort studies. These early risk factors analysed in same way as adult risk factors.	Age at menarche and breast cancer. Sunburn in childhood and melanoma. Age started smoking and lung cancer. (see section 3.4)	Validity of recalled information may be questionable. Mainly limited to events and habits in childhood, although information on height and weight has been collected in such studies.
Infant mortality rates by geographic area	Infant mortality rates (IMR) taken as proxy measure of conditions in pre-natal life and infancy. Early life effects inferred if IMR for defined geographic areas in the past correlate with adult mortality rates in the same areas decades later.	IMR by area in England and Wales in first part of century correlated with current coronary heart disease mortality. (see section 3.2.1)	Design cannot exclude possibility that correlation is due to socioeconomic confounding eg areas with high IMR in past were deprived, and because of continued deprivation have high adult mortality today.
Social or geographic mobility studies	Place of birth or residence or socio-economic circumstances in preadult life used as indirect measures of exposure. Association with adult disease risk examined controlling for adult place of residence or socioeconomic circumstances.	Socioeconomic position in childhood and coronary heart disease. Place of residence in childhood and cardiovacular mortality. (see section 3.2.2)	Only provides the most general and non-specific indication of independent effects of circumstances at different points in the life course.

Adult height	Taken as a cumulative measure of nutritional status and history of infection in childhood that may be correlated with adult outcomes.	Inverse association of adult height with ischaemic heart disease mortality and direct association with breast cancer. (see sections 3.2.4 and 3.3.2).	Adult height is a relatively indelible measure of processes that occurred in childhood (acting together with genes).
Anthropometric studies in childhood	Anthropometric data collected in special studies of children often initially designed to obtain information on growth for its own sake. Related to occurence of cancer or cardiovascular events in adult life usually by retrospective collection of event data.	Carnegie/Boyd-Orr study. (see section 3.2.4)	Depends upon identifying individual records from growth studies from at least 40-50 years ago which may be linked to subsequent occurence of disease in the study subjects.
Prenatal exposures and/ or nutrition	Information on size at birth, gestational age, complications of pregnancy etc. from obstetric records related to occurence of cancer or cardiovascular events in adult life usually by retrospective collection of event data.	Hertfordshire (UK) birth cohort and mortality from ischaemic heart disease. Obstetric records in Sweden traced in case-control study of breast cancer. (see sections 3.2.3.1 and 3.3.4).	Depends upon identifying historical series of obstetric records from at least 40–50 years ago which may be linked to subsequent occurence of disease in the study subjects.
Natural history studies from birth or childhood	Cohorts of subjects from birth or childhood examined and data collected on range of cardiovascular risk factors that are correlated with risk factor profiles in adult life and (more importantly) with markers of early cardiovascular disease (eg evidence of lesions in coronary arteries).	British 1946 Birth Cohort Study. Bogalusa Heart Study and Muscatine Studies. (see section 3.2.6).	Cohorts are still below the age at which cardiovascular events occur frequently. Remains unknown how far characteristics in childhood predict myocardial infarction or stroke.

A census-linkage study of intergenerational mobility from Sweden[21] found strong independent effects of childhood and adult socioeconomic conditions. The manual/non-manual CHD mortality rate ratio for childhood (OR = 1.99, 95% CI 1.30–3.05) was in fact greater than that for adulthood (OR = 1.77, 95% CI 1.17–2.67).

These mobility studies suggest that both place of origin and place of destination have independent influences on the risk of CHD in adult life. However, in themselves, they cannot exclude the alternative explanation that place of origin only matters in so far as, in combination with place of destination, it predicts risk factor levels in adult life. However, the relationship between size at birth and later risk of cardiovascular disease provides much more compelling evidence for preadult influences.

3.2.3 Growth in utero and infancy

Demonstrating an association between birthweight and CHD is arguably of greater significance than simply showing that size at birth is related to adult blood pressure or insulin resistance. These latter continuous outcomes are of importance in so far as they may mediate the association between exposures (such as in utero growth) and subsequent cardiovascular events.

It is difficult to assemble evidence linking growth in early life with cardiovascular events 50 or more years later, and only a few settings have been able to gather such data. Much of the evidence to date, comes from historical midwifery data from a large cohort of men and women[5] born in Hertfordshire, England between 1911 and 1930 and rediscovered by David Barker and colleagues.[5,22–27] They were able to extract data on maternal characteristics, birthweight, and progress throughout the infant's first 12 months, including weight at 1 year. From the 37 000 live singleton births originally identified, Barker's team were able to trace the mortality (1951–1992) experience of 16 000 subjects (43%). Despite criticisms concerning the relatively low rate of inclusion and the potential unrepresentativeness of identified subjects, it is difficult to see how the associations between birthweight or weight at 1 year with subsequent mortality among the traced subjects could be seriously biased.

3.2.3.1 Birth weight and weight at 1 year

Results from the Hertfordshire cohort reveal a decline in mortality risk from coronary heart disease (ICD9 codes 410-414) with increasing weight at birth in men and women (summarized in Table 3.2), with a suggestion in both sexes of a slight increase in risk in the heaviest birthweight group.[5] In contrast, weight at one year showed little association with CHD mortality in women, but a decline in risk with increasing weight for men. Causes other than cardio-vascular disease, taken in aggregate, showed no clear pattern of association with either weight at birth or at one year in either sex.

The Hertfordshire cohort has also been used to look at the association between prevalence of CHD and growth in utero and in infancy within a sample of 290 men who were still living in Hertfordshire and for whom weight at birth and at 1 year had been recorded.[25] The overall prevalence of CHD was 14%. There was a suggestion of a decrease in prevalence with birthweight over the first 4 categories, although overall the linear trend was not significant (see Table 3.3). However, there was a clearer trend ($p = 0.03$) of decreasing prevalence of CHD with increasing weight at 1 year.

Table 3.2 Rate ratios for coronary heart disease mortality among singleton men (ages 20–81) and women (ages 20–69) born in Hertfordshire in relation to birthweight and weight at one year

Birthweight (lbs)	Men (born 1911-30)	Women (born 1923-30)
≤ 5.5	1.00 (51)	1.00 (6)
6–	0.81 (118)	0.87 (19)
7–	0.80 (266)	0.81 (32)
8–	0.74 (266)	0.71 (23)
9–	0.55 (97)	0.52 (6)
≥ 10	0.65 (55)	0.59 (2)
p-value for trend	p < 0.0005	n.s.
Weight at 1 year (lbs)		
≤ 18	1.00 (68)	1.00 (14)
19–	0.79 (158)	0.59 (20)
21–	0.81 (305)	0.75 (32)
23–	0.62 (201)	0.52 (13)
25–	0.62 (98)	0.84 (7)
≥ 27	0.40 (23)	0.84 (2)
p-value for trend	p < 0.0001	n.s.

Figures in parentheses are numbers of deaths. n.s.—p > 0.05

Source : reference[5]

The association between early growth and left ventricular mass was also studied in this same subgroup. Increased mass (hypertrophy) is an established risk factor for CHD mortality. Analyses were based on 202 men after exclusion of those with valvular heart disease and those for whom echocardiographic data were inadequate.[26] As weight at 1 year increased there was a decrease in left ventricular mass (see Table 3.3). There was also a similar association between birthweight and left ventricular mass, although this was not significant. As with the finding for CHD mortality (Table 3.2), there was a decline in mass until the last birthweight category, which then showed a slight upturn.

A smaller but more elaborate cohort of births, from hospital obstetric records, born between 1907 and 1924 in Sheffield, Yorkshire, has also been

Table 3.3. Prevalence of coronary heart disease and left ventricular mass (g) among singleton men (mean age 67 years) born in Hertfordshire (1911–1930) in relation to birthweight and weight at one year

Birthweight (lbs)	Coronary heart disease prevalence (%) [N=290]		Left ventricular mass (g) [N=202]	
≤5.5	20	(10)	240	(8)
6–	21	(38)	207	(26)
7–	17	(84)	202	(63)
8–	6	(94)	201	(64)
9–	11	(5)	196	(32)
≥10	35	(7)	221	(9)
p-value for trend	p=0.9		p=0.3	
Weight at 1 year (lbs)				
≤18	27	(15)	239	(8)
19–	21	(47)	204	(31)
21–	14	(86)	212	(61)
23–	14	(85)	199	(64)
25–	6	(2)	191	(24)
≥27	9	(2)	190	(14)
p-value for trend	p=0.03		p=0.01	

Figures in parentheses are numbers of men.

Source : references [25,26]

collected by Barker and colleagues. Among 1586 singleton male births who could be traced, mortality from all cardiovascular disease was found to fall with increasing birthweight (see Table 3.4).[28] This effect was particularly strong for deaths occurring under 65 years of age. More recent analyses of the Sheffield cohort,[27] based on larger numbers of subjects, show that the association of birthweight with CHD mortality *per se* is similar to that presented in Table 3.4 for all cardiovascular disease.

The Sheffield cohort contains data not only on birthweight but also a number of other potential explanatory variables including head circumference, birth length, placental weight, gestational age, and mother's pelvic dimensions. The relationships between various combinations of these measures, such as ponderal index (birthweight/birth length^3) and placental to birthweight ratio with cause-specific mortality could be examined.[28] Of the various associations reported, head circumference was found to be inversely associated with cardiovascular mortality ($p=0.03$). Rates fell with increasing ponderal index ($p=0.05$), and were highest among men with the highest placental to birthweight ratio (i.e. large placenta compared to birthweight). Gestational age alone did not seem to be related to mortality from cardiovascular disease. As with the Hertfordshire study, it was not possible to adjust for socioeconomic position in adult life. Given the absence of clear prior hypotheses linking specific patterns of growth retardation with CHD mortality, the most important facet of the Sheffield findings was that they provided the first replication of the inverse association between cardiovascular disease mortality and birthweight observed in Hertfordshire.

Table 3.4. Rate ratios for all cardiovascular disease mortality among singleton men born in Sharoe Green Maternity Hospital, Sheffield (1907–1924) in relation to birth weight

Birthweight in lbs	<65 years	All ages (27-83 years)
≤5.5	1.00 (13)	1.00 (21)
6–	0.81 (34)	0.80 (61)
7–	0.89 (77)	0.88 (134)
8–	0.57 (36)	0.69 (73)
≥9	0.54 (14)	0.62 (27)
p-value for trend	p=0.02	p=0.06

Figures in parentheses are numbers of deaths.

Source : reference[28]

The association between birthweight and coronary heart disease has been reported from a further five settings, four of which are outside the UK. In four of the five, the inverse association found in Hertfordshire and Sheffield was confirmed. The one published study that fails to find this association is based on a follow up of a relatively small cohort of 855 men born in 1913 in Gothenburg, Sweden who were first examined at age 50 in 1963.[29] Information on birthweight and other factors was obtained from hospital obstetric records. The incidence of myocardial infarction (from hospital and clinic records) was found to *increase* with increasing birthweight ($p = 0.05$). No information was provided on the completeness of case ascertainment.

In contrast, an analysis of the incidence of CHDe in relation to self-reported birthweight among the 121 000 women recruited in 1976 aged 30–55 to the US Nurses Health Study,[30] found very similar results to the Hertfordshire and Sheffield studies. As shown in Table 3.5, the incidence of non-fatal CHD (defined as reported non-fatal myocardial infarction or coronary revascularization) declined with increasing birthweight until the last birthweight category when there was again a small upturn in risk. Adjustment for (unspecified) 'coronary risk factors' did not substantially alter these estimates.

A powerful approach to investigating the robustness of a potential etiological association is to see whether it can be found across a range of cultures and ethnic groups. Barker and colleagues have investigated whether fetal growth is related to CHD in a study of 517 singleton men and women born in a maternity hospital in Mysore, Southern India between 1934 and 1954.[31] They found the prevalence of CHD to decline with increasing birthweight, head circumference and birth length.

Table 3.5. Rate ratios for non-fatal coronary heart disease (age 30–71) among women in the US Nurses' Health Study in relation to self-reported birthweight

Birthweight in lbs	
≤5	1.00
5.0–	0.81
5.6–	0.80
7.1–	0.74
8.6–	0.55
>10	0.65
p-value for trend	p < 0.02

Source : reference[30]

Results from studies in Uppsala, Sweden have recently been reported that also suggest that CHD mortality declines with increasing birthweight.[32] In 1970, all men resident in Uppsala who were born between 1920 and 1924 were invited to take part in a study of cardiovascular risk factors. Overall 82% of those invited took part in the survey. Of these, the birthweights and birth lengths for 1335 (60%) were traced in the obstetric and midwives' records.[33,34] Mortality from CHD from 1970 to 1994 showed the same reverse J-shaped relationship with birthweight (Table 3.6). Because information on socioeconomic position, as well as on a large number of cardiovascular risk factors, was collected at the start of follow up in 1970, it has been possible to control for potential confounding by socioeconomic factors in adulthood and look at potential physiological mediators between size at birth and CHD mortality. Strikingly, however, control for socioeconomic circumstances at age 50, as well as blood pressure, body mass index, and smoking at age 50, had very little effect on the rate ratios.

Finally, in a study of middle aged men from Caerphilly in Wales, the incidence of coronary heart events (death and non-fatal myocardial infarction) was again inversely associated with birthweight.[35] This association was not effected by adjustment for socioeconomic position in childhood and adult life or by conventional cardiovascular risk factors measured on entry to study at ages 45–59 years. Strikingly, this association was only found amongst men in the top third of body mass index with no significant relationship between birthweight and CHD for those in the bottom two-thirds of the distribution.[36]

Cerebrovascular disease is a rarer event than CHD and hence the number of events available for analysis in the various cohort studies is small. Nevertheless, results based on the Sheffield, Hertfordshire, and Uppsala studies[27,32] suggest that there is an inverse association between size at birth and mortality from

Table 3.6. Rate ratios for coronary heart disease mortality (age 50–74) among Uppsala men born 1920–24 in relation to birthweight

Birthweight in grams [lbs]		
<3250 [<7.15]	1.00	(33)
3250– [7.15–]	0.86	(47)
3750– [8.25–]	0.63	(27)
4250+ [9.35+]	0.70	(9)
p-value for trend	p=0.09	

Figures in parentheses are numbers of deaths.

stroke. In Uppsala, this appears to be a step effect, between those individuals who were born weighing less than 3250 g at birth and the rest of the cohort.

3.2.3.2 Twin studies

Several studies have used mortality in twins to test the hypothesis that impaired fetal growth is associated with an increase in CHD, as twins tend to be lighter and smaller at birth than singletons. A study based on the Swedish twin registry[37] found that the mortality of twins from CHD was *not* higher than found in the Swedish population as a whole, and among males was in fact 0.85 of the national level (95% CI 0.79-0.92). These findings are thus not consistent with those from birth cohort studies described above. However, the association between height and cardiovascular disease was consistent with other studies (see below). Within monozygotic and dizygotic pairs the twins who were the shorter of the pair had higher mortality from CHD. Results from the Danish twin registry[38] revealed the same, finding no difference in mortality between twins and singletons after age 6, or between monozygotic twins and dizygotic twins, the former tending to have lower birthweights than the latter. This study, however, did not present any data on cause-specific rates. One possible explanation for the lack of consistency between the twin and cohort studies may be that the type of growth retardation experienced by twins is qualitatively different to other forms of intrauterine growth retardation.

3.2.3.3 Possible interpretations of early life associations

A summary of the studies that have reported associations between birthweight and CHD provided in Table 3.7. With the exception of the Gothenburg study,[29] all of them suggest a decline in risk with increasing birthweight. This effect is seen in men and women, and is found with mortality, prevalence and occurrence of CHD events. The Gothenburg study is the smallest of the studies that have looked at the incidence of myocardial infarctions or death from CHD. In the light of the relatively consistent patterns seen across the other studies this inconsistent observation may be spurious. A final assessment of this contrary finding will have to wait for the publication of a more detailed account of the findings.

How far can these results be explained by confounding by adult socio-economic position and circumstances? Not all of the studies were able to address this issue, as data on adult circumstances and risk factor profiles were not available. The Uppsala and US Nurses Health Study, however, are both based on cohorts recruited in adult life for whom information on socio-economic circumstances and potential physiological mediators were measured at the start of the follow up period. In the Uppsala study,[32] adjustment for socioeconomic factors and smoking had minimal effect on the strength of the association between birthweight and CHD mortality. In the Nurses Health Study,[5] the published results do not indicate the specific effect of adjustment for socioeconomic position. However, adjustment for unspecified cardio-vascular risk factors was described as having little effect. In the Hertfordshire mortality follow up, information on social class in adult life was not available for the cohort as a whole, and so adjustment for socioeconomic confounding was not possible. In the Hertfordshire prevalence survey of CHD,[25] the same form of association was seen within social class categories as in the data set overall and no relationship was found between socioeconomic variables and left ventricular mass. Thus the associations between birthweight and CHD do not appear to be seriously confounded by adult socioeconomic position and other adult life style factors.

The majority of studies also note a striking elevation in mortality risk in the highest birthweight group(s) giving overall a 'reverse J' shaped association. The three studies in which this is not apparent[28,31,35] do not provide separate estimates for weights over 9lb (4.08kg). A possible explanation for this observation is that the group of very heavy births include an appreciable proportion of macrosomic babies from diabetic mothers with poor glycaemic control in pregnancy. These infants may have an increased risk of death from a number of conditions, including CHD, either because of the long-term effects of being exposed to high levels of glucose in utero, or because they may inherit a tendency to be diabetic themselves, which carries with it an increased risk of CHD.

As many of the studies, including Hertfordshire, were confined to singleton births alone, the observed effects are independent of multiplicity at birth. The associations of CHD with other birth dimensions and parameters (e.g. ponderal index, placental to birthweight ratio), have only been examined in a minority of the studies. The significance of these other parameters as distinct from birthweight (with which most are highly correlated) is unclear as spurious associations may have arisen from making multiple comparisons. However, potential distinctions in biological growth patterns should be exploited where the data permits. To this extent, the Sheffield studies importantly suggest that it is disproportionate growth retardation rather than birthweight *per se* that is of importance for CHD.

The Hertfordshire study alone included information on size at birth and at one year. It is thus difficult to assess significance of growth in infancy as distinct from growth in utero. A possible reason for the more linear association between CHD mortality (in men at least) with weight at 1 year rather than with birthweight, may lie again with the macrosomic babies delivered to diabetic mothers with poor glycaemic control in pregnancy. Although birth-weight generally tends to predict weight at 1 year, macrosomic infants may be an exception if they are subject to a 'catch-down' growth phenomenon in the absence of the in utero stimulus of high maternal glucose levels. Their increased

Table 3.7. Summary of studies of coronary heart disease in relation to birthweight

Study	Number with birth weight	Period of birth	Source of information on birthweight	Outcome	Number of deaths /cases	Age at death / examination (years)	Form of association	Comment
Men								
Hertfordshire, UK [5]	10,141	1911–30	Midwives' records	CHD mortality	853	20–81	Reverse-J	See table 3.2
Hertfordshire, UK [25]	290	1920–30	Midwives' records	CHD prevalence	42	mean age 69	Reverse-J	See table 3.3
Sheffield, UK [28]	1,586	1907–24	Hospital	All cardio-vascular mortality	316	27–83	Inverse	See table 3.4
Gothenburg, Sweden [29]	855	1913	Hospital/ midwives' records	Myocardial infarctions	not stated	50–75	Direct	
Mysore, India [31]	266	1934–54	Hospital	CHD prevalence	25	38–60	Weak inverse	Results only given for men and women combined
Uppsala, Sweden [32]	1,335	1920–24	Hospital/ midwives' records	CHD mortality	116	50–74	Reverse-J	See table 3.6
Caerphilly, Wales [35]	1,258	1920–38	Self-reported or recall by mother/ female relative	Incident CHD	137	45–69	Inverse	Birthweight grouped into quartiles

Women

Hertfordshire, UK [5]	5,585	1923-30	Midwives' records	CHD mortality	88	20-69	Reverse-J	See table 3.2
Nurses Health Study, USA [30]	121,000	1921-46	Self-reported	Non-fatal CHD events	917	30-71	Reverse-J	See table 3.5
Mysore, India [31]	251	1934-54	Hospital	CHD prevalence	27	38-60	(see men)	Results only given for men and women combined

mortality, would thus not be concentrated in the top categories of weight at one year.

3.2.4 Growth in childhood and adolescence

Adult height has been found to be inversely associated with risk of CHD in studies in the UK,[39–42] Scandinavia,[18,43,44] Italy[45] and the United States[46–48] Although the majority of these studies are of men, the same thing is found for women.[42,44–46,48] This association has generally been interpreted as indicating a role for risk factors operating in childhood,[39] although several other explanations have been considered. Confounding is an obvious possibility as poor socioeconomic circumstances in childhood are associated with poor growth and lower socioeconomic position in later life, which increases the CHD risk (see Chapter 8, Section 8.2.3, for further discussion). Adjusting for socioeconomic position in adult life, however, reduces the strength of the association only slightly.[40,48,49] Adjustment for a wider range of adult cardiovascular risk factors such as cholesterol levels, blood pressure and family history of myocardial infarction also reduces, but does not abolish the height association.[41,46,47,50] It has been suggested that respiratory function, as measured by FEV_1 is the key mediator between height and CHD[41] although this finding has not been confirmed in another study that explicitly set out to test this hypothesis.[40] In summary, although adult risk factors explain some of the association between height and CHD, we still lack a clear view of the biological basis of any association between childhood circumstances that effect height and subsequent disease risk.

One possibility is that genetic factors underlie the association, although the finding that diminished height is still associated with CHD mortality among monozygotic twins provides strong evidence that either developmental or environmental factors are of importance.[37] Some of the height-CHD association may be explained by differential 'shrinkage'; morbidity preceding death from CHD could lead to a reduction in measured height (reverse causality).[49] Thus, one of the few studies that failed to find a decrease in CHD mortality with increasing height,[51] specifically excluded subjects with evidence of cardiovascular disease at recruitment.

Recent work has shown an inverse association between stature in *childhood* and later CHD mortality,[52] which cannot be explained by a reduction in measured height due to morbidity. This study traced mortality of several thousand children aged 2–14 who had detailed dietary assessments and were examined between 1937 and 1939 in 14 centres across England and Scotland. It found that the component of childhood stature that showed the strongest association with CHD mortality was leg length rather than trunk length. Leg length is thought to be particularly sensitive to postnatal environmental influences such as dietary intake.

As height in childhood and adult life are positively correlated with birthweight, it is important to clarify how far the height effect simply reflects differences in fetal growth. Two studies[40,46] have attempted to look at height effects adjusted for birthweight, but in both cases this adjustment had no substantial effect upon the association of height with CHD mortality. Larger studies are required to establish firmly that birthweight and attained adult height are independent risk factors for CHD. It is possible that growth in pre- and postnatal life both influence CHD risk through different pathways.

3.2.5 Infections in childhood

The notion that infection may play a role in the pathogenesis of atherosclerosis has existed since the beginning of this century, but was inconsistent with early clinical studies as cases with CHD paradoxically reported fewer past infections than controls (see Chapter 2, Section 2.4).

Recent studies[53–60] have noted elevated serum antibody levels for subjects with CHD and specifically for *Chlamydia pneumoniae*, a respiratory pathogen, and *Helicobacter pylori*, an enteric pathogen. Most of these studies have relied on measuring immunological markers of infection on cases with existing heart disease, hence infection could occur after disease onset or as a consequence due to reactivation (reverse causality). However some studies have been able to measure levels on stored blood samples and demonstrate that elevation preceded clinical heart disease.[55,60] Results from the Helsinki Heart study[55] found that associations between *Chlamydia pneumoniae* and incident heart disease were stronger for IgA than for IgG titres indicating chronic persistent rather than acute infection. Samples taken 6 months before the cardiac event showed stronger relationships than those taken at recruitment into the study indicating that infection was acquired in adulthood rather than childhood. Similarly, seropositivity amongst cases with heart disease increases with age (19% amongst 45–49 year olds to 35% amongst 60–65 year olds).[57]

In contrast, *Helicobacter pylori* is more likely to be acquired in childhood, with a quarter of current children under the age of 6 being positive for infection rising to over 50% by the age of 12 or older.[61,62] Children in the past are more likely to have experienced infection with *Helicobacter pylori*, as exposure is associated with poor housing conditions, overcrowding, and sharing a bed with parents[61,62] An earlier ecological study had noted that infant mortality from diarrhoea and enteritis, as opposed to pneumonia, was a strong predictor of subsequent CHD.[63]

Poor socioeconomic status increases the likelihood of both infection with *Helicobacter pylori* and CHD and therefore any observed associations may be due to confounding. Two studies have demonstrated that the association between *Helicobacter pylori* and heart disease was independent of adult social class and detailed measures of childhood conditions,[56,59] whilst a third, from the British Regional Heart Study, found that the relationship was greatly weakened after adjustment for adult social class and other conventional risk factors.[60] *Helicobacter pylori* infection is also associated with diminished childhood growth amongst girls but not boys.[64] It may therefore also help to partially explain the relationship between adult height and CHD.

Several biological mechanisms have been proposed to causally link *Helicobacter pylori* with CHD. Seropositivity has been associated with increases in fibrinogen, total leucocyte count, and C reactive protein,[56,65] although one other study has failed to demonstrate raised fibrinogen.[59] C reactive protein has also been shown to be associated with a worse lipid profile, although it is not clear whether elevation is merely a marker of atherogenesis or the effect of chronic infection on cytokines which could effect both C reactive protein and lipid metabolism.[65]

3.2.6 Early onset of atherosclerosis

There is an established body of evidence that suggests strongly that atherosclerosis (the process whereby arteries become narrowed and damaged by deposition of fatty material) starts in childhood.[66] Autopsy studies of young US soldiers killed in the Korean and Vietnam wars[67,68] found widespread macroscopic evidence of arteriosclerosis. These results provided part of the motivation[69] to set up prospective studies of cardiovascular risk factors in children and young adults, which have now accumulated up to 15 years follow up.[70]

The Bogalusa Heart Study[71] was set up in 1973 to explore the childhood precursors of cardiovascular disease. A multiethnic population of approximately 8000 children have been examined several times with measurements including blood pressure, anthropometry, lipids, echocardiography and life style factors. This study has clearly demonstrated tracking[72,73] and clustering[74] of cardiovascular risk factor levels, such as blood pressure and lipids, between childhood and young adult life, consistent with pre-adult influences on later disease. Whether childhood risk factors have more direct effects on atherosclerosis is less clear. However, autopsy examinations have demonstrated that the prevalence and extent of fatty streaks in the aorta of children under the age of 10 years are correlated with a variety of cardiovascular risk factors measured prior to their death, including total cholesterol and blood pressure,[75] although the pathological and prognostic significance of these fatty streaks has yet to be firmly established.

More compelling evidence for childhood risk factors being associated with the onset of atherosclerosis comes from a recent analysis from the Muscatine Study,[76,77] set up in 1971, which screened over 15,000 children aged 6–18 years. A subgroup of the full study, composed of 197 men and 187 women, who had been examined at least once in childhood (mean age 15, range 8–18) and once between age 20–34, attended a third screening (mean age 33, range 29-37). Ultrafast computed tomography was used to detect calcification of the coronary arteries: an established correlate of atherosclerotic disease.[78] This was found in 30% of men and 10% of women, and was positively associated with childhood weight, body mass index and waist–hip ratio, independently of risk factors measured at subsequent examinations.[79]

These longitudinal studies from childhood to adult life will yield increasingly valuable insights into the aetiology of CHD. However, as yet, the cohorts are too young to see the extent to which the preadult risk factors are actually predictive of cardiovascular events. The addition of data on size at birth to these cohorts would enable a number of important questions to be addressed, in particular how far blood pressure and serum lipids in childhood mediate the association between growth in utero and the development of CHD. It is intriguing to consider the possibility that impaired growth in utero or childhood, or early infection, may influence the tempo and extent of early atherosclerosis, and hence risk of CHD in later life.

3.3 Breast cancer

The aetiology of breast cancer well illustrates the influence of preadult exposures and circumstances on disease in later life. Of the wide range of risk factors investigated,[80] a number are particularly relevant in this respect. These include age at first birth, adult height, age at menarche, size at birth and other perinatal factors. While age at first birth is one of the most firmly established risk factors, the intriguing hypothesis that breast cancer has origins in utero remains highly speculative.[81]

3.3.1 Age at first birth

The classic multicentre breast cancer case control study, conducted by MacMahon and colleagues,[82] was the first study to demonstrate that breast cancer risk increases linearly with age at first birth. Women who had completed teenage pregnancies were the most protected of all. Since then, a large number of other studies conducted throughout the world have shown a linear increase in the risk of breast cancer with increasing age at first birth, independent of other known risk factors.[83]

3.3.2 Adult height

The significance of nutrition and diet in the aetiology of breast cancer has been an area of considerable debate.[84] However, there is a view that nutrition and growth in childhood may be of particular importance.[85] In support of this line of argument it is frequently observed that adult height is directly associated with risk of breast cancer,[84,86] independent of age at menarche and reproductive history.[87,88] It has been noted that the minority of studies that do not find this association have not measured height directly.[87]

Height is the end result of genetic influences and nutritional and other environmental factors. Nutrition in childhood may influence breast composition but may also be confounded with later adult dietary factors. Alternatively, Swanson and colleagues[88] speculate that height reflects a common hormonal milieu in childhood, unrelated to nutrition, which both increases growth and the susceptibility to later breast cancer risk. Genetic and environmental factors may simply result in height being related to absolute breast tissue mass, which itself may be a risk factor for breast cancer.[89–91]

3.3.3 Age at menarche

Menstruation usually begins between the ages of 10 and 13 years. There exists a strong body of evidence showing that a younger age at menarche is associated with an increased risk of breast cancer[83] independently of other established risk factors including parity, age at first birth, and age at menopause.[87,92] Age at menarche appears to be inversely related to weight, height, and measures of adiposity.[93] Young female athletes, with a relatively high lean/fat tissue ratio, have delayed menarche.[94]

Two possible mechanisms have been proposed to explain this association. Women with early menarche will be exposed to a larger cumulative number of monthly hormonal cycles of oestrogen, which might directly increase the risk of malignancy. Alternatively, early menarche may lead to higher levels of oestrogens throughout reproductive life, although direct evidence for this is lacking.[95]

3.3.4 Perinatal and in utero influences

More recently, it has been hypothesized that breast cancer originates in utero, with the level of fetal exposure to oestrogens determining risk of subsequent breast cancer.[81] Part of the evidence used to formulate this hypothesis[96] was the finding that women whose mothers were relatively old at the time of their birth had an increased risk of breast cancer. A hospital-based case control study of several cancer sites had found associations between cancer risk and the age of the mother and father.[97] In particular, consistent with a number of earlier reports, they found that a 10 year increase in maternal age was associated with a 24% increased risk of breast cancer (95% CI 9–41%). These data were interpreted as suggesting an aetiological role for prenatal factors, explained by oestrogen levels in pregnancy going up with maternal age,[96] although this left unexplained why a slightly smaller effect (19%) in the same direction was found for paternal age (95% CI 7–33%). Since these early reports, however, the association between parental age and breast cancer risk appears less certain, with no clear pattern emerging across the various studies that have looked at this issue.[98]

Perinatal characteristics have been treated as proxy measures for levels of in utero exposure to oestrogens, with high birthweight indicating high levels and pre-eclampsia low levels of exposure. One of the first papers to look at perinatal characteristics directly in relation to breast cancer was a small case control study in Hawaii.[99] This failed to find any statistically significant associations between risk of breast cancer and birthweight, parental age, birth rank, gestation, or pregnancy complications. If anything, risk declined with increasing birthweight. The authors, however, picked out a doubling of risk associated with a history of pre-eclampsia as worthy of further investigation. Since this initial report, the results of two other studies of perinatal factors and breast cancer have been published.[98,100]

In a Swedish case control study[100] of 458 breast cancers registered between 1958 and 1990, a positive but non-significant association was found with placental weight, but no simple gradient was seen with birthweight. Its one significant finding was a *reduction* in risk associated with a history of pre-eclampsia or eclampsia (OR = 0.24, 95% CI 0.09–0.70). This was in the direction predicted by the 'in utero' hypothesis, although strikingly in the opposite direction to the earlier Hawaiin study,[99] an inconsistency that was not commented upon. The situation has not been clarified with the publication of the most recent data from two US case control studies.[98] This found a suggestion of increasing risk with increasing birthweight in premenopausal women, while the opposite was found for postmenopausal women.

Finally, a Swedish study[101] found that the prevalence of mammographic patterns thought to be predictive of breast cancer increased with placental weight. However, no association was seen with a history of pre-eclampsia/ eclampsia. These data, however, provides relatively weak evidence, as the issue of the association between mammographic patterns (as distinct from putative lesions) and breast cancer risk is contentious.

In summary, therefore, the direct evidence to support the 'in utero' hypothesis for breast cancer is inconsistent and no more than suggestive. Future research should resist spawning other indirect proxy measures for in utero exposure to oestrogens, until a clearer picture emerges of the association between breast cancer risk and pre-eclampsia and birthweight.

3.4 Childhood exposures and other cancers

Evidence exists for preadult exposures and circumstances having a role in the aetiology of a number of other cancer sites. For example, sunburn is an established risk factor for cutaneous malignant melanoma. Although it does not appear that sunburn in childhood is more risky than in adulthood,[102] children in the US tend to be three times more exposed to the sun than adults.[103] Reducing sun exposure and sunburn in childhood will have an impact on melanoma in adult life by reducing total cumulative exposure. Similar arguments can be made about smoking in childhood and subsequent risk of smoking-related cancers.

Infections in childhood and in pregnancy may also play a role in the aetiology of other adult cancers, as recently reviewed.[104] The epidemiology of persistent hepatitis B infection (mainly acquired in childhood) parallels that of liver cancer in many populations.[104] *Helicobacter pylori* (see above), also largely acquired in childhood and associated with poor living conditions,[61,62] is a cause of chronic gastritis, that is itself a risk factor for stomach cancer.[105] This fits with the almost universal finding that stomach cancer rates are highest in the poorest and most deprived sections of a population.[106] However, there is no evidence that age at infection itself is a risk factor for stomach cancer, childhood being relevant only in so far as this appears to be when most infection with *Helicobacter pylori* is initially acquired.

3.4.1 Perinatal associations with testis, ovarian and prostate cancer

Some evidence has been found for perinatal and in utero factors being implicated in the aetiology of cancers of the testis, prostate, and ovary. As with breast cancer, these are hypothesized to involve in utero or perinatal exposure to sex hormones.

The incidence of testicular cancer peaks in the third decade of life, implying that there may important preadult factors involved in its aetiology. Attention was first focused on prenatal circumstances by a case control study published in 1979,[107] which identified excessive nausea or exposure to exogenous hormones during the index pregnancy or a history of undescended testis as risk factors. It was suggested that all three risk factors were markers of high in utero exposure to oestrogen at the time of differentiation of the testis. A history of undescended testis has been found to be associated with testicular cancer in many subsequent studies, while the findings regarding nausea and exogenous oestrogen exposure in pregnancy have been inconsistent.

Fetal growth has shown inconsistent relationships with risk of testicular cancer in several studies. Two US case control studies[108,109] have found an increased risk with impaired growth; the first found that men weighing less than 6 lb (2.7 kg) at birth had an odds ratio of 3.2 (95% CI 1.2–8.4) compared with the rest, whilst the second found men who weighed 5 lb (2.27 kg) or less had an odds ratio of 13.5 (95% CI 2.9–86.6) relative to those weighing 7.1–8.0 lb (3.2–3.63 kg). However, the most recent study[110] to look at this question found that those weighing 2500–3999g at birth had the lowest risk. Relative to this group, those weighing <2500g and >3999g had odds ratios of 2.59 (95%CI 1.05–6.38) and 1.58 (95%CI 1.10–2.29) respectively.

The use of exogenous oestrogens during pregnancy and prepregnancy body mass index have been associated with an increased risk of ovarian cancer before age 35.[111] This study concluded that in utero exogenous hormone exposure in the first trimester of pregnancy is associated with ovarian germ cell tumours in adolescence. This finding, however, has not been replicated. The Hertfordshire study (see Section 3.2.3.1) found that weight at 1 year was positively associated with risk of death from ovarian cancer.[112] These data were regarded as consistent with in utero imprinting of the fetal hypothalamus effecting patterns of gonadotrophin release. An alternative interpretation argues that sex hormones in utero effect both fetal growth and the number of ovarian tissue stem cells, hence risk of ovarian cancer.[113]

An increased risk of prostatic cancer has been associated with a history of maternal pre-eclampsia,[114] being delivered after 35 weeks gestation,[114] and increasing birthweight.[115]

In summary, the evidence linking in utero circumstances and cancers of the testis, ovary and prostate is sparse. The young age at onset of testicular cancer is the strongest indication for preadult influences. Interpretation of future results should take account of the fact that birthweight and maternal conditions such as pre-eclampsia only provide crude proxy measures for the in utero hormonal milieu (see Chapter 7).

3.5 Conclusions

3.5.1 Models and mechanisms

The simplest form of preadult influence is where exposure to an established risk factor is known to extend back into early life. Childhood, and even prenatal life,[116] may be important in that they mark the start of, or contribute to, the cumulative exposure to a carcinogenic influence. This is illustrated well with respect to sunburn in childhood and risk of malignant melanoma and hepatitis B infection and primary liver cancer (see Section 3.4).

Breast cancer provides a disease model where events at several different phases of the life course probably play an important role. The age at which menarche occurs is well established as a risk factor for breast cancer (Section

3.3.3). The probable reason for this association is that it marks the start of exposure to monthly hormonal cycles, or is correlated with long term levels of oestrogen exposure.

The hypothesized mechanism which results in risk going up as age at first birth increases (see Section 3.3.1) is rather different to that proposed for the menarche effect. Within tissues which undergo continual renewal, such as the breast, stem cells constitute a core population that give rise to differentiated progeny. Experimental and observational studies suggest that many tumours, in the breast and other organs, arise from irreversible changes to these stem cells.[117] There is a consensus that a first pregnancy results in a reduction in the number of breast tissue stem cells (from which malignancies are believed to arise) or in their sensitivity to insult.[118,119] This is a model in which a life course event (a woman's first birth), results in a permanent change to subsequent disease susceptibility.

It has also been proposed that the total complement of stem cells in different tissues is determined initially by circumstances in utero.[113,120] This may provide a general explanation for associations between perinatal factors and later cancers, although as discussed above the current epidemiological evidence for such associations is equivocal.

These considerations have parallels with the concept of 'biological programming' proposed to account for the observed effects of fetal growth on subsequent risk of cardiovascular disease, hypertension and non-insulin dependent diabetes.[121] The notion that the nutritional and hormonal milieu of the fetus may permanently alter the structure and function of the adult organism, and hence susceptibility to disease, was first proposed by Frienkel in 1979[122,123] in his theory of *fuel-mediated teratogenesis* (see also Chapter 7). Both Frienkel and subsequent workers have hypothesized that impaired fetal growth could result in a suboptimal number of cells in various organs, giving rise to functional deficits in later life, expressed as a greater susceptibility to disease. Thus, a possible deficit in the number of pancreatic β cells at birth could predispose to non-insulin dependent diabetes,[124] while a deficit in kidney nephrons could increase susceptibility to hypertension.[125] However, it is unlikely that cell number is the only way in which in utero circumstances might effect later disease. Permanent changes to the sensitivity of cells to endocrine signals is also likely to be important,[126] as well as other pathways yet to be uncovered.

Discussion of the mechanisms that may underlie the association between CHD and birthweight[127] have tended to focus upon the mediating role of in utero effects on cardiovascular risk factors such as insulin resistance or deficiency (see Chapter 4), blood pressure (see Chapter 6), fibrinogen[35,128] and cholesterol.[129] On this basis, one might expect that the strength of association of birthweight with CHD events would be attenuated after controlling for potential intermediaries such as blood pressure. However, as discussed in

Section 3.2.3.1, the few studies that have been able to do this[32,35] fail to note any substantive change in the strength of this association. Further studies of this sort are clearly required. However, it is possible that blood pressure and other cardiovascular risk factors in middle age are inadequate measures of the long-term effects of these influences as determined by in utero factors. It may be that adult risk of cardiovascular events is more influenced by the extent of early stage atherosclerotic lesions in childhood. These appear to be correlated with cardiovascular risk factor levels in childhood (see Section 3.2.6). If this is the case, then it maybe these childhood risk factor levels, rather than those in adult life, that are of importance in mediating the in utero effects on CHD.

The mechanisms that might underlie the association of height with CHD and breast cancer have already been discussed (see Sections 3.2.4 and 3.3.2 respectively). The few studies that have examined whether the effect of adult height is confounded by size at birth[40,46] have reached negative conclusions. Further work on this question is required. However, the nature and regulation of prenatal and postnatal growth are different, and it is very probable that the mechanisms underlying the associations of growth with later disease in these two periods will be different.

Finally, the role of genetic as distinct from environmental factors on the observed associations between growth and later disease has yet to be determined. For non-insulin dependent diabetes at least (see Chapter 4), there is a prima facie case to answer that genetic factors may be important. Of course, it is likely that these associations may ultimately be shown to involve both genetic and environmental components.

3.5.2 Public health implications

The work on preadult influences on cardiovascular disease and cancer has obvious relevance to our understanding of basic disease mechanisms. However, the public health implications of this work are less clear. This is particularly so with respect to in utero determinants of cardiovascular disease, where there has been a tendency to overemphasize the significance of improved maternal nutrition (see Chapters 7 and 12). Nevertheless, over the next few years, more firmly based public health conclusions are likely to arise from this work on preadult factors. What is already clear is that giving credence to preadult factors should not be regarded as undermining the importance of the classic adult risk factors. There is already evidence that for blood pressure,[33] non-insulin dependent diabetes[34] and CHD,[52] adult risk factors such as obesity powerfully potentiate the susceptibilities that appear to be established in utero. A framework that places early life–adult interactions at its centre is likely to be the most fruitful.

References

Those marked with an asterisk are especially recommended for further reading

1   Murray CJL and Lopez AD, eds. *Global comparative assessments in the health sector. Disease burden, expenditures and intervention packages.* Geneva: World Health Organisation, 1994.

2   Elo IT, Preston SH. Effects of early life conditions on adult mortality: a review. *Popul Index* 1992;**58**:186–212.

3   Marmot M and Elliott P, eds. *Coronary heart disease epidemiology: from aetiology to public health.* Oxford: Oxford University Press, 1992.

4   Wadsworth MEJ. *The imprint of time : childhood, history, and adult life.* Oxford: Clarendon Press, 1991.

5* Osmond C, Barker DJP, Winter PD. Early growth and death from cardiovascular disease in women. *Br Med J* 1993;**307**:1519–24.

6   Forsdahl A. Are poor living conditions in childhood and adolesence an important risk factor for arteriosclerotic heart disease ? *Br J Prev Soc Med* 1977;**31**:91–5.

7   Williams DRR, Roberts SJ, Davies TW. Deaths from ischaemic heart disease and infant mortality in England and Wales. *J Epidemiol Community Health* 1979;**33**:199–202.

8   Barker DJP, Osmond C. Infant mortality, childhood nutrition, and ischaemic heart disease in England and Wales. *Lancet* 1986;**i**:1077–81.

9   Barker DJP, Osmond C, Golding J. Height and mortality in the counties of England and Wales. *Ann Hum Biol* 1990;**17**:1–6.

10 Barker DJP, Osmond C, Golding J, Kuh D, Wadsworth MEJ. Growth in utero, blood pressure in childhood and adult life, and mortality from cardiovascular disease. *Br Med J* 1989;**298**:564–7.

11 Whincup PH, Cook DG, Adshead F *et al.* Cardiovascular risk factors in British children from towns with widely differing adult cardiovascular mortality. *Br Med J* 1996;**313**:79–84.

12 Ben-Shlomo Y, Davey Smith G. Deprivation in infancy and adult life : which is more important for mortality risk ? *Lancet* 1991;**337**:530–4.

13 Strachan DP, Leon DA, Dodgeon B. Mortality from cardiovascular disease among interregional migrants in England and Wales. *Br Med J* 1995;**310**:423–7.

14 Elford J, Philips AN, Thomson AG, Shaper AG. Migration and geographic variations in ischaemic heart disease in Great Britain. *Lancet* 1989;**i**:343–6.

15 Kaplan BH, Cassel JC, Tyroler HA, Cornoni JC, Kleinbaum DG, Hames CG. Occupational mobility and coronary heart disease. *Arch Intern Med* 1971;**128**:938–42.

16   Gillum RF, Paffenbarger RSJ. Chronic disease in former college students. XVII. Sociocultural mobility as a precursor of coronary heart disease and hypertension. *Am J Epidemiol* 1978;**108**:289–98.

17   Burr ML, Sweetnam PM. Family size and paternal unemployment in relation to myocardial infarction. *J Epidemiol Community Health* 1980; **34**:93–5.

18   Notkola V, Punsar S, Karvonen MJ, Haapakoski J. Socioeconomic conditions in childhood and mortality and morbidity caused by coronary heart disease in adulthood in rural Finland. *Soc Sci Med* 1985;**21**:517–23.

19   Kaplan GA, Salonen JT. Socioeconomic conditions in childhood and ischaemic heart disease during middle age. *Br Med J* 1990;**301**:1121–3.

20   Lynch JW, Kaplan GA, Cohen RD *et al*. Childhood and adult socioeconomic status as predictors of mortality in Finland. *Lancet* 1994;**343**: 524–7.

21   Vågerö D, Leon DA. Social class in childhood and adulthood : how do they influence mortality? *Lancet* 1994;343:1224–5.

22   Barker DJP, Winter PD, Osmond C, Margetts B. Weight in infancy and death from ischaemic heart disease. *Lancet* 1989;**ii**:577–80.

23   Fall CHD, Barker DJP, Osmond C *et al*. The relation of infant feeding to adult serum cholesterol and death from ischaemic heart disease. *Br Med J* 1992;**304**:801–5.

24   Fall CHD, Osmond C, Barker DJP *et al*. Fetal and infant growth and cardiovascular risk factors in women. *Br Med J* 1995;**310**:428–32.

25   Fall CH, Vijayakumar M, Barker DJ *et al*. Weight in infancy and prevalence of coronary heart disease in adult life. *Br Med J* 1995;**310**:17–9.

26   Vijayakumar M, Fall CH, Osmond C, Barker DJ. Birth weight, weight at one year, and left ventricular mass in adult life. *Br Heart J* 1995;**73**: 363–7.

27   Martyn CN, Barker DJP, Osmond C. Mothers' pelvic size, fetal growth and death from stroke in men. *Lancet* 1996;**348**:1264–8.

28   Barker DJP, Osmond C, Simmonds SJ, Wield GA. The relation of small head circumference and thinness at birth to death from cardiovascular disease. *Br Med J* 1993;**306**:422–6.

29   Eriksson M, Tibblin G, Cnattingius S. Low birthweight and ischaemic heart disease. *Lancet* 1994;**343**:731.

30   Rich Edwards J, Stampfer M, Manson J *et al*. Birthweight, breastfeeding and the risk of coronary heart disease in the Nurses' Health Study. *Am J Epidemiol* 1995;**141**:S78.

31   Stein CE, Fall CHD, Kumaran K *et al*. Fetal growth and coronary heart disease in South India. *Lancet* 1996;**348**:1269–73.

32   Koupilova I, Leon DA. Birth weight and mortality from ischaemic heart disease and stroke in Swedish men aged 50–70 years (abstract). *J Epidemiol Community Health* 1996;**50**:592.

33 Leon DA, Koupilová I, Lithell HO *et al.* Failure to realise growth potential in utero and adult obesity in relation to blood pressure in 50 year old Swedish men. *Br Med J* 1996;**312**:401–6.

34 Lithell HO, McKeigue PM, Berglund L *et al.* Relationship of birth-weight and ponderal index to non-insulin-dependent diabetes and insulin response to glucose challenge in men aged 50–60 years. *Br Med J* 1996; **312**:406–10.

35* Frankel S, Elwood P, Sweetnam P *et al.* Birthweight, adult risk factors and incident coronary heart disease: the Caerphilly study. *Public Health* 1996; **110**:139–43.

36 Frankel S, Elwood P, Sweetnam P *et al.* Birth weight, body mass index in middle age, and incident coronary heart disease. *Lancet* 1996;**348**: 1478–80.

37* Vågerö D, Leon DA. Is heart disease mortality elevated in a low birth weight population? A test of the foetal origins hypothesis based on the Swedish Twins Registry. *Lancet* 1994;**343**:260–3.

38 Christensen K, Vaupel JW, Holm NV, Yashin AI. Mortality among twins after age 6: fetal origins hypothesis versus twin method. *Br Med J* 1995;**310**:432–6.

39 Marmot MG, Shipley MJ, Rose G. Inequalities in death specific explanations of a general pattern? *Lancet* 1984;**i**:1003–6.

40 Yarnell JWG, Limb ES, Layzell JM, Baker IA. Height : a risk marker for ischaemic heart disease : prospective results from the Caerphilly and Speedwell heart disease studies. *Eur Heart J* 1992;**13**:1602–5.

41 Walker M, Shaper AG, Phillips AN, Cook DG. Short stature, lung function and risk of a heart attack. *Int J Epidemiol* 1989;**18**:602–6.

42 Watt GCM, Hart CL, Hole DJ *et al.* Risk factors for cardiorespiratory and all cause mortality in men and women in urban Scotland: 15 year follow up. *Scott Med J* 1995;**40**:108–12.

43 Allbeck P, Bergh C. Height, body mass index and mortality: Do social factors explain the association? *Public Health* 1992;**106**:375–82.

44 Waaler HT. Height, Weight and Mortality. *Acta Med Scand* 1984; **(Suppl 679)**:1–56.

45 D'Avanzo B, La Vecchia C, Negri E. Height and the risk of acute myocardial infarction in Italian women. *Soc Sci Med* 1994;**38**:193–6.

46* Rich Edwards JW, Manson JE, Stampfer MJ *et al.* Height and the risk of cardiovascular disease in women. *Am J Epidemiol* 1995;**142**: 909–17.

47 Hebert PR, Rich Edwards JW, Manson JE *et al.* Height and incidence of cardiovascular disease in male physicians. *Circulation* 1993;**88**: 1437–43.

48 Palmer JR, Rosenberg L, Shapiro S. Stature and the risk of myocardial infarction in women. *Am J Epidemiol* 1990;**132**:27–32.

49 Leon DA, Davey Smith G, Shipley M, Strachan DP. Adult height and mortality in London: early life, socioeconomic confounding or shrinkage? *J Epidemiol Community Health* 1995;**49**:5–9.

50 Davey Smith G, Shipley MJ, Rose G. Magnitude and causes of socio-economic differentials in mortality: further evidence from the Whitehall Study. *J Epidemiol Community Health* 1990;**44**:265–70.

51 Yao CH, Slattery ML, Jacobs DR *et al*. Anthropometric predictors of coronary heart disease and total mortality: Findings from the US railroad study. *Am J Epidemiol* 1991;**134**:1278–89.

52 Gunnell DJ, Davey Smith G, Frankel S *et al*. Childhood leg length and adult mortality-followup of the Carnegie Survey of diet and growth in prewar Britain. *J Epidemiol Community Health* 1996;**50**:580–1.

53 Mattila KJ. Viral and bacterial infections in patients with acute myocardial infarction. *J Intern Med* 1989;**225**:293–6.

54 Thom DH, Grayston JT, Siscovick DS *et al*. Association of prior infection with *Chlamydia pneumoniae* and angiographically demonstrated coronary artery disease. *JAMA* 1992;**268**:68–72.

55 Saikku P, Leinonen M, Tenkanen L *et al*. Chronic *Chlamydia pneumoniae* infection as a risk factor for coronary heart disease in the Helsinki Heart Study. *Ann Intern Med* 1992;**116**:273–8.

56 Patel P, Mendall MA, Carrington D *et al*. Association of *Helicobacter pylori* and *Chlamydia pneumoniae* infections with coronary heart disease and cardiovascular risk factors. *Br Med J* 1995;**311**:711–4.

57 Mendall MA, Carrington D, Strachan D *et al*. *Chlamydia pneumoniae*: risk factors for seropositivity and association with coronary heart disease. *J Infect* 1995;**30**:121–8.

58 Martin de Argila C, Boixeda D, Canton R. High seroprevalence of *Helicobacter pylori* infection in coronary heart disease. *Lancet* 1995; **346**:310.

59 Murray LJ, Bamford KB, O'Reilly DP *et al*. *Helicobacter pylori* infection: relation with cardiovascular risk factors, ischaemic heart disease, and social class. *Br Heart J* 1995;**74**:497–501.

60* Whincup PH, Mendall MA, Perry IJ *et al*. Prospective relations between *Helicobacter pylori* infection, coronary heart disease, and stroke in middle aged men. *Heart* 1996;**75**:568–72.

61 McCallion WA, Murray LJ, Bailie AG *et al*. *Helicobacter pylori* infection in children relation with current household living conditions. *Gut* 1996;**39**:18–21.

62 Mendall MA, Goggin PM, Molineaux N *et al*. Childhood living conditions and *Helicobacter pylori* seropositivity in adult life. *Lancet* 1992;**339**:896–7.

63 Buck C, Simpson H. Infant diarrhoea and subsequent mortality from heart disease and cancer. *J Epidemiol Community Health* 1982;**36**:27–30.

64   Patel P, Mendall MA, Khulusi S *et al. Heliobacter pylori* infection in childhood: risk factors and effect on growth. *Br Med J* 1994;**309**: 1119–23.

65   Mendall MA, Patel P, Ballam L *et al.* C reactive protein and its relation to cardiovascular risk factors: a population based cross sectional study. *Br Med J* 1996;**312**:1061–65.

66   Berenson GS, Srinivasan SR, Freedman DS *et al.* Atherosclerosis and its evolution in childhood. *Am J Med Sci* 1987;**294**:429–40.

67   Enos WF, Holmes RH, Beyer J. Coronary disease among United States soldiers killed in action in Korea: preliminary report. *JAMA* 1953; **152**: 1090–3.

68   McNamara JJ, Molot MA, Stremple JF. Cutting RT. Coronary artery disease in combat casualties in Vietnam. *JAMA* 1971;**216**:1185–7.

69*   Berenson GS, Wattigney WA, Bao W *et al.* Rationale to study the early natural history of heart disease: the Bogalusa Heart Study. *Am J Med Sci* 1995;**310 (Suppl 1)**:S22–8.

70   Lenfant C, Savage PJ. The early natural history of atherosclerosis and hypertension in the young: National Institutes of Health perspectives. *Am J Med Sci* 1995;**310 (Suppl 1)**:S3–7.

71   Berenson GS, MacMahan CA, Voors AW *et al. Cardiovascular Risk Factors in Children The Early Natural History of Atherosclerosis and Essential Hypertension.* New York: Oxford University Press, 1980.

72   Myers L, Coughlin SS, Webber LS. Prediction of adult cardiovascular multifactorial risk status from childhood risk factor levels. The Bogalusa Heart Study. *Am J Epidemiol* 1995;**142**:918–24.

73   Wattigney WA, Webber LS, Srinivasan SR, Berenson GS. The emergence of clinically abnormal levels of cardiovascular disease risk factor variables among young adults: the Bogalusa Heart Study. *Prev Med* 1995;**24**:617–26.

74   Bao W, Srinivasan SR, Wattigney WA, Berenson GS. Persistence of multiple cardiovascular risk clustering related to syndrome X from childhood to young adulthood. The Bogalusa Heart Study. *Arch Intern Med* 1994;**154**:1842–7.

75   Tracy RE, Newman WP, Wattigney WA, Berenson GS. Risk factors and atherosclerosis in youth autopsy findings of the Bogalusa Heart Study. *Am J Med Sci* 1995;**310 (Suppl 1)**:S37–41.

76   Lauer RM, Connor WE, Leaverton PE *et al.* Coronary heart disease risk factors in school children: the Muscatine Study. *J Pediatr* 1975;**86**: 697–706.

77   Lauer RM, Lee J, Clarke WR. Factors affecting the relationship between childhood and adult cholesterol levels: the Muscatine Study. *Pediatrics* 1988;**82**:309–18.

78   Eggen DA, Strong JP, McGill HCJ. Coronary calcification. Relationship

to clinically significant coronary lesions and race, sex, and topographic distribution. *Circulation* 1965;**32**:948–55.

79* Mahoney LT, Burns TL, Stanford W *et al.* Coronary risk factors measured in childhood and young adult life are associated with coronary artery calcification in young adults: the Muscatine Study. *J Am Coll Cardiol* 1996;**27**:277–84.

80 Kelsey JL. Breast cancer epidemiology : summary and future directions. *Epidemiol Rev* 1993;**15**:256–63.

81 Trichopoulos D. Hypothesis : does breast cancer originate in utero? *Lancet* 1990;**335**:939–40.

82 MacMahon B, Cole P, Lin TM *et al.* Age at first birth and breast cancer risk. *Bull WHO* 1970;**43**:209–21.

83 Kelsey JL, Gammon MD, John EM. Reproductive factors and breast cancer. *Epidemiol Rev* 1993;**15**:36–47.

84 Hunter DJ, Willett WC. Nutrition and breast cancer. *Cancer Causes Control* 1996;**7**:56–68.

85 de Waard F, Trichopoulos D. A unifying concept of the aetiology of breast cancer. *Int J Cancer* 1988;**41**:666–9.

86 Howe GR, Hirohata T, Hislop TG, et al. Dietary factors and risk of breast cancer: combined analysis of 12 case-control studies. *J Natl Cancer Inst* 1990;**82**:561–9.

87 De Stavola BL, Wang DY, Allen D *et al.* The association of height, weight, menstrual and reproductive events with breast cancer: results from two prospective studies on the island of Guernsey (United Kingdom). *Cancer Causes Control* 1993;**4**:331–40.

88 Swanson CA, Coates RJ, Schoenberg JB *et al.* Body size and breast cancer risk among women under age 45 years. *Am J Epidemiol* 1996;**143**:698–706.

89 Albanes D, Jones DY, Schatzkin A *et al.* Adult stature and risk of cancer. *Cancer Res* 1988;**48**:1658–62.

90 Albanes D, Winick M. Are cell number and cell proliferation risk factors for cancer? *J Natl Cancer Inst* 1988;**80**:772–5.

91 Trichopoulos D, Lipman RD. Mammary gland mass and breast cancer risk. *Epidemiology* 1992;**3**:523–6.

92 Hsieh CC, Trichopoulos D, Katsouyanni K, Yuasa S. Age at menarche, age at menopause, height and obesity as risk factors for breast cancer: associations and interactions in an international case-control study. *Int J Cancer* 1990;**46**:796–800.

93 Moisan J, Meyer F, Gingras S. A nested case-control study of the correlates of early menarche. *Am J Epidemiol* 1990;**132**:953–61.

94 Frisch RE, Gotz Welbergen AV, McArthur JW *et al.* Delayed menarche and amenorrhea of college athletes in relation to age of onset of training. *JAMA* 1981;**246**:1559–63.

95 Bernstein L, Pike MC, Ross RK, Henderson BE. Age at menarche and oestrogen concentrations of adult women. *Cancer Causes Control* 1991; **2**:221–5.

96 Trichopoulos D. Is breast cancer initiated in utero? *Epidemiology* 1990; **1**:95–6.

97 Janerich DT, Hayden CL, Thompson WD. Epidemiologic evidence of perinatal influence in the aetiology of adult cancers. *J Clin Epidemiol* 1989;**42**:151–7.

98 Sanderson M, Williams MA, Malone KE *et al*. Perinatal factors and the risk of breast cancer. *Epidemiology* 1996;**7**:34–7.

99 Le Marchand L, Kolonel LN, Myers BC, Mi MP. Birth characteristics of premenopausal women with breast cancer. *Br J Cancer* 1988;**57**: 437–9.

100 Ekbom A, Trichopoulos D, Adami HO *et al*. Evidence of prenatal influences on breast cancer risk. *Lancet* 1992;**340**:1015–8.

101 Ekbom A, Thurfjell E, Hsieh CC *et al*. Perinatal characteristics and adult mammographic patterns. *Int J Cancer* 1995;**61**:177–80.

102 Whiteman D, Green A. Melanoma and sunburn. *Cancer Causes Control* 1994;**5**:564–72

103 Truhan AP. Sun protection in childhood. *Clin Pediatr Phila* 1991;**30**: 676–81.

104 Hall AJ, Peckham CS. Infections in childhood and pregnancy as a cause of adult disease: methods and examples. *Brit Med Bull* (in press).

105 EUROGAST Study Group. An international association between *Helicobacter pylori* infection and gastric cancer. *Lancet* 1993;**341**:1359–62.

106 Leon DA. *Longitudinal Study: Social distribution of cancer, 1971–75*. OPCS Series LS No. 3. London: HMSO, 1988.

107 Henderson BE, Benton B, Jing J *et al*. Risk factors for cancer of the testis in young men. *Int J Cancer* 1979;**23**:598–602.

108 Depue RH, Pike MC, Henderson BE. Estrogen exposure during gestation and risk of testicular cancer. *J Natl Cancer Inst* 1983;**71**:1151–5.

109 Brown LM, Pottern LM, Hoover RN. Prenatal and perinatal risk factors for testicular cancer. *Cancer Res* 1986;**46**:4812–6.

110 Akre O, Ekbom A, Hsieh CC. Testicular nonseminoma and seminoma in relation to perinatal characteristics. *J Natl Cancer Inst* 1996;**88**:883–9.

111 Walker AH, Ross RK, Haile RW, Henderson BE. Hormonal factors and risk of ovarian germ cell cancer in young women. *Br J Cancer* 1988;**57**: 418–22.

112 Barker DJ, Winter PD, Osmond C *et al*. Weight gain in infancy and cancer of the ovary. *Lancet* 1995;**345**:1087–8.

113 Lipworth L, Trichopoulos D *et al*. Weight gain in infancy and cancer of the ovary. *Lancet* 1995;**345**:1515.

114 Ekbom A, Hsieh CC, Lipworth L *et al.* Perinatal characteristics in relation to incidence of and mortality from prostate cancer. *Br Med J* 1996;**313**:37–341.

115 Tibblin G, Eriksson M, Cnattingius S, Ekbom A. High birthweight as a predictor of prostate cancer risk. *Epidemiology* 1995;**6**:423–4.

116 Yamasaki H, Loktionov A, Tomatis L. Perinatal and multigenerational effect of carcinogens: possible contribution to determination of cancer susceptibility. *Environ Health Perspect* 1992;**98**:39–43

117 Editorial. Stem cells in neoplasia. *Lancet* 1989;**i**:701–2.

118 Moolgavkar SH, Day NE, Stevens RG. Two-stage model for carcinogenesis: Epidemiology of breast cancer in females. *J Natl Cancer Inst* 1980;**65**:559–69.

119 Albrektsen G, Heuch I, Tretli S, Kvale G. Breast cancer incidence before age 55 in relation to parity and age at first and last births : A prospective study of one million Norwegian women. *Epidemiology* 1994;**5**:604–11.

120* Trichopoulos D, Lipworth L. Is cancer causation simpler than we thought, but more intractable? *Epidemiology* 1995;**6**:347–9.

121 Lucas A. Programming by early nutrition in man. In: Bock GR, Whelan J, eds. *The childhood environment and adult disease. Ciba Foundation Symposium 156.* Chichester: Wiley, 1991;38–50.

122 Freinkel N, Metzger BE. Pregnancy as a tissue culture experience : the critical implications of maternal metabolism for fetal development. In: *Pregnancy metabolism, diabetes and the fetus. Ciba Foundation Symposium No. 63.* Amsterdam: Excerpta Medica, 1979;3–23.

123 Freinkel N. Banting Lecture 1980 : Of pregnancy and progeny. *Diabetes* 1980;**29**:1023–35.

124 Hales CN, Barker DJP, Clark PMS *et al.* Fetal and infant growth and impaired glucose tolerance at age 64. *Br Med J* 1991;**303**:1019–22.

125 Mackenzie HS, Brenner BM. Fewer nephrons at birth: a missing link in the aetiology of essential hypertension? *Am J Kidney Dis* 1995;**26**:91–8.

126 Aerts L, Pijnenborg R, Verhaeghe J *et al.* Fetal growth and development. In: Dornhorst A, Hadden DR, eds. *Diabetes and pregnancy: an international approach to diagnosis and management.* John Wiley & Sons Ltd, 1996; 77–97.

127* Barker DJP. Fetal origins of coronary heart disease. *Br Med J* 1995;**311**:171–4.

128 Barker DJP, Meade TW, Fall CHD *et al.* Relation of fetal and infant growth to plasma fibronogen and factor VII concentrations in adult life. *Br Med J* 1992;**304**:148–52.

129 Barker DJP, Hales CN, Fall CHD *et al.* Type 2 (non-insulin dependent) diabetes mellitus, hypertension and hyperlipidaemia (syndrome X); relation to fetal growth. *Diabetologia* 1993;**36**:62–7.

4 Diabetes and insulin action

Paul McKeigue

This chapter reviews the evidence that the risk of non-insulin dependent diabetes in adult life may be set by nutrition and growth in fetal life. Two studies in England have found a strong inverse association between birthweight and the prevalence of glucose intolerance in later life. The association of reduced size at birth with non-insulin dependent diabetes has since been confirmed in three other populations, although the relationship was less strong than in the original studies of English populations, and the form of the relationship was non-linear. Other studies in children and young adults have shown that plasma glucose levels after oral glucose challenge are inversely related to birthweight. Recent studies suggest that glucose intolerance is related more strongly to thinness at birth, measured by low ponderal index, than to low birthweight. This association is not accounted for by known predictors of diabetes such as obesity. Although the association between glucose intolerance and birthweight depends on adjusting for body mass index, this does not apply to the association of glucose intolerance with thinness at birth. Suggestions that the association can be accounted for by selective survival of low birthweight infants genetically predisposed to diabetes are not compatible with historical data on infant mortality rates.

The association between size at birth and diabetes could be mediated through impairment of insulin secretion, resistance to the action of insulin in lowering blood glucose levels, or both. Although there is experimental evidence that severe under-nutrition in early life can lead to impaired insulin secretion, epidemiological studies have failed to demonstrate that reduced size at birth predicts impaired β-cell function in normoglycaemic individuals. Such studies have found instead that thinness at birth predicts resistance to insulin-mediated glucose uptake and defects in muscle fuel utilization. However, there is as yet no experimental model in which undernutrition in utero causes insulin resistance in adult life. In the general population, insulin resistance commonly occurs as part of a cluster of physiological disturbances including hypertension and lipid disturbances. Although reduced size at birth predicts both insulin resistance and hypertension, it does not predict the lipid disturbances usually associated with insulin resistance and obesity: thus the insulin resistance syndrome is not simply a 'small baby syndrome'.

The association of thinness at birth with insulin resistance and glucose intolerance in adult life could have a genetic or an environmental explanation. Because insulin regulates fetal growth, it is at least plausible that the association results from a primary genetic defect in insulin action. It may be possible to test this by studying how the association varies between sets of relatives who share genes and maternal environment to varying extents. It has been suggested also that the high rates of non-insulin dependent diabetes in some non-European populations such as Native Americans result from under-nutrition in early life: this 'thrifty phenotype' hypothesis has been proposed as an alternative to the usual 'thrifty genotype' explanation. However, there is compelling evidence from studies of migrants and admixed populations that differences in diabetes prevalence between high risk and low risk populations are at least partly attributable to genetic factors. Whatever the physiological and molecular basis of the association between reduced size at birth and glucose intolerance in adult life, prevention and control of obesity in adult life is likely to be the most effective measure to reduce the risk of diabetes in those who were thin at birth.

4.1 Introduction

Non-insulin dependent diabetes has long been recognized as a common disease in obese sedentary adults.[1] The prevalence increases almost exponentially with age: in high risk populations such as urban Indians, the prevalence is about 5% by age 40 years,[2,3] whereas in low risk populations such as northern Europeans this prevalence is not reached until about age 55 years.[3] Central deposition of body fat,[3] low physical activity,[4] and a family history of non-insulin-dependent diabetes[5] predict the disease independently of weight for height. Suggestions that early malnutrition could predispose to diabetes were based on clinical descriptions of malnutrition-associated diabetes and animal experiments in which undernutrition in early life produced lasting impairment of the insulin response to glucose.[6] It was therefore a natural extension of the fetal origins hypothesis to explore the possibility that reduced size at birth would predict the development of impaired glucose tolerance and non-insulin dependent diabetes in later life. This depends on being able to trace records of size at birth from at least 50 years ago, unless the risk of diabetes in the population under study is so high that the disease is common before this age.

4.2 Epidemiological studies relating glucose tolerance to size at birth

Five studies have examined the relation of size at birth to impaired glucose tolerance or non-insulin dependent diabetes in later life (Table 4.1).

4.2.1 Hertfordshire

In this study 408 of 1157 men born in Hertfordshire between 1920 and 1930 underwent glucose tolerance tests at a mean age of 64 years.[7] Glucose intolerance was defined by a 2 h glucose of 7.8 mmol/l or more. There was a linear inverse relationship between prevalence of glucose intolerance and birthweight, from 14% prevalence in the highest two birthweight categories to 36% in the lowest two birthweight categories. Adjustment for body mass index strengthened the relationship: the adjusted odds ratios for prevalence in the highest birthweight category compared with the lowest was 6.6. There was an equally strong relationship between glucose intolerance and weight at 1 year.

4.2.2 Preston

Oral glucose tolerance tests were administered to 266 men and women born in a hospital in Preston between 1935 and 1943, at a mean age of 50 years.[8] Prevalence of glucose intolerance showed a linear inverse relationship to birthweight. There was a similar relationship with ponderal index. Gestational age at birth (estimated from the date of last menstrual period) was similar in those with and without glucose intolerance. In a further regression analysis with 2 h glucose as the dependent variable, both shortness at birth (defined by a high ratio of head circumference to birth length), and thinness at birth (defined by low ponderal index) independently predicted diabetes.

Table 4.1 Studies relating diabetes or impaired glucose tolerance to size at birth

Population	N	Age	Outcome	Measurement of size at birth	Form of relation	Odds ratio highest/ lowest categories
Hertfordshire men[7]	468	64	IGT/new NIDDM	Birthweight	Linear	6.6*
Preston adults[8]	266	46–54	IGT/new NIDDM	Birthweight	Linear	6.4*
Pima-American adults[12]	1179	20–39	NIDDM	Birthweight	U-shaped	3.8*
US male health professionals[11]	22693	61	Diagnosed NIDDM	Birthweight (recalled)	Non-linear	1.9
Uppsala men[10]	1093	60	NIDDM	(i) birthweight (ii) ponderal index	Stepwise Stepwise	1.9, 2.3* 4.4*

* adjusted for body mass index

4.2.3 Uppsala

At age 50 years 2322 men living in the municipality of Uppsala who were born between 1920 and 1924 were examined.[9] Fasting samples were taken from all participants, and an intravenous glucose tolerance test was performed on the last 1692 participants. The 2139 participants who were still resident in Uppsala were invited for re-examination 10 years later (at age 60 years), and oral glucose tolerance tests were performed on all those whose fasting glucose was 5.7 mmol/l or higher. Birthweight records were traced for 61% of the 2200 men who had been born in Sweden and examined in 1970-73.[10]

When prevalence of diabetes at age 60 years was compared across the four birthweight groups, there was a stepwise increase in diabetes prevalence in the lowest birthweight category (less than 3.25 kg). This association was statistically significant only when adjusted for body mass index. There was a stronger stepwise association of diabetes with low ponderal index: prevalence of diabetes was three times higher in the lowest quintile of ponderal index than in the other four quintiles. This association was independent of body mass index. There was no clear relationship between prevalence of diabetes and birth length: prevalence was highest in the top and bottom quintiles of birth length, and the variation between quintiles was just statistically significant at $p = 0.05$.

4.2.4 US male health professionals

A survey of 22 693 men who had participated in the Health Professionals Follow-up Study were surveyed by questionnaire at a mean age of 61 years.[11] Five groupings of recalled birthweight were defined. With the middle group (birthweight 7–8.4 lb (3.2–3.8 kg)) as referent category, the odds ratio for diabetes was 1.9 in those in the lowest birthweight group (birthweight <5 lb (2.5 kg)) and 1.4 in the next highest birthweight group (5.5–6.9 lb (2.5–3.1 kg)). At higher levels of birthweight there was no trend in diabetes prevalence.

4.2.5 Native Americans

In Pima Native Americans the prevalence of diabetes is high even before the age of 40 years, and cohort studies with diabetes as an end point can be undertaken on young adults. 1179 Pimas whose birthweights had been recorded between 1965 and 1972 were examined between ages 20 and 39 years.[12] There was a U-shaped relationship between birthweight and the prevalence of diabetes. Prevalence of diabetes was raised only in those with birthweight less than 2.5 kg or more than 4.5 kg. Although the odds ratio for diabetes in those with low birthweight compared with those with normal birthweight was 3.8, the excess risk associated with low birthweight accounted for only 6% of all cases in the population. When maternal diabetes was included in the model, the excess prevalence in the high birthweight group was no longer significant.

4.2.6 Studies in young adults and children

These studies of glucose intolerance in older adults have been supplemented by other studies of fasting or post-load glucose levels in younger adults or children, for whom records of size at birth are more likely to be available (Table 4.2). As we do not know whether raised glucose levels in children predict diabetes in later life, these studies do not provide direct evidence of a relationship between size at birth and the risk of diabetes. In 40 men aged 21 years who had been born in a Southampton hospital, there was an inverse relationship between birthweight and glucose levels at 30 minutes after an oral glucose load.[13] In contrast, a study in San Antonio, Texas, found no associations of birthweight with fasting or 2 h glucose in 541 Mexican-Americans and Anglos examined at a mean age of 32 years, after adjusting for age, sex, and ethnicity.[14]

Two studies in children have measured glucose levels at 30 minutes after oral glucose challenge. In Pune, India, 379 4 year old children whose birthweights had been recorded in hospital were studied.[15] The 30-min glucose levels were inversely correlated with birthweight in those who had been on the routine postnatal wards, but not in those who had been admitted to the special care baby unit. In Salisbury, England, 30-minute glucose levels were inversely related to ponderal index but not to birthweight in a sample of 250 7 year old children.[16] As an alternative to measuring plasma glucose, glycated haemoglobin levels can be used as a measure of average plasma glucose levels. In a Jamaican study 659 children who were born in the University Hospital were

Table 4.2 Studies relating glucose levels in children and young adults to size at birth

Population	N	Age	Outcome	Measurement
Southampton men[13]	40	21	30-min glucose	Birthweight
Mexican-American adults[14]	541	31	Fasting glucose	Birthweight
Pune children[15]	379	4	30-min glucose	Birthweight
Salisbury children[16]	250	7	30-min glucose	Ponderal index
Jamaican children[17]	659	6–16	Glycated haemoglobin	Birth length

examined at ages from 6 to 16 years.[17] Children who were shorter at birth had thicker triceps skinfolds and higher glycated haemoglobin levels.

4.2.7 Summary

A consistent finding in these studies is that in populations of European descent, where gestational diabetes is uncommon, there is a consistent association of reduced size at birth with raised glucose levels in children and with glucose intolerance in adults. Where measurements of birth length are available, the association of glucose intolerance with low ponderal index is generally stronger than the association with low birthweight. In populations at high risk for diabetes, such as Native Americans or Mexican-Americans, the inverse relationship between glucose intolerance and size at birth is less clear, and the relationship may be U-shaped or flat. A possible explanation for this reversal of the direction of association is that in high risk populations the prevalence of glucose intolerance in pregnancy is high. The infants of these mothers will be large at birth because of fetal hyperinsulinaemia, and will also be predisposed to develop diabetes in adult life because of the genes inherited from their mothers and possibly also because raised glucose levels in fetal life lead to permanent impairment of glucose homeostasis. If this explanation is correct, restricting the analysis to infants of mothers who were unlikely to have had glucose intolerance during pregnancy, for instance by excluding older mothers and those who were later diagnosed diabetic, would strengthen the inverse relationship between prevalence of diabetes and size at birth in populations where gestational diabetes is common.

4.3 Can selective survival or confounding account for the association?

One of the criticisms of the fetal origins hypothesis has been that the association between glucose intolerance and birthweight depends to some extent on adjustment for adult body mass index.[18] Body mass index is strongly related to prevalence of diabetes, and also has a weak positive correlation ($r = 0.1$) with birthweight.[10] Associations adjusted for body mass index are difficult to interpret because of uncertainties about what underlying physiological variables are adjusted for. Weight for height indexes a combination of factors including fat mass, lean tissue mass and skeletal proportions. Adiposity probably underlies the association of glucose intolerance with raised body mass index, whereas it is possible that lean tissue mass underlies the correlation of adult body mass index with birthweight. If so, then at any level of body mass index the percentage body fat would be higher in those who were small at birth than in those who were large at birth. Adjusting for body mass index could thus produce an association between diabetes and low birthweight simply because of confounding by adiposity. This argument does not apply to the association with ponderal index shown in Uppsala, as ponderal index at birth is uncorrelated with adult body mass index. Low ponderal index may be a more specific indicator of fetal malnutrition than is low birthweight.[19]

Others have suggested that the inverse association between fetal growth and diabetes could be accounted for by an inverse association between genetic susceptibility to diabetes and mortality among low birthweight infants:[12,20] in other words, that low birthweight infants are more likely to survive if they are genetically predisposed to diabetes. The Uppsala results are not consistent with this explanation: when the men in this cohort were born in 1920–24, the infant mortality rate in Uppsala County was around 60 per 1000 live births, similar to the national rate for Sweden.[21] Even if all these deaths had occurred in the lowest quintile of ponderal index among infants who were not susceptible to diabetes, such selection at birth could account only for a prevalence ratio for diabetes in adults of 1.3 in the lowest quintile compared to the other four quintiles. This contrasts with the observed prevalence ratio of 3.0.

4.4 Insulin resistance or impaired insulin secretion?

Plasma glucose levels are regulated by the β-cells of the pancreatic islets, which sense the glucose level in the extracellular fluid and respond to raised levels by secreting insulin. Insulin lowers plasma glucose by stimulating uptake of glucose from the blood (mainly by skeletal muscle) and by suppressing production of glucose by the liver. Failure to keep plasma glucose down to normal levels implies either that the secretion of insulin is inadequate, or that there is resistance to the action of insulin in lowering plasma glucose. To explain the association between reduced fetal growth and glucose intolerance, Hales and colleagues initially suggested that inadequate fetal nutrition might impair the development of the endocrine pancreas:[7] on this hypothesis the pathways of association between low birthweight and non-insulin-dependent diabetes would be as in Fig. 4.1.

More recent work has led the Southampton–Cambridge group to suggest instead that the association between glucose intolerance and reduced size at birth may be mediated through an effect of malnutrition in fetal life leading to thinness at birth and insulin resistance in adult life.[22,23] The pathways by which this would give rise to an association between thinness at birth and non-insulin dependent diabetes are shown in Fig. 4.2. This is in line with other evidence that insulin resistance has a primary role in the pathogenesis of non-insulin dependent diabetes.[24] Thus insulin resistance measured by euglycaemic clamp or intravenous glucose tolerance test predicts diabetes in high risk groups such as Pima Americans[25] or first-degree relatives of those

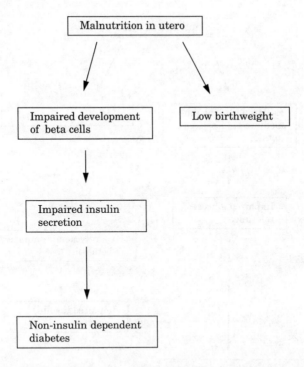

Figure 4.1 How impaired β-cell function could mediate an effect of malnutrition in utero on reduced size at the risk of diabetes in adult life

with non-insulin-dependent diabetes.[26] Obesity and central obesity, which are strongly associated with insulin resistance, predict diabetes in the general population.[27] Defects in β-cell function, such as loss of the acute insulin response to glucose challenge, are seen in people with impaired glucose tolerance and non-insulin dependent diabetes, but may be a consequence of hyperglycaemia rather than a primary cause of it.[24] Raised glucose levels are toxic to the β-cell,[28] and impairment of the acute insulin response can be induced experimentally in animals by raising glucose levels just above the normal range for 2 days.[29]

The relationship between size at birth and the risk of diabetes in adult life is complicated in high risk populations by the effects of glucose intolerance during pregnancy. Maternal hyperglycaemia causes fetal hyperinsulinaemia which in turn promotes fetal growth, especially in subcutaneous fat depots.[30] Experimental studies suggest that maternal hyperglycaemia itself affects glucose homeostasis. Induction of hyperglycaemia in female rats leads to glucose intolerance, insulin resistance and impaired β-cell function in the adult offspring,[31,32] an effect which is transmissible from one generation to the next.[33] In Pima Americans, the risk of diabetes is much higher in the offspring of mothers who were diabetic during pregnancy than in the offspring of

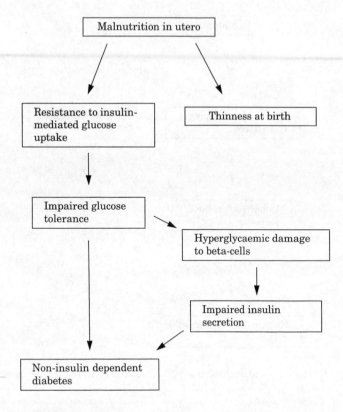

Figure 4.2 How resistance to insulin-mediated glucose uptake could mediate an effect of malnutrition in utero on the risk of diabetes in adult life

mothers who developed diabetes subsequently.[34] Maternal glucose intolerance will thus generate a positive association between size at birth and risk of diabetes in adult life. In populations where gestational diabetes is common, this will tend to obscure any inverse association between size at birth and diabetes risk unless the analysis is restricted to those whose mothers were at low risk of gestational diabetes.

4.4.1 Experimental studies of malnutrition in early life

There is considerable experimental evidence for the hypothesis that malnutrition in early life leads to impaired β-cell function. Protein-restricted diets administered to rats from weaning until 6 weeks of age cause impairment of the insulin secretory response to glucose and glucose intolerance, which persists after refeeding.[6,35] Similar effects have been reported when rats are exposed to protein restriction in utero, followed by a normal diet from birth to adult life.[36]

The hypothesis that malnutrition in early life leads to insulin resistance does not have such clear experimental support. There is some evidence for an effect of malnutrition after weaning. In comparison with controls, rats fed energy restricted diets from weaning until 6 weeks of age have a delayed and exaggerated insulin secretory response to glucose as adults, suggesting that they are insulin resistant.[35] In contrast, adult rats exposed in utero to restriction of protein in the diets of their mothers clear an intravenous glucose load more rapidly than controls.[37,38] The basis of this effect appears to be that production of glucose from glycogen by the liver is reduced in rats exposed to protein restriction in utero. This effect has been demonstrated under basal conditions[38] and when the liver is perfused with glucagon which stimulates glucose production.[39] In one of these studies, insulin action was measured directly by the euglycaemic clamp.[38] Basal glucose uptake was slower in rats exposed to protein restriction in utero than in controls, but there was no difference in insulin-stimulated glucose uptake between the two groups. Thus there is as yet no clear experimental evidence that malnutrition in fetal life can cause impairment of insulin-mediated glucose uptake sufficient to account for the observed relationship between size at birth and diabetes in humans.

4.4.2 Relation of size at birth to measures of beta-cell function and insulin sensitivity

The hypothesis that malnutrition in early life could impair the development of the endocrine pancreas is compatible with the known timing of differentiation and growth of this tissue. Studies of human fetal and infant autopsy material indicate that the differentiation of β-cells occurs over a critical period beginning with the second trimester in utero and finishing by 6 months postnatally.[40] Studies of children malnourished in infancy have shown lower insulin responses to glucose[41] and amino acids.[42] Williams et al.[43] found that small for gestational age infants had lower stool chymotrypsin activity at 14 days after birth than controls, suggesting possible dysfunction of the exocrine pancreas.

In epidemiological studies, deficient β-cell function has been inferred from impairment of the acute insulin response to glucose challenge, or from raised levels of proinsulin and split proinsulin. In Hertfordshire men aged 64 years[7] and in Southampton men aged 21 years[13] there was no relationship of insulin levels at 30 min after a glucose load with birthweight or weight at 1 year. In the Hertfordshire men, there was an inverse relationship between weight at 1 year and the fasting level of plasma 32-33 split proinsulin after adjusting for body mass index.[7] The raised fasting split proinsulin was interpreted as an indicator of β-cell dysfunction, although subsequent studies from the same group have shown that raised proinsulin levels correlate well with insulin resistance.

The most generally accepted measure of β-cell function in humans is the acute insulin response to intravenous glucose challenge, which has been validated in baboons against measurements of β-cell mass at autopsy.[44] Epidemiological studies in Preston adults[22] and Uppsala men[10] have failed to demonstrate that reduced size at birth predicts impairment of the acute insulin response. In Uppsala the measurements of insulin response were recorded 10 years before the participants were tested for diabetes, and the relationship between size at birth and diabetes could thus be analysed with insulin response as an intervening variable. In such analyses, adjusting for acute insulin response at age 50 years strengthened the relationship between reduced size at birth and diabetes at age 60 years, which is not consistent with the hypothesis that the relationship is mediated through impairment of β-cell function.

The most direct evidence for the alternative hypothesis—that the relationship is mediated through insulin resistance—comes from a study of Preston adults, in which insulin resistance was measured by the short insulin tolerance test.[23] An inverse relation was found with ponderal index but not birthweight, head circumference or gestational age. The relationship was present within each stratum of body mass index. Other studies have used insulin levels, either in the fasting state or 1–2 h after an oral glucose load, as a proxy measure of insulin resistance in non-diabetic individuals (Table 4.3). In non-diabetic Mexican-Americans aged 32 years, both fasting and 2 h insulin levels were inversely related to birthweight.[14] In Uppsala, fasting and 60-minute insulin levels in the intravenous glucose tolerance test were used as proxy measures of insulin resistance in non-diabetic men. Insulin levels were inversely correlated with birthweight and with ponderal index. The strongest relationship was between 60 min insulin and ponderal index, and the association was restricted to men in the highest tertile for body mass

Table 4.3 Studies relating insulin resistance or insulin levels to size at birth in non-diabetic adults

Population	N	Age	Outcome	Measurement
Southampton men[13]	40	21	30-min insulin	Birthweight
Mexican-American adults[14]	541	31	Fasting and 2 h insulin	Birthweight
Preston adults[23]	103	47-55	Insulin tolerance test	Ponderal index
Uppsala men[10]	1032	50	Insulin at 60 min after intravenous glucose	Ponderal index
Salisbury children[16]	250	7	Fasting insulin	Ponderal index
Pune children[15]	379	4	30-min insulin	Birthweight

index. This interaction between the effects of thinness at birth and overweight in adult life was statistically significant. Adjusting for fasting and 60 min insulin at age 50 years reduced the strength of association between low ponderal index at birth and diabetes at age 60, but did not fully account for it. Inverse assocation between insulin levels and size at birth have also been found in children, although the validity of insulin levels as proxy measures of insulin resistance in children is unknown. In 4 year old children in Pune, India, there was a significant inverse relationship between insulin levels at 30 minutes after a glucose load and birthweight,[15] but in seven-year old children in Salisbury, England no relationship was found between insulin levels and size at birth.[16]

These results are consistent with the hypothesis suggested by the South-ampton group that a specific association of thinness at birth with insulin resistance underlies the association between reduced size at birth and non-insulin-dependent diabetes. Because the inverse association between ponderal index and raised postload insulin level is strongest in overweight individuals, who account for most new cases of diabetes, a weak overall association between low ponderal index and insulin resistance is compatible with a strong association between low ponderal index and diabetes. However, the interaction found between raised body mass index and low ponderal index in Uppsala men at age 50 remains to be confirmed in other studies.

4.5 Physiological basis of insulin resistance in adults who were thin at birth

Most insulin-mediated glucose disposal is accounted for by the ability of skeletal muscle to take up glucose and store it as glycogen. If thinness at birth is associated with resistance to insulin-mediated glucose uptake, there must presumably be some structural or functional defect in skeletal muscle which accounts for this. The absence of any relation of plasma triglycerides or non-esterified fatty acids with size at birth suggests that the link with insulin resistance is not mediated by disordered regulation of lipid metabolism.[45] The Southampton group have used several innovative approaches to study the physiological basis of the defect in insulin-mediated glucose uptake in those who were thin at birth.

Taylor studied 25 women selected to cover a wide range of birthweight and ponderal index at birth, using phosphorus-31 magnetic resonance spectroscopy.[46] A constant heavy workload was applied to a forearm muscle (flexor digitorum superficialis) to test anaerobic glycolysis, and to a calf muscle (gastrocnemius) to test oxidative metabolism. In response to forearm exercise, fatigue was more rapid and the rise in adenosine diphosphate levels in the forearm was greater in women who were thin at birth. They suggested that thinness at birth might be associated with a reduced ability to generate adenosine triphosphate by anaerobic glycolysis. The half-time of muscle reoxygenation was measured by near-infrared spectroscopy of haemoglobin during metabolic recovery from ischaemic finger exercise.[47] Women who had been thin at birth showed higher reoxygenation rates. Reoxygenation rates correlated strongly ($r = 0.6$) with rates of phosphocreatinine depletion and ADP accumulation in the magnetic resonance study. They suggested that this increased oxygenation in women who had been thin at birth could be a compensatory response to a defect in anaerobic glycolysis.

In Preston adults, adult muscle mass was correlated with birthweight but not with ponderal index: thus the association with insulin resistance is not explained by alterations in muscle mass.[48] Lower capillary density in muscle has been suggested as a possible mechanism which could impair insulin-mediated glucose disposal. However, no relation of thinness at birth with the density of capillaries in the gastrocnemius muscle, or with the percentage of Type I (slow-twitch) muscle fibres was found when biopsy specimens were examined.[47] Glycogen synthase is the enzyme which converts glucose to glycogen, and in the general population insulin sensitivity is correlated with postprandial glycogen synthase activity.[49] When this was measured in the muscle biopsies, glycogen synthase activity correlated with insulin sensitivity measured by short insulin tolerance test and with central obesity, but not with size at birth.[50] These findings suggest that the reduced insulin-mediated glucose uptake in adults who were thin at birth may have a different physiological mechanism from the insulin resistance that is commonly associated with obesity, and may be part of a more general alteration of fuel utilization in skeletal muscle.

4.6 Relation of fetal growth to central obesity and plasma lipids

In the general population, insulin resistance is strongly associated with raised plasma triglyceride levels, low high-density lipoprotein levels, and a central pattern of obesity in which a high proportion of body fat is deposited in intra-abdominal depots.[51] The mechanism of these associations is not well understood, but both the insulin resistance and the lipid disturbances are ameliorated or reversed by weight loss,[52] which suggests that obesity has a primary role. Production of triglyceride by the liver is regulated by the supply of non-esterified fatty acids from lipolysis in fat cells. Because intra-abdominal fat depots are drained by the portal vein, the size of these portal fat stores is likely to exert a strong influence on hepatic triglyceride production.

The waist–hip girth ratio is a crude measure of central obesity; the correlation with measurements by computed tomography of the proportion of total body fat that is in intra-abdominal depots is about 0.6.[53] In Hertfordshire men[54] and in Preston adults,[8] there was an inverse relation between birthweight and waist–hip ratio, even though body mass index is positively correlated with both birthweight and waist–hip ratio. In a subsequent study of 93 Preston adults aged 50 there was no relation between size at birth and waist–hip ratio.[45] Waist-hip ratio is not a pure measure of body fat distribution, and depends also on skeletal proportions. Thus a high waist–hip ratio in those who were small at birth could be a consequence of small pelvic diameter rather than intra-abdominal obesity. Further studies with direct measurements using computed tomography or magnetic resonance imaging to measure intra-abdominal fat directly are required to establish whether there is any relationship between body fat distribution and size at birth. Low birthweight does not predict raised triglyceride or low HDL cholesterol,[10,45] which are closely related to central obesity.

4.7 Small baby syndrome or insulin resistance syndrome?

The clustering in the population of physiological disturbances associated with insulin resistance—hyperinsulinaemia, glucose intolerance, hypertension, elevated plasma triglyceride and low high-density lipoprotein cholesterol—is now considered as a distinct syndrome.[55,56] Barker and colleagues have shown that when glucose intolerance, hypertension, and lipid disturbances are combined to define a single binary trait, there is a strong inverse relationship between birthweight and the prevalence of this trait in middle age, with an odds ratio of 18 between the highest and the lowest categories.[57] They suggested that impaired fetal growth could account for the clustering of glucose intolerance, hypertension and lipid disturbances in the population, and that the insulin resistance syndrome should therefore be renamed 'small baby syndrome'.[57] In other studies which have examined the associations of size at birth with glucose intolerance, hypertension and disturbances of plasma lipid levels separately, with diabetic individuals excluded,[10,14,45] reduced fetal growth has been found to predict hyperinsulinaemia, glucose intolerance, and hypertension but not to predict the lipid abnormalities characteristic of the insulin resistance syndrome—elevated triglyceride and low high-density lipoprotein cholesterol levels—which are correlated with central obesity. It is thus possible to distinguish two patterns of clustering: a 'small baby syndrome' characterized by hypertension, insulin resistance and glucose intolerance, and a central obesity syndrome characterized by raised triglyceride levels, low high-density lipoprotein cholesterol, insulin resistance, and glucose intolerance.

4.8 Does the association have a genetic or an environmental explanation?

Hales and colleagues have interpreted the association between glucose intolerance and reduced fetal growth in terms of a causal pathway from inadequate nutrition in early life to impairment of the ability to maintain glucose homeostasis in later life[7,58] (Fig. 4.1). If the relationship between reduced size at birth and diabetes in adult life were mediated through impaired β-cell function, this would be the most plausible explanation as there is experimental evidence that malnutrition in utero causes impairment of β-cell function. The demonstration of associations between reduced fetal growth and impairment of insulin action, however, means that genetic explanations for the association between reduced size at birth and glucose intolerance are also plausible. Insulin regulates fetal growth, so that a primary defect in insulin action would reduce growth in utero and also predispose to glucose intolerance in later life. The pathways by which this would produce an association between reduced size at birth and non-insulin dependent diabetes are shown in Fig. 4.3. Such a mechanism would be consistent with clinical observations that human infants with rare genetic defects causing severe insulin resistance are small at birth.[59] An experimental model is provided by mice in which the gene for insulin receptor substrate-1 (a postreceptor mediator of insulin action) has been destroyed: in comparison with their normal littermates, these mice are 30% lighter at birth and more resistant to insulin-stimulated glucose uptake as adults.[60] In contrast no experimental model for undernutrition in fetal life causing insulin resistance has been established.

4.8.1 Genetic influences on birthweight in humans

One argument against genetic explanations for associations with size at birth has been that genetic effects on size at birth are weak in comparison to the effects of maternal environment. The strength of genetic effects on a continuous trait is measured by the heritability (the proportion of variance attributable to genetic factors). Morton (1955) concluded from data on twins and half-sibs that the effects of maternal environment on birthweight were more important than the effects of fetal genotype.[61] In his study, however, the intraclass correlation coefficient for birthweight in 168 pairs of paternal half-sibs was 0.10, which is consistent with additive genetic effects accounting for 40% of the variance in birthweight. An alternative means of estimating heritability while controlling for the effects of maternal environment is to compare the intraclass correlation between full sibs with the intraclass correlation between maternal half-sibs (or the offspring of female monozygotic twins, who are genetically maternal half-sibs). Applying this method to a study of the offspring of a large Norwegian twin panel[62] yields an estimate

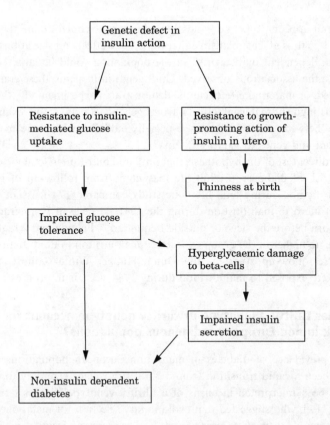

Figure 4.3 How a primary genetic defect in insulin action could generate an association between birth and diabetes in adult life

of about 40% for the heritability of birthweight. Thus although it is likely that maternal environment accounts for at least half the variation in birthweight, the genetic effects on birthweight are sufficiently large for genetic explanations of associations between size at birth and other traits to be plausible.

4.8.2 Genetic influences on non-insulin dependent diabetes risk

The strength of genetic influences on a binary trait such as non-insulin dependent diabetes can be measured by the recurrence risk ratio: the ratio of risk in relatives of a case to risk in the general population. The recurrence risk ratio for non-insulin dependent diabetes in siblings of cases is about 5.[5] Studies of recurrence risk in half-sibs, which would distinguish genetic from maternal environmental effects, are not available. Other evidence for genetic influences on diabetes risk comes from ethnic differences, as discussed below. Some of the genetic influence on diabetes is likely to be mediated through central obesity, and this trait appears to be more closely under genetic control than obesity in general.[63] It is thus at least plausible that the genetic effects on size at birth and non-insulin dependent diabetes risk in the population could be large enough to generate the associations observed. Until genes influencing these traits can be identified, or maternal effects can be demonstrated experimentally, the only way to distinguish maternal effects from genetic effects is by examining covariance between sets of relatives, especially half-sibs, who share maternal environment and genes to varying extents.

A more direct test of the hypothesis that impaired nutrition in fetal life causes increased risk of diabetes in adult life may come from follow-up of groups exposed to famine during fetal life. One study compared 174 Russian adults exposed in utero to malnutrition during the 1941–42 siege of Leningrad with controls born before the siege or outside Leningrad.[64] Fasting and 2 h glucose levels were no higher in the group exposed to malnutrition in utero than in the controls. A follow-up study of the Dutch Hunger Winter cohort, whose mothers were exposed to malnutrition during 1944–45,[65] is in progress.

4.8.3 Does thrifty phenotype or thrifty genotype account for high risk in non-European indigenous populations?

The high prevalence of diabetes in many non-European populations where there has been a rapid transition from a rural subsistence economy to urban living has been interpreted in terms of a 'thrifty genotype'.[66] This term was coined by Neel, who suggested that evolutionary selection for metabolic traits which help people to survive famine might lead to increased frequency of genes which predispose to the development of diabetes in urban societies. Hales and Barker have suggested as an alternative explanation that the high rates of diabetes in these populations result from undernutrition in fetal and infant life, followed by relative overnutrition later.[58] They cite the high rates of diabetes recorded in Nauru,[67] where there has been a recent transition from undernutrition to relative affluence, as an example. Other evidence, however, points strongly to genetic influences underlying the high rates of diabetes in such populations. One line of evidence comes from migrant studies.[68] Prevalence of diabetes is uniformly high (around 20% in those aged over 35 years) in Indian populations overseas whose migration occurred during the mid-nineteenth century.[69] While it is plausible that an effect of maternal environment could persist over one or two generations after migration, it is unlikely that such an effect would persist five or six generations after migration as an exposure specific to Indians. In Singapore, for instance, a rapid transition to affluence has been shared by all three of the main ethnic groups (Chinese, Malays and Indians) but the prevalence of diabetes is much higher in Indians than in Chinese.[70] In several of the populations at high risk of diabetes, it has been reported that prevalence of diabetes is lower in those of mixed descent than in those without admixture from other populations at lower risk. In Nauru, for instance, prevalence of diabetes in those who had genetic markers of non-Nauruan admixture was found to be less than one-quarter of the prevalence in those without evidence of admixture.[71] Admixture in this population resulted mainly from unions between Nauruan women and European sailors: thus admixture introduced European genes but not European maternal environment. Similar relationships between diabetes and admixture have been reported for Pima-Americans.[72] It is of course possible that ethnic differences in the risk of diabetes could be a consequence of ethnic differences in fetal growth which have a genetic basis: average ponderal index at birth has been reported to be lower in the infants of Indian than European mothers in England. Such an explanation, however would still assign a primary role to genetic influences.

4.9 Conclusions

Recent studies support the hypothesis that thinness at birth is associated with insulin resistance and consequently with increased risk of non-insulin dependent diabetes. It remains to be established whether this relationship is mediated by genetic or environmental influences. The association of maternal glucose intolerance with increased size at birth and increased risk of diabetes in later life may account for the U-shaped associations seen in populations at high risk of non-insulin dependent diabetes is common. The relationship between obesity and insulin resistance appears to be at least as strong in those who were thin at birth as in those who were not thin at birth. This suggests that whatever the mechanism of the association, control of obesity is likely to be effective in reducing the risk of diabetes in individuals who were thin at birth. Although it is not practicable to test this directly in randomized trials with diabetes incidence as outcome measure, it is possible to study the effect of weight loss on insulin sensitivity as an intermediate variable.

References

Those marked with an asterisk are especially recommended for further reading.

1 Sharma P. Caraka Samhita (circa 200 BC) with English translation. Varanasi, India: Chaukambha Orientalia, 1981; 274–5.

2 Ramachandran A, Jali MV, Mohan V, Snehalatha C, Viswanathan M. High prevalence of diabetes in an urban population in south India. *Br Med J* 1988;**297**:587–90.

3   McKeigue PM, Pierpoint T, Ferrie JE, Marmot MG. Relationship of glucose intolerance and hyperinsulinaemia to body fat pattern in South Asians and Europeans. *Diabetologia* 1992;**35**:785–91.

4   Helmrich SP, Ragland DR, Leung RW, Paffenbarger RS. Physical activity and reduced occurrence of non-insulin dependent diabetes mellitus. *N Engl J Med* 1991;**325**:147–52.

5   Kobberling J, Tillil H. Empirical risk figures for first degree relatives of non-insulin dependent diabetics. In: Kobberling J, Tattersall R, eds. *The Genetics of Diabetes Mellitus* London: Academic Press, 1982:201–9.

6   Swenne I, Crace CJ, Milner RD, Milner RDG. Persistent impairment of insulin secretory response to glucose in adult rats after limited period of protein-calorie malnutrition early in life. *Diabetes* 1987;**36**:454–8.

7* Hales CN, Barker DJP, Clark PMS, et al. Fetal and infant growth and impaired glucose tolerance at age 64. *Br Med J* 1991;**303**:1019–22.

8* Phipps K, Barker DJP, Hales CN, Fall CHD, Osmond C, Clark PMS. Fetal growth and impaired glucose tolerance in men and women. *Diabetologia* 1993;**36**:225–8.

9   Lithell H, Aberg H, Selinus I, Hedstrand H. The primary preventive study in Uppsala: fatal and non-fatal myocardial infarction during a 10-year follow-up of a middle-aged male population with treatment of high risk individuals. *Acta Med Scand* 1984;**215**:403–9.

10* Lithell HO, McKeigue PM, Berglund L, Mohsen R, Lithell U, Leon DA. Relationship of size at birth to non-insulin dependent diabetes and insulin levels in men aged 50-60 years. *Br Med J* 1996;**312**:406–10.

11 Curhan GC, Willett WC, Rimm EB, Stampfer MJ. Birthweight and adult hypertension and diabetes mellitus in US men (abstract). *Am J Hypertens* 1996;**9**: 11A.

12* McCance DR, Pettitt DJ, Hanson RL, Jacobson LTH, Knowler WC, Bennett PH. Birthweight and non-insulin dependent diabetes: thrifty genotype, thrifty phenotype or surviving small baby genotype? *Br Med J* 1994;**308**:942–5.

13 Robinson S, Walton RJ, Clark PM, Barker DJP, Hales CN, Osmond C. The relation of fetal growth to plasma glucose in young men. *Diabetologia* 1992;**35**:444–6.

14 Valdez R, Athens MA, Thompson GH, Bradshaw BS, Stern MP. Birthweight and adult health outcomes in a biethnic population in the USA. *Diabetologia* 1994;**37**:624–31.

15 Yajnik CS, Fall CH, Vaidya U, *et al.* Fetal growth and glucose and insulin metabolism in four-year-old Indian children. *Diabet Med* 1995; **12**:330–6.

16 Law CM, Gordon CM, Shiell AW, Barker DJP, Hales CN. Thinness at birth and glucose tolerance in seven year old children. *Diabet Med* 1995; **12**:24–9.

17   Forrester TE, Wilks RJ, Bennett FI, et al. Fetal growth and cardiovas-
      cular risk factors in Jamaican schoolchildren. *Br Med J* 1996;**312**:156–60.
18   Paneth N, Susser M. Early origin of coronary heart disease: the 'Barker
      hypothesis'. *Br Med J* 1995;**310**:411–2.
19   Miller H, Hassanein K. Fetal malnutrition in White newborn infants:
      maternal factors. *Pediatrics* 1973;**52**:504–12.
20   Zimmet PZ. The pathogenesis and prevention of diabetes in adults—
      genes, autoimmunity, and demography. *Diabet Care* 1995;**18**:1050–64.
21   Sjolin S. Infant mortality in Sweden. In: Wallace HM, ed. *Health care of
      mothers and children in national health services: implications for the United
      States*. Cambridge, Massachusetts: Ballinger, 1975:229–40.
22   Phillips DIW, Hirst S, Clark PMS, Hales CN, Osmond C. Fetal growth
      and insulin secretion in adult life. *Diabetologia* 1994;**37**:592–6.
23*   Phillips DIW, Barker DJP, Hales CN, Hirst S, Osmond C. Thinness at
      birth and insulin resistance in adult life. *Diabetologia* 1994;**37**:150-4.
24*   Yki-Jarvinen H. Evidence for a primary role of insulin resistance in the
      pathogenesis of Type 2 diabetes. *Ann Med* 1990;**22**:197–200.
25   Lillioja S, Mott DM, Spraul M, *et al.* Insulin resistance and insulin
      secretory dysfunction as precursors of non-insulin dependent diabetes
      mellitus: prospective studies of Pima Indians. *N Engl J Med* 1993;**329**:
      1988–92.
26   Martin BC, Warram JH, Krolewski AS, Bergman RN, Soeldner JS,
      Kahn CR. Role of glucose and insulin resistance in development of type 2
      diabetes mellitus: results of a 25-year follow-up study. *Lancet* 1992;**340**:
      925–9.
27   Lundgren H, Bengtsson C, Blohme G, Lapidus L, Sjostrom L. Adiposity
      and adipose tissue distribution in relation to incidence of diabetes in
      women: results from a prospective population study in Gothenburg,
      Sweden. *Int J Obes* 1989;**13**:413–23.
28   Leahy JL, Bonner-Weir S, Weir GC. Beta-cell dysfunction induced by
      chronic hyperglycemia: current ideas on mechanism of impaired glucose-
      induced insulin secretion. *Diabet Care* 1992;**15**:442–55.
29   Leahy JL, Cooper HE, Weir GC. Impaired insulin secretion associated
      with near normoglycaemia: study in normal rats with 96-h in vivo glucose
      infusions. *Diabetes* 1987;**36**:459–64.
30   Freinkel N. Of pregnancy and progeny. *Diabetes* 1980;**29**:1023–35.
31   Aerts L, Sodoyez Goffaux F, Sodoyez JC, Malaisse WJ, Van Assche FA.
      The diabetic intrauterine milieu has a long-lasting effect on insulin
      secretion by β cells and on insulin uptake by target tissues. *Am J Obstet
      Gynecol* 1988;**159**:1287–92.
32   Grill V, Johansson B, Jalkanen P, Eriksson UJ. Influence of severe
      diabetes mellitus early in pregnancy in the rat: effects on insulin sensi-
      tivity and insulin secretion in the offspring. *Diabetologia* 1991;**34**:373–8.

33 Gauguier D, Bihoreau MT, Ktorza A, Berthault MF, Picon L. Inheritance of diabetes mellitus as consequence of gestational hyperglycemia in rats. *Diabetes* 1990;**39**:734–9.

34 Pettitt DJ, Aleck KA, Baird HR, Carraher MJ, Bennett PH, Knowler WC. Congenital susceptibility to NIDDM: role of intrauterine environment. *Diabetes* 1988;**37**:622–8.

35 Crace CJ, Swenne I, Milner RDG. Long term effects on glucose-tolerance and insulin secretory response to glucose following a limited period of severe protein or energy malnutrition in young-rats. *Upsala J Med Sci* 1991;**96**:177–83.

36 Dahri S, Snoeck A, Reusensbillen B, Remacle C, Hoet JJ. Islet function in offspring of mothers on low-protein diet during gestation. *Diabetes* 1991;**40**:115–20.

37 Langley SC, Browne RF, Jackson AA. Altered glucose tolerance in rats exposed to maternal low-protein diets in utero. *Comp Biochem Physiol* 1994;**109**:223–9.

38* Holness MJ. Impact of early growth-retardation on glucoregulatory control and insulin action in mature rats. *Am J Physiol* 1996;**33**:E 946–54.

39 Ozanne SE, Smith GD, Tikerpae J, Hales CN. Altered regulation of hepatic glucose output in the male offspring of protein-malnourished rat dams. *Am J Physiol* 1996;**33**:E 559–64.

40 Rahier J, Wallon J, Henquin JC. Cell populations in the endocrine pancreas of human neonates and infants. *Diabetologia* 1981;**20**:540–6.

41 James WP, Coore HG. Persistent impairment of insulin secretion and glucose tolerance after malnutrition. *Am J Clin Nutr* 1970;**23**:386–9.

42 Milner RD. Metabolic and hormonal responses to oral amino acids in infantile malnutrition. *Arch Dis Child* 1971;**46**:301–5.

43 Williams SP, Durbin GM, Morgan MEI, Booth IW. Catch-up growth and pancreatic function in growth-retarded neonates. *Arch Dis Child* 1995;**73**:F 158–61.

44 McCulloch DK, Koerker DJ, Kahn SE, Bonner-Weir S, Palmer JP. Correlations of in vivo beta cell function tests with beta cell mass and pancreatic insulin content in streptozotocin-treated baboons. *Diabetes* 1991;**40**:673–9.

45 Phillips DIW, McLeish R, Osmond C, Hales CN. Fetal growth and insulin resistance in adult life: role of plasma triglyceride and nonesterified fatty acids. *Diabet Med* 1995;**12**:796–801.

46* Taylor DJ, Thompson CH, Kemp GJ, et al. A relationship between impaired fetal growth and reduced muscle glycolysis revealed by P-31 magnetic resonance spectroscopy. *Diabetologia* 1995;**38**:1205–12.

47 Thompson CH, Stein C, Caddy S, et al. Fetal growth and insulin resistance in adult life: role of skeletal muscle microcirculation and oxygenation (abstract). *Diabetologia* 1995;**38**:A 136.

48 Phillips DIW. Relation of fetal growth to adult muscle mass and glucose-tolerance. *Diabet Med* 1995;**12**:686–90.

49 Kida Y, Esposito Del Puente A, Bogardus C, Mott DM. Insulin resistance is associated with reduced fasting and insulin- stimulated glycogen synthase phosphatase activity in human skeletal muscle. *J Clin Invest* 1990;**85**:476–81.

50 Phillips DIW, Borthwick AC, Stein C, Taylor R. Fetal growth and insulin resistance in adult life: relationship between glycogen synthase activity in adult skeletal muscle and birth weight. *Diabet Med* 1996; **13**:325–9.

51 Stern MP, Haffner SM. Body fat and hyperinsulinaemia as risk factors for diabetes and cardiovascular disease. *Arteriosclerosis* 1986;**6**: 123–30.

52 Olefsky JM, Reaven GM, Farquhar JW. Effects of weight reduction on obesity: studies of carbohydrate and lipid metabolism. *J Clin Invest* 1974; **53**:64–76.

53 Seidell JC, Oosterlee A, Thijssen MAO, et al. Assessment of intra-abdominal and subcutaneous abdominal fat: relation between anthropometry and computed tomography. *Am J Clin Nutr* 1987;**45**:7–13.

54 Law CM, Barker DJP, Osmond C, Fall CHD, Simmonds SJ. Early growth and abdominal fatness in adult life. *J Epidemiol Community Health* 1992;**46**:184–6.

55 Reaven GM. Role of insulin resistance in human disease. *Diabetes* 1988; **37**:1595–607.

56 DeFronzo RA, Ferrannini E. Insulin resistance: a multifaceted syndrome responsible for NIDDM, obesity, hypertension, dyslipidemia, and atherosclerotic cardiovascular disease. *Diabet Care* 1991;**14**:173–94.

57 Barker DJP, Hales CN, Fall CHD, Osmond C, Phipps K, Clark PMS. Type 2 (non-insulin-dependent) diabetes mellitus, hypertension and hyperlipidaemia (syndrome X): relation to reduced fetal growth. *Diabetologia* 1993;**36**:62–7.

58 Hales CN, Barker DJP. Type 2 (non-insulin-dependent) diabetes mellitus —the thrifty phenotype hypothesis. *Diabetologia* 1992;**35**:595–601.

59* Gluckman PD. The role of pituitary hormones, growth factors and insulin in the regulation of fetal growth. *Oxford Rev Reprod Biol* 1986; **8**:1–60.

60 Tamemoto H, Kadowaki T, Tobe K, et al. Insulin resistance and growth retardation in mice lacking insulin receptor substrate-1. *Nature* 1994; **372**:182–6.

61 Morton NE. The inheritance of human birth weight. *Ann Hum Genet* 1955;**20**:125.

62 Magnus P. Further evidence for a significant effect of fetal genes on variation in birth weight. *Clin Genet* 1984;**26**:289–96.

63   Perusse L, Despres JP, Lemieux S, Rice T, Rao DC, Bouchard C. Familial aggregation of abdominal visceral fat level: results from the Quebec Family Study. *Metabolism* 1996;**45**:378–82.

64   Yudkin JS, Stanner S, Bulmer K, et al. Is cardiovascular risk related to intrauterine starvation—the Leningrad Siege Study (abstract). *Diabetes* 1996;**45 (suppl 2)**:193A.

65   Ravelli GP, Stein ZA, Susser MW. Obesity in young men after famine exposure in utero and early infancy. *N Engl J Med* 1976;**295**:349–53.

66   Neel JV. Diabetes mellitus: a 'thrifty' genotype rendered detrimental by 'progress'. *Am J Hum Genet* 1962;**14**:353–62.

67   Dowse GK, Zimmet PZ, Finch CF, Collins VR. Decline in incidence of epidemic glucose intolerance in Nauruans—implications for the thrifty genotype. *Am J Epidemiol* 1991;**133**:1093–104.

68   Taylor R, Zimmet P. Migrant studies in diabetes epidemiology. In: Mann JI, Pyorala K, Teuscher A, eds. *Diabetes in epidemiological perspective.* Edinburgh: Churchill Livingstone, 1983:58–77.

69   McKeigue PM, Miller GJ, Marmot MG. Coronary heart disease in South Asians overseas: a review. *J Clin Epidemiol* 1989;**42**:597–609.

70   Hughes K, Yeo PPB, Lun KC, et al. Cardiovascular diseases in Chinese, Malays and Indians in Singapore. II. Differences in risk factor levels. *J Epidemiol Community Health* 1990;**44**:29–35.

71   Serjeantson SW, Owerbach D, Zimmet P, Nerup J, Thoma K. Genetics of diabetes in Nauru: effects of foreign admixture, HLA antigens and the insulin-gene-linked polymorphism. *Diabetologia* 1983;**25**:13–7.

72   Knowler WC, Williams RC, Pettitt DJ, Steinberg AG. Gm3;5,13,14 and type 2 diabetes mellitus: an association in American Indians with genetic admixture. *Am J Hum Genet* 1988;**43**:520–6.

5 Respiratory and allergic diseases

David P Strachan

Respiratory illnesses are caused by a sometimes complex interaction of infection, allergy, mucus hypersecretion, reversible bronchospasm, and irreversible airflow obstruction. Cigarette smoking is a powerful and partially reversible influence on the risk of mucus hypersecretion, reversible and irreversible airflow obstruction, and should be the priority in any preventive programme. However, not all smokers appear to be prone to disabling or fatal airflow obstruction and cofactors including impaired prenatal and postnatal lung growth, genetic antitrypsin deficiency, and dietary antioxidant deficiency may determine which smokers are most susceptible. In the past, high levels of outdoor air pollution were associated with increased morbidity and mortality among bronchitic patients, but the role of outdoor or indoor air pollution as a determinant of the prevalence of obstructive lung disease remains uncertain.

As smoking becomes less common, allergic sensitization and other influences on adult asthma may attain greater relative importance. A role for dietary factors in adult asthma and chronic airflow obstruction has been suggested but not consistently confirmed by observational or experimental studies. There is suggestive but not conclusive evidence that the risk of allergy may to some extent be programmed in early childhood, by early allergen exposure and/or exposure to infectious illnesses (the latter being protective). Although childhood chest infections are closely associated with subsequent asthma, the direction of cause and effect here remains a matter for debate.

5.1 Introduction

Respiratory disease poses a substantial public health problem in terms of premature death, disability, hospital admissions, primary care contacts, loss of productivity, and interference with work and schooling.[1] Much of this disease burden is thought to relate to five broadly defined clinical syndromes:

(a)   *Respiratory infections*, often of a viral nature, affecting all ages but more severe in the very young and the elderly.

(b)   *Atopy*, characterised by elevated levels of circulating immunoglobulin E and cutaneous hypersensitivity on skin prick testing with common aeroallergens.

(c)   *Reversible airflow obstruction*, embracing 'wheezy bronchitis' in early life, 'extrinsic (allergic) asthma' of children and young adults, and 'intrinsic (non-allergic) asthma', typically of later onset

(d)   *Chronic mucus hypersecretion*, characterised by persistent cough and phlegm, used by the British Medical Research Council to define 'chronic bronchitis'.

(e)   *Irreversible airflow obstruction*, the main cause of death and severe disability from chronic respiratory disease,[2] and an important predictor of all-cause mortality, even among lifelong non-smokers.[3,4]

These syndromes are interconnected by a complex web of associations and putative causal relationships (Fig. 5.1). Lower respiratory illnesses in infancy (a) have been proposed as a cause of a chronic wheezing tendency (c),[5,6]

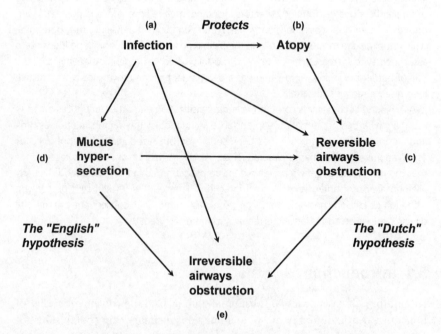

Figure 5.1 Postulated relationships between different forms of respiratory and allergic disease.

chronic cough and phlegm (d),[5,7] irreversible impaired ventilatory function (e)[5,8] and related mortality.[9] An alternative explanation for these associations could be that they reflect a longstanding tendency to all forms of chest illness, perhaps related to impaired lung development[10] and/or asthma (c).[11] Although viral infections (a) are an immediate cause of many wheezing attacks[12] (c), it has been suggested that early infection may protect against the development of allergic sensitization (b).[13]

The association between atopy (b) and extrinsic asthma (c) is well established, but the role of atopic history in the other wheezing syndromes is less clear.[10,14] Asthma[11] and airways responsiveness[15] (c) are associated with chronic productive cough (d). Irreversible airflow obstruction (e) has been postulated as the end result of chronic airway irritation and inflammation (d)— the so-called 'English hypothesis'[16]—or related primarily to the asthmatic tendency (c)—the 'Dutch hypothesis'.[17] Although much of the excess mortality among asthmatic adults (c) is due to deaths certified as chronic bronchitis or emphysema, rather than asthma,[18] the true degree of overlap between these syndromes remains in dispute.[19]

These relationships are further complicated by interactions with causal factors. Thus, active smoking is established as a powerful cause of mucus hypersecretion (d)[16] and progressive decline of ventilatory function (e),[14,16] but asthmatics and those with non-specific airways hyperreactivity may be particularly susceptible to these effects.[14] Smoking can also trigger asthmatic attacks (c) and increase the risk of atopic sensitization to some occupational allergens (b).[20] A wide range of other factors have been related to one or more of the respiratory syndromes, including birthweight, family size and structure, passive smoking, urban air pollution, diet, occupation, and socioeconomic circumstances in childhood and adult life. A life course approach to the epidemiology of respiratory disease thus seems appropriate.

This chapter addresses the independent and combined effects of perinatal, childhood and adult lifestyle factors on the development of both allergic and non-allergic lung disease.

5.2 Development of ventilatory function

The emergence of severe impairment of ventilatory function, as measured by marked reductions in spirometric indices such as forced expiratory volume in one second (FEV_1) and peak expiratory flow rate (PEFR), is the end result of many years of decline in function from maximal levels attained during early adulthood. The risk of disabling airflow obstruction in later adult life is believed to be influenced by the maximum level attained through lung growth and by the rate of functional decline throughout adulthood (Fig. 5.2).

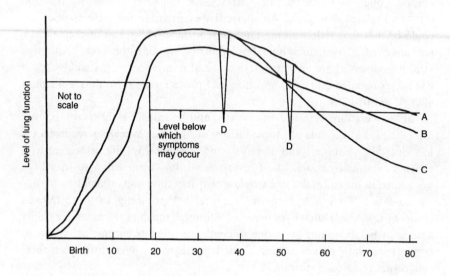

Figure 5.2 Schematic representation of the life course of ventilatory function measurements such as forced expiratory volume in one second.
Footnotes:
A = normal growth and decline.
B = impaired prenatal or postnatal growth, leading to reduced maximal function and increased risk of later disability and death from chronic respiratory disease despite a normal rate of decline.
C = normal growth but accelerated decline, leading to premature disability and risk of death from chronic respiratory disease.
D = episodes of reversible airflow obstruction, which may be superimposed on any of curves A, B or C.

5.2.1 Lung growth

The factors influencing lung growth are not fully understood but may include both prenatal and postnatal exposures.[21] Ventilatory function is reduced among children of low birthweight,[22,23] whether this is due to prematurity or intrauterine growth retardation. Maternal smoking during pregnancy is currently the most important remediable influence on intrauterine growth and lung function abnormalities in the offspring of smoking mothers are apparent shortly after birth.[24] Premature infants who require prolonged artificial ventilation appear to be at particular risk of later lung function abnormalities.[25]

Maternal smoking and neonatal intensive care are unlikely to have influenced the lung development of today's adults who have survived to middle and old age. Nevertheless, low birthweight predicted both lower FEV_1 and mortality from chronic obstructive lung disease among men born in

Hertfordshire during 1911–1930.[26] Weight at 1 year of age was less strongly associated with adult FEV_1, although the study had insufficient statistical power to distinguish conclusively the effects of prenatal and postnatal growth. Among the British 1958 birth cohort, FEV_1 measured at 35 years of age was positively related to both birthweight (after exclusion of premature deliveries) and to height at age 7, adjusting for adult height, smoking, and socioeconomic status in both childhood and adult life.[27] This suggests that both prenatal and postnatal lung growth may influence the 'capital investment' of ventilatory function in early adult life which is subject to 'depreciation' with advancing age.

5.2.2 Functional decline

The progressive and irreversible decline in ventilatory function throughout adult life is commonly due to pulmonary emphysema, a widespread destruction of alveolar ducts and walls, which is thought to result from an imbalance between destructive and repair forces in the peripheral lung and smaller airways. The environmental factors which may influence this balance favourably or unfavourably are discussed in a later section of this chapter.

Superimposed upon the irreversible component may be episodes of reversible airways narrowing related to asthma (Fig. 5.2). The propensity to asthma attacks is usually associated with measurable airflow reductions on inhalation of provocation agents such as histamine or methacholine. This non-specific bronchial hyperresponsiveness (BHR) is widely believed to relate to chronic inflammatory processes in the airways which may be initiated or sustained in atopic individuals by allergen exposure. If this inflammation persists it is thought that remodelling of the airway tissues may lead to a degree of irreversible airflow obstruction which may thus predispose to disabling or fatal chronic obstructive lung disease. Such a link between reversible and irreversible airways obstruction was first proposed by Dutch workers in the 1960s[17] and since termed the 'Dutch hypothesis'.

There has been considerable debate about the relationship between BHR and accelerated decline in adult ventilatory function.[14,28] Confusion arises because BHR in adults without asthma may be related to cigarette smoking, itself a powerful risk factor for rapid lung function decline. In cross-sectional studies, BHR is most closely associated with atopy and 'extrinsic' asthma in younger adults and with smoking and 'intrinsic' asthma in older age groups.[29] The increased BHR of older smokers is almost invariably associated with reduced baseline FEV_1, so it is possible that irreversible airways obstruction alone may increase BHR, perhaps through distortions of airway geometry.[30]

Burrows and colleagues have proposed that it may be useful to consider two major causes of persistent airflow obstruction in middle aged and elderly subjects.[19] One type, associated with asthma and atopy mainly in non-smokers, is that to which the Dutch hypothesis applies most clearly. The other, with a worse prognosis, occurs in non-atopic cigarette smokers among whom bronchial hyperresponsiveness may be a consequence, rather than a cause, of accelerated lung function decline. This distinction may be relevant to the subsequent discussion of effects of childhood chest illness on chronic respiratory disease in adults. The clearest way to disentangle which comes first is to perform repeat measures of BHR and lung function over the life course.

5.3 Childhood chest illness, lung development and adult lung disease

An association between chest illness in childhood and both chronic respiratory morbidity and impaired ventilatory function in later life has emerged in several studies.[5] This could reflect lung damage due to early episodes of chest infection, a longstanding susceptibility to all forms of lung disease, or continuity of socioeconomic circumstances or environmental exposure[31] (Fig. 5.3)

Two historical cohort studies, in Hertfordshire[26] and Derbyshire,[32] suggest that lower respiratory illness in the first year of life is associated with later

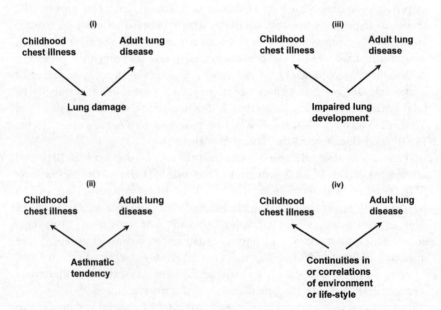

Figure 5.3 Four possible explanations for the association of childhood chest illness and adult respiratory disease.

cough, phlegm and impaired ventilatory function, independent of smoking habit and social class (model (i), Fig.5.3). Illnesses after the first year did not appear to pose a risk, supporting the idea of a critical period of influence for infection. Mortality from chronic respiratory disease was associated with early bronchitis and pneumonia in Hertfordshire.[26] These studies, together with ecological correlations,[9,33] have been interpreted as evidence of persistent lung damage from chest infections in infancy. However, a prospective study of the British 1946 birth cohort found that there was no significant independent effect of bronchitis, bronchiolitis or pneumonia before 2 years of age on peak expiratory flow rate at age 36, although early chest illnesses were independently associated with lower respiratory illness, phlegm and asthma or wheeze in adulthood.[34] When all respiratory illnesses up to 10 years of age were considered, a significant effect on PEFR was found for bronchitis and pneumonia,[8] but not for whooping cough.[35]

Asthmatic children often have a history of early chest illnesses which in past decades might have been labelled as bronchitis or pneumonia. The direction of cause and effect is a matter of debate,[31] but it has been suggested that the asthmatic trait might form a continuity between childhood and adult life and increase the susceptibility to both early chest illness and adult morbidity (model (ii), Fig.5.3).[11] Supporting evidence comes from studies of whooping cough—although asthmatic children are more common among those with a history of whooping cough, the onset of wheezing symptoms usually precedes the whooping cough illness.[36] Two long-term follow up studies confirm that although the majority of wheezy children grow out of their asthma, those that do not are at increased risk of cough and phlegm in their early twenties.[11,37] A retrospective American study also suggested that the respiratory problems in childhood which were associated with adult obstructive airways disease were those in the category of 'chronic or recurrent airway disease' (consistent with childhood asthma) rather than 'severe acute respiratory illness'.[38] On the other hand, the association of early chest illness and adult respiratory symptoms in the British 1946 birth cohort was independent of asthma history.[34]

The influences of early and later onset asthma or wheezy bronchitis on adult ventilatory function were studied at age 34–35 in the British 1958 cohort. Ventilatory function of young adults who had 'outgrown' a childhood wheezing tendency did not differ from that of healthy controls,[39] consistent with findings from Melbourne.[40] Young adults reporting wheeze in the past year at examination had lower levels of ventilatory function, the reduction being greater for those with childhood wheezing of earlier onset. These differences persisted after inhalation of salbutamol, suggesting a degree of irreversible airflow obstruction. Two longitudinal studies have suggested progressive deterioration in ventilatory function (as measured by FEV_1/FVC ratio) among adolescents with persistent asthma[41] or bronchial hyperresponsiveness.[42] These findings would be consistent with cumulative airway damage resulting from chronic inflammation in the bronchi of asthmatic individuals.

Infants with small airways are prone to early respiratory illnesses[43,44] which usually do not progress to chronic asthma.[44] It has thus been suggested that the link between early childhood chest illness and chronic respiratory disease in adults may arise from host susceptibility related to impaired prenatal lung growth, rather than from continuities in disease or lung damage from early infectious illnesses (model (iii), Fig.5.3).[10] The results of the 1958 cohort study offer only limited support for this hypothesis, in that FEV_1 at age 35 was slightly lower among children with transient early wheezing illness than among controls, although the dominant effect was of persistent asthma (ie. model ii).[39]

Marked seasonal fluctuations in many respiratory viruses and the greater vulnerability of young infants together imply that babies born in the autumn are at substantially greater risk of developing viral bronchiolitis, bronchitis, and pneumonia than those born in the spring. If these early infections had direct long term consequences for lung function or respiratory symptoms, then these outcomes should also be more common among autumn births. This was not found in several large datasets,[45] arguing that host susceptibility related to airways reactivity (model (ii)) or lung development (model (iii)), rather than lung damage (model (i)), may be the more important factor underlying the association of early chest illness with later lung disease and respiratory mortality.

5.4 Allergic sensitization

The ability to generate an immunoglobulin E (IgE) response to common inhaled proteins (aeroallergens) such as pollens, house dust mite faeces, or pet dander is consistently related to asthma and bronchial hyperresponsiveness in cross-sectional surveys of older children[46] and adults.[29] This atopic tendency may be assessed directly by skin prick tests or by measurement of serum IgE levels or imputed (less reliably) from a history of hay fever, allergic rhinitis, or eczema. Both the incidence and prognosis of asthma throughout childhood and early adult life are strongly influenced by atopy.[47]

Although there is undoubtedly a genetic component to atopy, environmental exposures are important in its expression. There is growing evidence that the process of allergic sensitization may be influenced by events during a critical period in early childhood, or on the first contact with the sensitizing allergen. Three possibilities have been considered: early growth, early allergen exposure, and early infection.[48]

In the Preston study, Godfrey et al.[49] measured levels of serum IgE among men and women aged about 50 years whose weight and dimensions at birth had been recorded in unusual detail. Raised IgE levels were positively correlated with head circumference and weight at birth, independent of circumstances in adult life. Head circumference was found to be the more influential factor, with no significant effect of birthweight at any given head circumference. They speculated that prenatal undernutrition of the thymus may influence subsequent IgE production and allergic sensitization, but there is as yet no evidence linking neonatal head circumference to allergen-specific IgE production or clinically apparent allergic disease.

The relative immaturity of the immune system in early infancy, has led to widespread speculation that allergen exposure in the first few months of life may enhance the risk of later sensitization. A number of studies have reported month of birth variations in sensitization to grass or tree pollens but despite some striking results[50] the evidence overall is inconsistent, both between and within studies.[45,48] If programming by early allergen exposure does occur, it is clearly a matter of degree, since sensitization can occur to occupational allergens encountered for the first time in adult life, as discussed in a later section of this chapter.

Several studies have shown that children from large families are at reduced risk of developing hay fever,[13,51,52] eczema,[13,52] and allergic sensitization to common aeroallergens.[51,53,54] Older siblings appear to exert a stronger protective effect than younger siblings[51-53] and offspring of more affluent families are at increased risk of hay fever and allergic sensitization.[53,55] Such observations led to speculation that infection acquired by household contact in early childhood might protect against allergic sensitization.[13,55]

Recent advances in our understanding of human immunological development[56] have suggested a possible mechanism for such a protective effect. Production of IgE responses and symptomatic atopic disease are associated with the presence of allergen-specific thymus-derived helper 2 (Th2) lymphocytes, whereas in non-atopic individuals non-pathogenic responses to the same antigens are mediated by Th1 cells. Th1 and Th2 cells are thought to develop in early life from uncommitted precursors and the direction of differentiation can be influenced by the levels of cytokines prevailing at the time of challenge with antigen. The 'natural' immune response to bacterial and viral infections increases the production of cytokines which selectively enhance the development of Th1-type lymphocytes, and suppress Th2-type differentiation.[57]

Direct evidence of a protective effect of early infection is still awaited.[51,58] The critical period during which programming by infection may occur is also uncertain. The suggestion that the first month of life is especially important[59] has been tested specifically and is not supported by the epidemiological evidence.[51] It is likely that a stable pattern of allergen-specific IgE response may evolve over a number of years,[60] in relation to repeated exposures to allergen, offering multiple 'windows of opportunity' for infection acquired from siblings and playmates to influence the cytokine environment of developing thymus-derived lymphocytes.

5.5 Later influences on adult respiratory disease

5.5.1 Tobacco smoking

Tobacco smoking is the dominant influence on respiratory symptoms related to chronic mucus hypersecretion, irreversible airflow obstruction and asthma. The evidence implicating smoking and the benefits of smoking cessation have been extensively reviewed[61,62] and only the salient points are reiterated here. Cough, phlegm, wheeze, and breathlessness are much more common among individuals and populations who smoke and are reduced when they quit the habit. The decline of ventilatory function is slowed, but not reversed, by smoking cessation. These benefits have been determined largely from observational studies but are supported by the results of two randomized controlled trials of antismoking advice.[63,64] Unfortunately, these lack the statistical power to demonstrate a reduction in respiratory mortality.

Although most smokers develop chronic mucus hypersecretion, only a minority develop disabling airflow obstruction, and the rate of decline of ventilatory function throughout adult life varies greatly.[14,16,28,30] A rare but powerful risk factor for accelerated decline is genetically determined α_1-antitrypsin deficiency.[65] Smokers with the abnormal PiZ α_1-antitrypsin genotype rapidly develop severe emphysema and usually die in their thirties or forties. Non-smokers with α_1-antitrypsin deficiency have a survival curve closer to that of smokers in the general population.

5.5.2 Diet

α_1-Antitrypsin is one of several lung antiprotease enzymes which are defence mechanisms against destructive proteolytic enzymes released in the lung on exposure to tobacco smoke. These antiproteases are inactivated by oxidants and this has led to speculation that antioxidants may improve the protease–antiprotease balance and thus protect against emphysema. By analogy with genetic α_1-antitrypsin deficiency, this protective effect might be more evident in smokers. A few cross-sectional studies have found lower levels of lung function in subjects consuming less fruit and vegetables,[66-68] although this effect appears in both smokers and non-smokers and it has been difficult to exclude residual confounding by socioeconomic factors. Studies are inconsistent regarding the association of dietary antioxidants and respiratory symptoms.[66,69]

A link between dietary sodium and reversible airflow obstruction was first suggested from a regional correlation of asthma mortality and salt purchases in England and Wales.[70] This was supported by observations of a correlation of urinary sodium excretion and non-specific bronchial hyperresponsiveness,[71] and reduction in BHR on dietary salt restriction.[72] All these effects were evident in males, but not in females, a difference which remains unexplained.

A later study did not confirm the association of BHR sodium excretion,[73] but suggested that dietary magnesium might protect against BHR and wheezing in adults.[74] With recent reports that fish oil may also have a protective role,[75] further studies investigating the role of nutritional factors in the aetiology of chronic respiratory disease can be expected.

5.5.3 Socioeconomic status

It has long been recognised that there is a strong association between poor socioeconomic status and both mortality and general practice consultations for adult respiratory disease in Britain.[76] Although much of this may be attributable to social class differences in smoking behaviour, population surveys have shown associations of socioeconomic status with symptoms of mucus hypersecretion[77,78] and measures of ventilatory function,[79] independent of current smoking habit. Furthermore, bronchitis mortality showed a strong social class gradient long before there was any substantial variation in smoking behaviour by social class.[80] Socioeconomic gradients may reflect upbringing and living conditions in childhood or life style and environment in adult life. Indeed, continuity of socioeconomic circumstances may be a further factor underlying associations between respiratory morbidity in childhood and adult life (model (iv), Fig.5.3). Among the British 1946 birth cohort, strong associations emerged between indices of socioeconomic deprivation in child-hood (particularly domestic crowding) and adult ventilatory function, measured as peak expiratory flow rate.[34] However, chronic cough and PEFR were also related to current socioeconomic circumstances, as indicated by housing tenure.[8] More specific studies of socially mobile individuals are required to distinguish reliably between influences in childhood and later life.

5.5.4 Occupational exposures

Marked social class trends are apparent in women (classified by their husband's occupation) as well as men, suggesting that specific occupational exposures play only a small part in explaining socioeconomic differentials. Nevertheless, a causal link between occupational dust exposure and mucus hypersecretion is generally acknowledged[77,81] and allergic sensitization to proteins and low molecular weight chemicals encountered in the workplace accounts for a small proportion of adult-onset asthma.[82] Smoking seems to promote allergic sensitization to some,[20] but not all,[83] occupational allergens. The role of dust and fumes in the aetiology of progressive airflow obstruction remains controversial. The best evidence emerges from longitudinal studies of workers in specific occupations, which suggest that exposures to a variety of inorganic dusts and to sulphur dioxide are consistently related to more rapid decline in FEV_1, whereas exposure to other fumes such as chlorine is not.[84]

5.5.5 Outdoor pollution

A more widespread source of inhaled particles and sulphur dioxide is combustion of fossil fuels, and throughout the past century there has been concern that urban air pollution may initiate or exacerbate chronic respiratory disease.[85] The following discussion will concentrate on disease initiation, since it is of greater relevance to the life course approach. Historically there was a geographical correlation between particulate pollution and chronic respiratory disease mortality in Britain,[86] but this became less marked after control of pollution in the 1960s.[87] Nevertheless, studies of communities exposed to lower levels of pollution in the USA during the 1970s show correlations of particulate exposure with both reduced FEV_1[88] and physician-diagnosed bronchitis.[89] Recent British reviews have concluded that the possibility of chronic effects on respiratory health at levels of particulates below 100 µg/m^3 annual average cannot be excluded,[90] although it is impossible to distinguish the effects of current low level exposure from past exposure to higher levels of air pollution.[91]

There have been few longitudinal studies addressing cumulative pollution exposure in relation to adult respiratory disease. The most comprehensive of these is the British 1946 birth cohort, who were exposed as children to high levels of smoke and sulphur dioxide pollution in urban areas, but as adults to much lower levels. Air pollution exposure in childhood was estimated from domestic coal consumption in the area of residence during wartime coal rationing. Although childhood chest illnesses were more common in highly polluted areas,[92] the effect of early pollution on symptoms of cough and phlegm at age 21 was small.[7] At age 36, air pollution exposure from age 2 to 11 years was significantly associated with lower respiratory illnesses over the preceding 16 years, but not with phlegm, wheeze, asthma or reduced PEFR, after adjustment for current smoking, socioeconomic status, parental history of bronchitis and history of asthma or chest illness before age 2 years.[34] It is arguable that the last two of these might be intermediate factors, rather than confounders, but this analysis suggests that long-term consequences are difficult to demonstrate, even from days when particulate and sulphur dioxide pollution levels were orders of magnitude higher than are currently experienced in Britain.

While in the past research and policy focused on the link between chronic bronchitis and smoke and sulphur dioxide ('old-fashioned winter pollutants'), more recently public concern has concentrated on asthma and the possible hazards of 'new' pollutants such as nitrogen oxides, ozone, and diesel particles, which are related to vehicle emissions. The evidence relating outdoor air pollution to asthma has been extensively reviewed.[93] Although other factors are likely to be more important than air pollution in the initiation of asthma, there are two lines of evidence which suggest outdoor pollution exposure should not be entirely dismissed.

Two studies in Japan have suggested a higher prevalence of wheezing[94] and allergic rhinitis[95] among non-smoking adults living close to busy roads, and it has been suggested that either diesel exhaust particles or nitrogen oxides, or both, may potentiate allergic sensitization. On the other hand, no association with local traffic density was found in a large study of general practitioner consultations for asthma in east London,[96] and no excess of respiratory symptoms has emerged in studies of groups with heavy occupational exposure to traffic fumes.[93]

Well designed cohort studies among Seventh Day Adventists in California have found a significantly higher incidence of asthma and chronic respiratory symptoms among persons with high cumulative exposure to particulates and ozone.[97,98] These studies are especially valuable because the study group avoid smoking for religious reasons, removing an important potential confounding variable.

5.5.6 Indoor pollution

The Seventh Day Adventist studies[98] are among the more convincing to demonstrate an adverse effect of home or workplace exposure to environmental tobacco smoke on chronic respiratory disease in adults. This emphasises that throughout life, indoor environments contribute a much greater proportion of personal pollutant exposure than does outdoor air. Nitrogen dioxide, although generated by motor vehicles, is often found at higher levels indoors than outdoors, due to emissions from unvented gas or paraffin appliances. Few studies have investigated the effects of indoor NO_2 on respiratory health in adults. The findings with respect to chronic cough and phlegm and lung function are inconsistent, possibly because the presence of a gas cooker has been used as a crude surrogate for personal NO_2 exposure. However, a recent study suggested substantial adverse effects of gas cooking on allergic sensitization, asthma, and ventilatory function, each of which were greater in women.[99] In one small study where NO_2 exposure was measured, there was also a significant association with spirometric measurements in non-smoking women at entry to the study, but not with the rate of subsequent lung function decline.[100] These results suggest that indoor air quality deserves greater emphasis in future studies of the chronic respiratory effects of air pollution exposure.

5.6 Conclusion

Respiratory and allergic diseases are well suited to the life course approach. It is evident that events early in the development of the lung and immune system may influence susceptibility to later infectious, allergenic, or toxic challenges to the airways. The critical periods during which these early influences may operate are poorly defined, but probably include both prenatal and postnatal development. The complex relationships between early infectious illness and later lung disease may prove particularly difficult to disentangle. While early intervention offers exciting prospects for prevention in the future, there is ample scope to modify the risk at later ages. Control of tobacco smoking remains the highest priority, but diet and indoor air pollution may also prove to be remediable influences worthy of attention. As smoking becomes less common, allergic sensitization and other influences on adult asthma may attain greater relative importance.

References

Those marked with an asterisk are especially recommended for further reading.

1   Anderson HR, Esmail A, Hollowell J, Littlejohns P, Strachan D. Lower respiratory disease. In Stevens A, Raftery J, eds. *Health Care Needs Assessment. The epidemiologically based needs assessment reviews. Volume 1.* Oxford: Radcliffe Medical Press, 1994:256–340.

2* Peto R, Speizer FE, Cochrane AL, Moore F, Fletcher CM, Tinker CM, Higgins ITT, Gray RG, Richards SM, Gilliland J, Norman-Smith B. The relevance in adults of airflow obstruction, but not of mucus hypersecretion, to mortality from chronic lung disease. *Am Rev Respir Dis* 1983;**128**:491–500.

3   Lange P, Nyboe J, Appleyard M, Jensen G, Schnohr P. Spirometric findings and mortality in never smokers. *J Clin Epidemiol* 1990;**43**:867–73.

4   Strachan DP. Ventilatory function, height and mortality among lifelong non-smokers. *J Epidemiol Community Health* 1992;**46**:66–70.

5* Samet JM, Tager IB, Speizer FE. The relationship between respiratory illness in childhood and chronic air-flow obstruction in adulthood. *Am Rev Respir Dis* 1983;**127**:508–23.

6   McConnochie KM, Roghmann KJ. Bronchiolitis as a possible cause of wheezing in childhood: new evidence. *Pediatrics* 1984;**74**:1–10.

7   Colley JRT, Douglas JWB, Reid DD. Respiratory disease in young adults: influence of early childhood lower respiratory tract illness, social class, air pollution and smoking. *Br Med J* 1973;**iii**:195–198.

8   Britten N, Davies JMC, Colley JRT. Early respiratory experience and subsequent cough and peak expiratory flow rate in 36 year old men and women. *Br Med J* 1987;**297**:1317–20.

9   Barker DJP, Osmond C. Childhood respiratory infection and adult chronic bronchitis in England and Wales. *Br Med J* 1986;293:1271–5.

10* Silverman M. Out of the mouths of babes and sucklings. Lessons from early childhood asthma. *Thorax* 1993;**48**:1200–4.

11   Strachan DP, Anderson HR, Bland JM, Peckham CS. Asthma as a link between chest illness in childhood and chronic cough and phlegm in young adults. *Br Med J* 1988;**296**:890–3.

12   Busse WW. The relationship between viral infections and onset of allergic diseases and asthma. *Clin Exp Allergy* 1989;**19**:1–9

13   Strachan DP. Hay fever, hygiene and household size. *Br Med J* 1989; **299**:1259–60.

14*   O'Connor GT, Sparrow D, Weiss ST. The role of allergy and nonspecific airways responsiveness in the pathogenesis of chronic obstructive pulmonary disease. *Am Rev Respir Dis* 1989;**140**:225–52.

15   Woolcock AJ, Peat JK, Salome CM, Yan K, Anderson SD, Schoeffel RE, McCowage G, Killalea T. Prevalence of bronchial hyperresponsiveness and asthma in a rural adult population. *Thorax* 1987;**42**: 361–8.

16   Fletcher CM, Peto R, Tinker CM, Speizer FE. *The natural history of chronic bronchitis and emphysema. An 8-year study of working men in London.* Oxford: Oxford University Press, 1976.

17   Orie NGM, Sluiter HJ, de Vries K, Tammerling GJ, Witkop J. The host factor in bronchitis. In Orie NGM, Sluiter HJ, eds. *Bronchitis*. Assen: Royal van Gorcum, 1961:43–59.

18   Markowe HLJ, Bulpitt CJ, Shipley MJ, Rose G, Crombie DL, Fleming DM. Prognosis in adult asthma: a national study. *Br Med J* 1987;**295**: 949–52.

19   Burrows B, Bloom JW, Traver GA, Cline MG. The course and prognosis of different forms of chronic airways obstruction in a sample from the general population. *N Engl J Med* 1987;**317**:1309–14.

20   Venables KM, Topping MD, Howe W, Luczynska CM, Hawkins R, Newman Taylor AJ. Interaction of smoking and atopy in producing specific IgE antibody against a hapten protein conjugate. *Br Med J* 1985; **290**:201–4.

21   Sly PD, Willet K. Developmental physiology. In Silverman M, ed. *Childhood asthma and other wheezing disorders*. London: Chapman & Hall, 1995:55–66.

22   Chan KN, Noble-Jamieson CM, Elliman A, Bryan EM, Silverman M. Lung function in children of low birthweight. *Arch Dis Child* 1989; **64**:1284–93.

23   Rona RJ, Gulliford MC, Chinn S. Effects of prematurity and intrauterine growth on respiratory health and lung function in childhood. *Br Med J* 1993;**306**:817–20.

24   Hanrahan JP, Tager IB, Segal MR, Tosteson TD, Castile RG, van Vunakis H, Weiss ST, Speizer FE. The effect of maternal smoking during pregnancy on early infant lung function. *Am Rev Respir Dis* 1992;**145**: 1129–35.

25 de Kleine MJK, Roos CM, Voorn WJ, Jansen HM, Koppe JG. Lung function 8-18 years after intermittent positive pressure ventilation for hyaline membrane disease. *Thorax* 1990;**45**:941–6.

26* Barker DJP, Godfrey KM, Fall C, Osmond C, Winter PD, Shaheen SO. Relation of birthweight and childhood respiratory infection to adult lung function and death from chronic obstructive lung disease. *Br Med J* 1991;**303**:671–5.

27 Strachan DP, Griffiths JM, Anderson HR, Johnston IDA. Association of intrauterine and postnatal growth with ventilatory function in early adult life. *Thorax* 1994;**49**:1052P.

28 Pride NB, Burrows B. Development of impaired lung function: natural history and risk factors. In Calverley P, Pride N, eds. *Chronic obstructive pulmonary disease*. London: Chapman & Hall, 1995:69–91.

29 Burney PGJ, Britton JR, Chinn S, Tattersfield AE, Papacosta AE, Kelson MC, Anderson F, Corfield DR. Descriptive epidemiology of bronchial reactivity in an adult population: results from a community study. *Thorax* 1987;**42**:38–44.

30 Pride NB, Taylor RG, Lim TK, Joyce H, Watson A. Bronchial hyperresponsiveness as a risk factor for progressive airflow obstruction in smokers. *Bull Eur Physiopathol Respir* 1987;**23**:369–75.

31 Strachan DP. Do chesty children become chesty adults? *Arch Dis Child* 1990;**65**:161–2.

32 Shaheen SO, Barker DJP, Shiell AW, Crocker FJ, Wield GA, Holgate ST. The relationship between pneumonia in early childhood and impaired lung function in late adult life. *Am Rev Respir Dis* 1994;**149**:616–9.

33 Barker DJP, Osmond C, Law CM. The intrauterine and early postnatal origins of cardiovascular disease and chronic bronchitis. *J Epidemiol Community Health* 1989;**43**:237–40.

34* Mann SL, Wadsworth MEJ, Colley JRT. Accumulation of factors influencing respiratory illness in members of a national birth cohort and their offspring. *J Epidemiol Community Health* 1992;**46**:286–92.

35 Britten N, Wadsworth J. Long term sequelae of whooping cough in a nationally representative sample. *Br Med J* 1986;292:441–4

36 Johnston IDA, Anderson HR, Lambert HP, Patel S. Respiratory morbidity and lung function after whooping cough. *Lancet* 1983;**ii**:1104–8.

37 Martin AJ, Landau LI, Phelan PD. Asthma from childhood at age 21: the patient and his disease. *Br Med J* 1982;**284**:380–2.

38 Burrows B, Knudson RJ, Lebowitz MD. The relationship of childhood respiratory illness to adult obstructive lung disease. *Am Rev Respir Dis* 1977;**115**:751–60.

39* Strachan DP, Griffiths JM, Anderson HR, Johnston IDA. Ventilatory function in British adults after asthma and wheezing illness at ages 0–35. *Am J Respir Crit Care Med* 1996;**154**:1629–35.

40 Kelly WJW, Hudson I, Raven J, Phelan PD, Pain MCF, Olinsky A. Childhood asthma and adult lung function. *Am Rev Respir Dis* 1988; **138**:26–30.

41 Weiss ST, Tosteson TD, Segal MR, Tager IB, Redline S, Speizer FE. Effects of asthma on pulmonary function in children. A longitudinal population-based study. *Am Rev Respir Dis* 1992;**145**:58–64.

42 Sherrill D, Sears MR, Lebowitz MD, Holdaway MD, Hewitt CJ, Flannery EM, Herbison GP, Silva PA. The effects of airway hyperresponsiveness, wheezing and atopy on longitudinal pulmonary function in children: a 6-year follow-up study. *Pediat Pulmonol* 1992;**13**:78–85.

43 Tager IB, Hanrahan JP, Tosteson TD, Castille RG, Brown RW, Weiss ST, Speizer FE. Lung function, pre- and post-natal smoke exposure, and wheezing in the first year of life. *Am Rev Respir Dis* 1993;**147**:811–7.

44 Martinez FD, Wright AL, Taussig LM, Holberg C, Halonen M, Morgan WJ, Group Health Medical Associates. Asthma and wheezing in the first six years of life. *N Engl J Med* 1995;**332**:133–8.

45 Strachan DP, Seagroatt V, Cook DG. Chest illness in infancy and chronic respiratory disease in later life: an analysis by month of birth. *Int J Epidemiol* 1994;**23**:1060–8.

46 Burrows B, Sears MR, Flannery EM, Herbison GP, Holdaway MD. Relationship of bronchial responsiveness assessed by methacholine to serum IgE, lung function, symptoms and diagnosis in 11 year old children. *J Allergy Clin Immunol* 1992;**90**:376–85.

47 Strachan DP, Butland BK, Anderson HR. The incidence and prognosis of asthma and wheezing illness from early childhood to age 33 in a national British cohort. *Br Med J* 1996;**312**:1195–9.

48 Strachan DP. Is allergic disease programmed in early life? *Clin Exp Allergy* 1994;**24**:603-5.

49 Godfrey KM, Barker DJP, Osmond C. Disproportionate fetal growth and raised IgE concentration in adult life. *Clin Exp Allergy* 1994;**24**:641–8.

50 Björkstén F, Suoniemi I, Koski V. Neonatal birch pollen contact and subsequent allergy to birch pollen. *Clin Allergy* 1980;**10**:585–91.

51 Strachan DP, Taylor EM, Carpenter RG. Family structure, neonatal infection and hay fever in adolescence. *Arch Dis Child* 1996;**74**:422–6.

52 Golding J, Peters T. Eczema and hay fever. In Butler N, Golding J, eds. *From birth to five. A study of the health and behaviour of Britain's five-year-olds.* Chapter 12. Oxford: Pergamon Press, 1986:171–86.

53 Strachan DP, Harkins LS, Johnston IDA, Anderson HR. Childhood antecedents of allergic sensitization in young British adults. *J Allergy Clin Immunol* 1997;**99**:1–12.

54 von Mutius E, Martinez FD, Fritzsch C, Nicolai T, Reitmar P, Thiemann HH. Skin test reactivity and number of siblings. *Br Med J* 1994;**308**: 692-5.

55* Strachan DP. Epidemiology of hay fever: towards a community diagnosis. *Clin Exp Allergy* 1995;**25**:296-303.

56 Holt PG. A potential vaccine strategy for asthma and allied atopic diseases during early childhood. *Lancet* 1994;**344**:456–8.

57 Romagnani S. Human TH1 and TH2 subsets: regulation of differentiation and role in protection and immunopathology. *Int Arch Allergy Immunol* 1992;**98**:279–85.

58 Backman A, Björkstén F, Ilmonen S, Juntunen K, Suoniemi I. Do infections in infancy affect sensitization to airborne allergens and development of allergic disease? *Allergy* 1984;**39**:309–15.

59 Martinez FD. Role of viral infections in the inception of asthma and allergies during childhood: could they be protective? *Thorax* 1994;**49**: 1189–91.

60 Hattevig G, Kjellman B, Björkstén B. Appearance of IgE antibodies to ingested and inhaled allergens during the first 12 years of life in atopic and non-atopic children. *Pediatr Allergy Immunol* 1993;**4**:182–6.

61* United States Department of Health and Human Services, Public Health Service. *The health consequences of smoking: chronic obstructive lung disease. A report of the Surgeon General.* Washington, DC: US Government Printing Office, 1984.

62* United States Department of Health and Human Services, Public Health Service. *The health benefits of smoking cessation. A report of the Surgeon General.* Washington, DC: US Government Printing Office, 1990.

63 Rose G, Hamilton PJS. A randomised controlled trial of the effect on middle-aged men of advice to stop smoking. *J Epidemiol Community Health* 1978;**32**:275–81.

64 Kuller LH, Ockene JK, Townsend M, Browner W, Meilahn E, Wentworth D. The epidemiology of pulmonary function and COPD mortality in the Multiple Risk Factor Intervention Trial. *Am Rev Respir Dis* 1989; **140**:S76–81.

65 Larsson C. Natural history and life expectancy in severe alpha-1-antitrypsin deficiency, PiZ. *Acta Med Scand* 1978;**204**:345–51.

66 Strachan DP, Cox BD, Erzinclioglu SW, Walters DE, Whichelow MJ. Ventilatory function and winter fresh fruit consumption in a random sample of British adults. *Thorax* 1991;**46**:624–9.

67 Schwartz J, Weiss ST. Relationship between dietary vitamin C intake and pulmonary function in the First National Health and Nutrition Examination Survey (NHANES I). *Am J Clin Nutr* 1994;**59**:110–4.

68 Britton JR, Pavord ID, Richards KA, Knox AJ, Wisniewski AF, Lewis SA, Tattersfield AE, Weiss ST. Dietary antioxidant vitamin intake and lung function in the general population. *Am J Respir Crit Care Med* 1995;**151**:1383–7.

69   Schwartz J, Weiss ST. Dietary factors and their relation to respiratory symptoms. *Am J Epidemiol* 1990;**132**:67–76.

70   Burney P. A diet rich in sodium may potentiate asthma. Epidemiologic evidence for a new hypothesis. *Chest* 1987;**6 (Suppl)**:143S–8S.

71   Burney PG, Britton JR, Chinn S, Tattersfield AE, Platt HS, Papcosta AO, Kelson MC. Response to inhaled histamine and 24 hour sodium excretion. *Br Med J* 1986;**292**:1483–6.

72   Burney PG, Neild JE, Twort CH, Chinn S, Jones TD, Mitchell WD, Bateman C, Cameron IR. Effect of changing dietary sodium on the airway response to histamine. *Thorax* 1989;**44**:36–41.

73   Britton J, Pavord I, Richards K, Knox A, Wisniewski A, Weiss S, Tattersfield A. Dietary sodium intake and the risk of airway hyper-reactivity in a random adult population. *Thorax* 1994;**49**:875–80.

74   Britton J, Pavord I, Richards K, Wisniewski A, Knox A, Lewis S, Tattersfield A, Weiss S. Dietary magnesium, lung function, wheezing and airway hyperreactivity in a random adult population sample. *Lancet* 1994;**344**:357–62.

75   Britton J. Dietary fish oil and airways obstruction. *Thorax* 1995;**50 (Suppl 1)**:S11–5.

76   Strachan DP. Epidemiology: a British perspective. In Calverley P, Pride N, eds. Chronic obstructive pulmonary disease. London: Chapman & Hall, 1995:47–68.

77   Dean G, Lee PN, Todd GF, Wicken AJ, Sparks DN. Factors related to respiratory and cardiovascular symptoms in the United Kingdom. *J Epidemiol Community Health* 1978;**32**:86–96.

78   Respiratory Diseases Study Group of the College of General Practitioners. Chronic bronchitis in Great Britain. *Br Med J* 1961;**ii**:973–8.

79   Cox BD. Blood pressure and respiratory function. (in) Cox BD, Blaxter M, Buckle ALJ, Fenner NP, Golding JF, Gore M, Huppert FA, Nickson J, Roth M, Wadsworth MEJ, Whichelow M. *The health and lifestyle survey. Preliminary report of a nationwide survey of the physical and mental health, attitudes and lifestyle of a random sample of 9003 British adults.* London: Health Promotion Research Trust, 1987:17–33.

80   Registrar-General for England and Wales. *Decennial supplement for 1921. Occupational mortality.* London: HMSO, 1931.

81   Morgan WKC. Industrial bronchitis. *Br J Ind Med* 1978;**35**:285–91.

82   Newman Taylor AJ. Occupational asthma. *Thorax* 1980;**35**:241–45.

83   Chang-Yeung M. Occupational asthma. *Chest* 1990;**98 (Suppl 5)**:148–61.

84   Becklake MR. Occupational exposures: evidence for a causal association with chronic obstructive pulmonary disease. *Am Rev Respir Dis* 1989; **140**:S85–9.

85   Collis EL. The general and occupational prevalence of bronchitis and its relation to other respiratory diseases. *J Ind Hyg Toxicol* 1923;5:264–76.

86   Gardner MJ, Crawford MD, Morris JN. Patterns of mortality in middle and old age in the county boroughs of England and Wales. *Br J Prev Soc Med* 1969,**23**.133-40.

87   Chinn S, Florey CDV, Baldwin IG, Gorgol M. The relationship of mortality in England and Wales 1969-73 to measurements of air pollution. *J Epidemiol Community Health* 1981;**35**:174-9.

88   Chestnut LG, Schwartz J, Savitz DA, Burchfiel CM. Pulmonary function and ambient particulate matter: epidemiological evidence from NHANES I. *Arch Environ Health* 1991;**46**:135-44.

89   Schwartz J. Particulate air pollution and chronic respiratory disease. *Environ Res* 1993;**62**:7-13.

90   Department of Health Advisory Group on the medical aspects of air pollution episodes. *Second report: sulphur dioxide, acid aerosols and particulates.* London: HMSO, 1992.

91* Department of Health Committee on the medical effects of air pollutants. *Non-biological particles and health.* London: HMSO, 1995.

92   Douglas JWB, Waller RE. Air pollution and respiratory infection in children. *Br J Prev Soc Med* 1966;**20**:1-8.

93* Department of Health Committee on the medical effects of air pollutants. *Asthma and outdoor air pollution.* London: HMSO, 1995.

94   Nitta H, Sato T, Nakai S, Maeda K, Aoko S, Ono M. Respiratory health associated with exposure to automobile exhaust. I. Results of cross-sectional studies in 1979, 1982 and 1983. *Arch Environ Health* 1993; **48**:53-8.

95   Ishizaki T, Koizumi K, Ikemori R, Ishiyama Y, Kushibiki E. Studies of prevalence of Japanese cedar pollinosis among the residents in a densely cultivated area. *Ann Allergy* 1987;**58**:265-70.

96   Livingstone AE, Shaddick G, Grundy C, Elliott P. Do people living near inner city main roads have more asthma needing treatment? A case-control study using routine general practice data. *Br Med J* 1996;**311**:676-7.

97   Abbey DE, Lebowitz MD, Mills PK, Petersen FF, Beeson L, Burchette RJ. Long-term ambient concentrations of particulates and oxidants and development of chronic disease in a cohort of nonsmoking California residents. *Inhalation Toxicology* 1995;**7**:19-34.

98   Greer JR, Abbey DE, Burchette RJ. Asthma related to occupational and ambient air pollutants in nonsmokers. *J Occup Med* 1993;**35**:909-15.

99   Jarvis D, Chinn S, Luczynska C, Burney P. Association of respiratory symptoms and lung function in young adults with use of domestic gas appliances. *Lancet* 1996;**347**:426-31.

100 Fischer P, Remjin B, Brunekreef B, van der Lende R, Schouten J, Quanjer P. Indoor air pollution and its effect on pulmonary function of adult non-smoking women. II: Associations between nitrogen dioxide and pulmonary function. *Int J Epidemiol* 1985;**14**:221-6.

6 Blood pressure and hypertension

Peter Whincup and Derek Cook

Blood pressure is a major risk factor for cardiovascular disease. Blood pressure in adult life, rather than blood pressure earlier in the life course, is the critical influence on cardiovascular risk. The patterns of blood pressure seen in middle age emerge in the individual in the first years of life and in the population during childhood or adolescence. These patterns are substantially reversible, and closely related to development of variations in body mass. Factors influencing blood pressure in middle age, particularly body mass and potassium intake, are also related to blood pressure in childhood and adolescence, again in a reversible way. Fetal factors (particularly related to birthweight) may have a long term influence on adult blood pressure. However, the effect of fetal factors appears to be smaller than that of factors acting in adult life and the underlying causes and mechanisms have yet to be defined.

6.1 Introduction

High blood pressure is a major risk factor for coronary heart disease and stroke, diseases of middle and later life. The conventional view of high blood pressure in recent decades is that it is, with specific exceptions, a condition of middle and later life (30 years +).[1-3] The search for aetiological factors, reflecting this view, has concentrated on factors operating in adult life.[4] Body mass and alcohol intake are strong determinants of blood pressure in middle age;[4-7] other factors, including electrolyte intake[4-6,8-10] and possibly physical activity and psychosocial factors,[11,12] also play a part. However, in recent years there has been increasing interest in the possibility that high blood pressure may have its origins in childhood[13] or even in utero.[14]

In defining whether the earlier phases of the life course, including early adult life (20–29 years), late childhood and adolescence (10–19 years), early childhood (1–9 years), infancy, and the intrauterine period are influencing blood pressure, it is important to recognize that the blood pressure in middle age and beyond (30 years +), rather than blood pressure earlier in the life course, is the main determinant of cardiovascular risk. A strong and consistent relation between casual adult blood pressure and cardiovascular risk has been demonstrated in many observational studies; taking the effects of random variation and regression to the mean into account, a 10 mmHg increase in diastolic pressure in middle age (equivalent to an 18 mmHg increase in systolic pressure) is associated with a doubling in risk of stroke and a 50% increase in coronary risk.[15] More importantly, comparisons of the reduction in cardiovascular risk observed in the major therapeutic trials of blood pressure reduction in middle age with the reduction expected on the basis of observational data relating blood pressure to cardiovascular risk[16,17] suggest that a therapeutic blood pressure reduction of 5–6 mmHg in diastolic pressure (equivalent to a 10–14 mmHg reduction in systolic pressure) in adult life achieves all the expected reduction in stroke incidence and at least two-thirds of the expected reduction in coronary incidence in 5 years. This emphasizes that the risks associated with elevated blood pressure are substantially reversible in middle life.

In considering the influence of factors operating during the earlier stages of the life course, the crucial question is whether such factors have an independent effect on adult blood pressure and, if so, whether such effects are reversible. Three approaches can be taken. First, one can attempt to define the point at which the variations in blood pressure seen in middle age first emerge. Second, one can examine the stage in the life course at which factors known to influence blood pressure in adult life begin to act. Third, one can examine whether factors operating at specific stages during the life course have specific effects on adult blood pressure. However, before addressing these questions, the problem of defining blood pressure and hypertension in population studies will be briefly addressed.

6.2 Defining blood pressure and hypertension in population-based studies

Blood pressure, both in adult life and during childhood, follows a continuous, unimodal distribution in the population.[1] Moreover, the relationship between blood pressure and cardiovascular risk is continuous and graded across a wide range of blood pressures.[15] For the epidemiologist, the distinction between normal and high blood pressure is quantitative rather than qualitative, and average blood pressures are used in preference to estimates of the prevalence of hypertension using arbitrary thresholds. Moreover, blood pressure variation occurs at two levels—within-population and between-population (particularly on a geographic basis). Variation in blood pressure within a population is likely to have a substantial genetic component, with estimates of heritability ranging from 30–60%.[18] In contrast, the results of studies of migration suggest that differences in the average blood pressure of different populations have a strong environmental basis (see Chapter 10).[19,20]

6.3 Development of adult patterns of blood pressure variation

6.3.1 Variation between individuals

The point at which the variations in blood pressure between individuals observed in middle age emerge has been extensively studied in all periods between infancy and middle age life, although few studies have covered the whole period. Consistency of blood pressure ranking ('tracking') has been described during the first year of life,[21] and at all stages in the life course thereafter.[22] However, the degree of consistency is weak. The tracking (correlation) coefficient for measurements of systolic pressure made at a 1 year interval rises from 0.1 or so in the first 2 years to about 0.4 between 3 and 4 years[23] and continues to rise during childhood. Although temporarily diminished during the period of rapid adolescent growth,[24] the coefficient rises to about 0.7 at the end of the second decade, and remains reasonably stable thereafter.[22]

That blood pressure 'tracks' from an early age suggests that at least some degree of stability in the balance of genetic and environmental determinants of blood pressure is present from early in the life course. However, the proportion of variation not accounted for by previous blood pressure measurements is very high in childhood (more than 80%) and even in adulthood it remains high (50% or more). Although some unexplained variation is explained by imprecision of blood pressure measurement and regression to the mean (the tendency for outlying measurements to be closer to the mean on repeated assessment), blood pressure rank appears to be changeable, especially in childhood. Variation in weight gain and growth rate, which are strongly related to blood pressure change, are likely to play an important part in the changes which occur.[25,26]

6.3.2 Variation between populations

Although geographic variations in blood pressure between populations have been well described for many years,[27] the point during the life course at which differences in blood pressure between population groups emerge has been little studied. Many authors have assumed that variations in blood pressure between populations emerge during middle age,[2] and that mean blood pressures in childhood and early adult life (up to 30 years) do not differ between populations.[3] However, there have been few systematic attempts to study variation in the mean blood pressure levels of children and young adults from different populations, or to relate them to average blood pressure levels in the same populations in middle age. A standardized measurement study of 8–9 year old children in 13 European countries[28] and a review of published studies on blood pressure in children[29] both suggested marked variation in average blood pressure levels between populations in childhood, but relations with adult blood pressure or cardiovascular mortality were not explored. The Intersalt Study made standardized measurements of blood pressure in men and women aged between 20 and 59 years in 52 different populations from 32 countries. Examining published data from the study,[30] it is apparent that mean blood pressure levels at 20–29 years vary markedly between populations, and are strongly related to levels at 50–59 years (Fig. 6.1), although level at 20–29 years is not strongly related to subsequent *change* in pressure.[31] This suggests that blood pressure differences of the middle aged pattern are apparent at 20–29 years. The strong correlation between mean blood pressure levels and published stroke mortality data for 19 of the 32 countries in that study ($r = 0.40$) makes between-centre observer bias an unlikely explanation for the finding. Strong associations have also been observed between mean systolic blood pressure levels at 15–19 years and those at 50–59 years, in 35 separate studies including data on men and 28 on women.[31] Comparable data for younger subjects are sparse. However, in the Tokelau Island Migrant Study, marked differences between the mean blood pressures of Tokelauan children

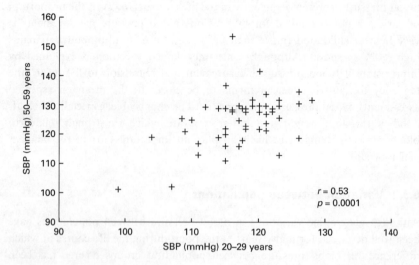

Figure 6.1 Systolic blood pressure (males) at 20–29 years and 50–59 years in 52 different population groups. Based on published Intersalt data.[30]

(aged 2–14 years) on Tokelau and New Zealand were observed from 2 years upwards[32] which paralleled adult differences and were not due to selection bias.[33] However, these remarkable findings in younger children require further substantiation in other populations, and at present it seems more likely that population differences are emerging in late childhood and adolescence rather than in early childhood. This is also consistent with the timing of emergence of adult blood pressure differences between socioeconomic groups, which are apparent in adolescence[34,35] but not at 7 years.[31] Differences in blood pressure of black and white American children have been reported in adolescence[34,35] and less consistently in younger children down to the later years of the first decade.[36] Factors operating between populations which may account for these differences are likely to include obesity and to a lesser extent diet, particularly intakes of sodium, potassium and alcohol.[4,5] Fetal factors (q.v.) are an unlikely explanation for these population differences; populations with particularly low blood pressure have characteristics which suggest that average birthweights are likely to be low rather than high.[37]

The reversibility of population differences in blood pressure can be investigated using data from studies which have examined the effect of migration between populations with different mean blood pressure levels. These studies have consistently shown that subjects moving to higher blood pressure populations, even when middle aged, experience a rise in blood pressure compared with non-migrants, which begins within a month of migration and becomes more marked during the first 2 years after migration (see Chapter 10).[38-41] Few studies have been able to examine the effect of migration to a low blood pressure setting. However, there is evidence, from a study of Australian aborigines reverting from a Western life style to a traditional life style[42] and from a study of British middle aged men migrating from regions of Britain with higher average blood pressure levels to those with lower levels,[20] that blood pressure may fall on migration as well as rise, although this requires confirmation in other settings.

6.4 Environmental influences on adult blood pressure—do they begin to act before adult life?

A second approach to studying the development of blood pressure and hypertension during the life course is to consider whether factors which influence blood pressure in middle age also do so earlier in life and, if so, whether the effects are reversible. Such questions can only be usefully addressed about factors which are consistently and causally related to blood pressure in middle age. Factors considered include body mass, alcohol intake, and dietary sodium and potassium. Dietary intakes of calcium and magnesium and physical activity are excluded because their relations with blood pressure in adults are inconsistent or weak[43] or have been difficult to establish.[44]

6.4.1 Body size

Body mass (weight for height, body mass index) is related to blood pressure at all stages of the life course. The association between weight and blood pressure is apparent at birth[21] and persists through childhood and adolescence into adult life, although it becomes weaker in late middle age.[13] Although the mechanisms of the association between obesity and blood pressure are not fully understood, the relation is likely to be causal. Moreover, the distribution of fat is important, with central obesity being particularly associated with raised blood pressure and hyperinsulinaemia both in adults[45] and in children.[46] Progressive weight gain in adult life, particularly on a diet high in saturated fat, is a consistent feature of populations at high risk of cardiovascular disease, particularly coronary heart disease.[47] Several studies have shown that weight in childhood, adolescence or early adult life predicts blood pressure in middle age.[13,47] However, there is considerable evidence suggesting that the influence of body mass on blood pressure is at least partly reversible. Although earlier weight is positively related to blood pressure, both in children and adults, adjustment for current weight abolishes (and may even reverse) the association with earlier weight (Table 6.1). In longitudinal studies, weight change is strongly related to changes in blood pressure, both in adults[48,49] and in children.[25,26] Moreover, controlled studies of weight loss both in adults and in children have suggested that the effects of body mass on blood pressure are reversible.[50] At present therefore it seems likely that the effects of obesity before middle age are theoretically reversible, even if this does not often occur in practice.

Could size or weight gain at particular periods in infancy or childhood have an important long term effect on blood pressure? The possibility that growth during early childhood might have long term effects on blood pressure has been postulated,[51] particularly as a possible explanation of the relationship between low birthweight and higher subsequent blood pressure (q.v.). However, supporting evidence is so far lacking.[52] On the other hand, it has been suggested that poor vertical growth in childhood may be an independent determinant of raised blood pressure in later life,[53] a finding which requires further exploration. Although growth later in childhood, particularly at adrenarche and at puberty, is strongly related to blood pressure rise,[13] it is not clear whether the timing and extent of growth at these periods have long term effects on attained blood pressure which are independent of later growth and attained adult size. This possibility requires critical examination in existing and future studies.

Table 6.1 Weight at 5–7 years and blood pressure at 9–11 years, showing effect of adjustment for weight at 9–11 years (males)

Adjustment for weight at 9–11 years	Systolic			Diastolic		
	Regression coefficient (mmHg/kg)	Standard error	p value	Regression coefficient (mmHg/kg)	Standard error	p value
No	1.62	0.23	<0.0001	0.38	0.15	0.01
Yes	−0.22	0.40	0.58	−0.30	0.27	0.27

Based on 543 subjects
Source: Two Towns Study[87]

Weight at 36 years and blood pressure at 43 years showing effect of adjustment for weight at 43 years (males)

Adjustment for weight at 43 years	Systolic			Diastolic		
	Regression coefficient (mmHg/kg)	Standard error	p value	Regression coefficient (mmHg/kg)	Standard error	p value
No	0.08	0.04	0.03	0.14	0.03	<0.0001
Yes	−0.21	0.08	0.009	−0.18	0.06	0.004

Based on 1,342 subjects
Source: MRC National Survey of Health and Development[70]

6.4.2 Alcohol intake

Alcohol intake is strongly related to blood pressure both in middle age and in young adults.[7,54] Because alcohol intakes are particularly high in young adults in many developed countries, alcohol is a very important determinant of blood pressure in early adult life[54] although its role in younger subjects is likely to be limited. However, the effects of alcohol intake on blood pressure in middle age appear to be reversible[55] and there is no evidence that alcohol intake before middle age has any sustained effect on later blood pressure.

6.4.3 Sodium intake

A positive relationship between sodium intake and blood pressure in adults, with an increase of approximately 0.03-0.06 mmHg in systolic pressure per

1 mmol increase in daily sodium intake, has been established both by observational studies[5,8,9] and by intervention trials.[10] In adults there is considerable evidence that the strength of the association between salt intake and blood pressure becomes stronger with increasing age between 20 and 59 years.[9,56] In children it has been difficult to demonstrate associations between salt intake and blood pressure. Although Cooper et al.[57] found a weak positive association between sodium excretion and blood pressure in 73 11–14 year old boys (each producing seven repeat 24 h urine samples) the finding was not replicated[58] or reproduced experimentally.[59] Similarly, no association was observed in 887 8-9 year old children.[28] The absence of an association between sodium intake and blood pressure in childhood is consistent with the findings of a study comparing observational and experimental effects of changes in salt intake in adults, suggesting that a short-term reduction in salt intake achieves all the blood pressure reduction expected on the basis of observational data.[8-10] This implies that any effect of sodium intake on blood pressure before adult life is likely to be reversible. However, the position in neonates is less clear. Hofman et al.[60] reported that a 6 month period of sodium restriction in newborns produced a reduction in systolic pressure of 2.1 mmHg at the end of the intervention. Although the effect was not sustained 6 months later,[61] a difference of 3.6 mmHg at 15 years of age has recently been reported.[62] This raises the possibility that sodium restriction early in the life course has a long term effect on blood pressure. However, this observation, based on follow up of only 35% of the original cohort without data on current sodium intake, has still to be substantiated. A trial of early postnatal sodium restriction in premature neonates showed no long term effect on blood pressure.[63]

6.4.4 Potassium intake

An inverse relation between potassium intake and blood pressure has been demonstrated in adults, both by observational studies[4-6] and by experimental studies.[64] In observational studies the relationship between potassium intake and blood pressure appears to become more marked with age.[64] Unlike sodium, similar (i.e. inverse) associations between potassium intake and blood pressure have been described in young adults and in children;[64,65] a high potassium intake may also be related to a smaller rate of rise in blood pressure with age in children and adolescents.[66] A physiological basis for the greater importance of potassium in blood pressure control in young subjects has been described.[67]

High maternal potassium intake in pregnancy may be related to lower blood pressure levels in offspring, although this remains an observational finding and the longer term effects are unclear.[68] However, as in the case of sodium, it appears from experimental studies in middle age that the hypotensive effect of potassium supplementation on blood pressure is reversible.[64] There is no evidence at present to suggest that potassium intake before middle age has long term effects on blood pressure level.

6.5 Factors which may act at specific points in the life course with long term effects on blood pressure

6.5.1 Fetal and infant factors and blood pressure

The finding that low birthweight was related to a higher subsequent mean blood pressure led to the suggestion that early life factors might have a long term effect on blood pressure. This observation has now been made in many studies,[69] including several different British adult populations of men and women—a national cohort study[70] as well as specific studies in Hertfordshire,[14] Preston[71] and Sheffield[72]—and a study of Swedish men.[73] The association is not dependent on adjustment for adult body size and appears to be independent of alcohol intake and social class in adults,[71,72] although the adequacy of adjustment has been questioned.[74] Moreover, similar but weaker associations have also been described in children aged between 3 and 11 years, independent of social class, parity and maternal blood pressure—but only after adjustment for current body size.[70, 75-77] Although such adjustment has been criticized, it may be reasonable in children, in whom birthweight and current size (particularly height) are still associated, and given that these associations become weaker with increasing age. The inverse birthweight-blood pressure association is not, however, apparent at adolescence, even after current size adjustment.[78,79] It has been suggested that the disruption of blood pressure tracking during puberty may provide an explanation for the absence of the inverse association at this age.[14] However, although tracking is attenuated in puberty it certainly does not disappear.[24] Moreover, the birthweight-blood pressure association at 10-11 years appears to be stronger in girls than boys,[70,80] again suggesting that a more specific explanation for the absence of the association in adolescence must be sought. Other potential markers of the intrauterine environment have also been studied, but without convincing results. Maternal age is not consistently related to blood pressure.[75,77,81] Birth rank has also been examined. Higher mean blood pressures have been described in firstborn or single children both in childhood[75,77] and in adult life,[82,83] although not in all studies.[81] The association is not however likely to have an intrauterine origin; childhood blood pressure is related as strongly to number of younger as older siblings, suggesting that postnatal factors are more important.[77]

6.5.2 Does the birthweight–blood pressure relationship represent 'programming'?

It has been argued that the presence of an independent association between birthweight and blood pressure in middle age may represent 'programming' (see Chapter 1),[84] in this case specifically involving long term effects on vascular structure and function, particularly perhaps arterial compliance.[72] However, while the finding may be consistent with the possibility of 'programming', it does not provide conclusive evidence. Two other lines of evidence could support the possibility of programming. First, it has been suggested that the birthweight–blood pressure relation becomes stronger (is 'amplified') with increasing age and, second, it has been suggested that more specific markers of fetal growth at particular phases of pregnancy may be particularly related to blood pressure. Each of these issues will be examined in turn.

Evidence for the amplification of the birthweight blood pressure relationship was first provided by Law et al., who examined one longitudinal and three cross-sectional studies relating birthweight to blood pressure at different ages and suggested that the birthweight–blood pressure relationship appeared to become stronger with age from childhood onwards.[52] However, the comparison, based mainly on cross-sectional rather than longitudinal data, provided only indirect evidence of amplification. Moreover, the extent of amplification has appeared less striking as more data have become available, although the fall in systolic pressure for a 1 kg increase in birthweight may still increase from 2 mmHg in childhood to 4–5 mmHg in adult life.[69] Undoubtedly some amplification of the birthweight blood pressure relationship must occur in early childhood, because it is not present at birth (when weight is *positively* related to blood pressure[21]) but is present by 3 years of age.[85,86] In older children, some direct evidence for the possibility of amplification has been provided by a longitudinal study of 540 children followed between 5–7 and 9–11 years, in whom the relation between birthweight and blood pressure almost doubled in strength.[87] However, this effect was almost entirely seen in girls and has not been confirmed in a larger study of children of a similar age.[80] Although further evidence from longitudinal studies is needed to clarify the degree of amplification, it should be recognized that amplification *per se* may not be sufficient evidence of programming, because the combination of tracking and dispersion of the blood pressure distribution with age are sufficient to amplify the association between birthweight and blood pressure.[85]

Since programming implies a disturbance at a critical period of development, attempts have been made to identify specific markers of impaired fetal growth which are more closely related to elevated blood pressure. The association between birthweight and blood pressure has reported to be stronger in term offspring (in which low birthweight is predominantly a result of impaired growth rather than prematurity) in two studies.[71,73] However, the relations between birthweight and blood pressure in children are similar in term and preterm offspring and adjusting birthweight for gestational age does not strengthen the association.[77,87] Two more specific markers, thinness at birth (i.e. a low weight/height^3) and shortness at birth (i.e. a low length/head circumference) were reported to be associated with particularly high adult levels of blood pressure in the Preston study.[88] However, neither of these markers, thought to be linked to fetal undernutrition in the second and third trimesters respectively, has been substantiated in later studies in adults,[72,73] nor in studies of children.[80] In the Preston study, increasing placental weight and a high placental weight : birthweight ratio were both linked to particularly high mean blood pressure levels,[71] suggesting that fetal undernutrition might underlie the association between placental size and blood pressure.[14] However, these findings were strongly dependent on the results in a small subgroup of individuals with particularly low birthweight and high placental weight. Moreover, the association between placental size and blood pressure, although supported by some studies[76,89] has not been replicated in several others, either in adults[72,73] or in children.[87,90] At present, therefore, no more specific marker of size at birth has been consistently found to relate more closely to blood pressure than birthweight. However, it has recently been reported that low birthweight is more strongly related to blood pressure when associated with a greater attained adult height.[73] This may imply that failure to express full growth potential in utero is the factor most closely related to adult blood pressure, a possibility which requires further investigation.

A further uncertainty about the contribution of programming concerns the underlying aetiology. Variation in birthweight is largely environmentally determined[91,92] and Barker has suggested that maternal undernutrition underlies the elevation of blood pressure and other cardiovascular consequences of small size at birth.[14] Animal studies have provided some support for this possibility, showing, for example, that protein restriction in pregnant rats is associated with higher blood pressure levels in offspring,[93] and also raising the possibility that failure of fetal protection against maternal glucocorticoids might play an important role.[94] However, the importance of maternal nutrition on offspring blood pressure in humans has still to be proven. Maternal starvation during pregnancy has very limited effects on the birthweight of offspring, and then only in the third trimester;[95] trials of protein supplementation have tended to reduce, rather than increase, birthweight.[96] However, in a study of the relation between maternal diet and offspring blood pressure 40 years later, it was found that either a high carbohydrate intake combined with a low protein intake, or a low carbohydrate intake with a high protein intake, were associated with the higher mean blood pressure levels among offspring.[97] Maternal anaemia, which is associated with a greater placental weight and a higher placental ratio, has also been implicated as a possible nutritional marker.[98] However, other studies have failed to confirm any relationship between either haemoglobin concentration or mean corpuscular volume and placental size[99,100] or blood pressure in children.[100] Moreover, since physiological haemodilution during pregnancy (leading to lower maternal haemoglobin concentration) is particularly marked in high birthweight pregnancies,[101] there is a contradiction between the hypotheses that low birthweight and low maternal haemoglobin concentration during pregnancy are both risk factors for later cardiovascular risk.[100] Maternal smoking does not appear to be involved in the process, having no consistent effect on offspring blood pressure, with or without birthweight adjustment.[100] The case for a relationship between maternal nutrition and blood pressure in offspring has therefore still to be proven. There is at present no suggestion that different feeding practices immediately after birth have any long term effect on blood pressure.[75,102]

6.5.3 Fetal factors and adult factors

If intrauterine factors are important long term influences on blood pressure, how important are they when compared with factors operating later in the life course, particularly obesity? Studies presenting data on the strength of both relationships are shown in Table 6.2. In all studies except the 1946 Birth Cohort, the strength of the associations between weight (body mass index) and blood pressure exceed those of birthweight by a factor of 2 or more—a difference not likely to be accounted for by differences in measurement precision. Moreover, in the Uppsala study the effect of low birthweight appeared to be particularly marked in subjects with the highest body mass index in middle age; evidence of interaction was particularly strong in taller men.[73] This implies that the expression of the birthweight effect may occur primarily in the presence of adult obesity, further emphasizing the dominance of the adult factor. However, corresponding effects have not yet been observed in other studies either in adults or children, so the finding requires further substantiation. A further possible complication to the interrelations of fetal and adult factors is posed by Ravelli's observation that undernutrition in utero during the first two trimesters of pregnancy is followed by an increased prevalence of obesity in adult life,[103] and by Law's finding that low birthweight is related to higher levels of central obesity in adult life.[104] This raises the possibility that the association between low birthweight and adult blood pressure might be explained by a relationship between low birthweight and adult obesity. However, this is not supported by data from the studies of birthweight and blood pressure in adults so far reported, in which the birthweight-blood pressure relationships were either unaffected or strengthened by adjustment for adult obesity and in which the relations between birthweight and adult obesity tend to be positive rather than inverse.[70-73]

Table 6.2 Comparison of the influence of birthweight (kg) and current weight (kg) on systolic blood pressure at different ages

| Study (reference) | Different ages | | | | | Systolic pressure effect (mmHg) | | |
	Age group (years)	N	Comparative grouping	Sex	Weight	Birthweight	Weight:Birthweight
Law et al.[76]	4	405	Fourths	M & F	3.7	−2.6	1.4
Whincup et al.[75]	5–7	3591	Standardized regression effect	M & F	3.11	−0.98	3.2
Whincup et al.[77]	5–7	3396	Standardized regression effect	M & F	2.90	−0.96	3.0
Barker et al.[70]	10	9921	Thirds	M F	5.1 5.3	−0.4 −1.3	12.8 4.1
Whincup et al.[87]	9–11	1335	Standardized regression effect	M & F	4.50	−1.4	3.2
Barker et al.[70]	36	3259	Thirds	M F	2.0 0.8	−2.5 −1.9	0.8 0.4
Barker et al.[71]	46–54	449	Fourths	M & F	10.0+	−5.0*	2.0
Leon et al.[73]	50	1333	Thirds/Fourths	M	9.9+	−2.7	3.7

* Not adjusted for placental weight
+ Body mass index; data on weight not available

6.6 Conclusions

The study of potential determinants of blood pressure acting at different stages in the life course need to focus on their effects on blood pressure in middle age as the main influence on cardiovascular risk. Differences in blood pressure between individuals are apparent from very early in life; those between populations probably appear during late childhood or adolescence. Individual determinants of blood pressure in middle age (body mass and potassium intake particularly) have similar effects on blood pressure at younger ages. The early appearance of these patterns, although theoretically reversible, is important from a public health viewpoint because it is closely linked to the conditioning of dietary behaviour, which is occurring during childhood and adolescence[105] and may be difficult in practice to reverse in middle age.

The potential importance of the associations between size at birth and later blood pressure is that, once established, they may represent irreversible influences on adult blood pressure. However, although this is a possibility, the underlying relationships have not yet been clarified and the role of maternal nutrition, particularly in humans, remains conjectural. Moreover, the associations are considerably weaker than those of adult body mass index and may be dependent on the presence of adult obesity, emphasizing the primacy of adult influences. If supported by further evidence, programming would have important implications for our approaches to the prevention of hypertension in adult life, focusing attention on maternal nutrition, both preconceptually and during pregnancy.[14] Further research should clarify the influence of maternal nutrition on size at birth and blood pressure in offspring, identify specific elements of size at birth which are most strongly related to blood pressure and establish the extent to which the birthweight-blood pressure association is being amplified in contemporary children and young adults.

References

Those marked with an asterisk are especially recommended for further reading.

1   Pickering GW. *High blood pressure* (2nd Edition). London, Churchill, 1968.
2   Peart WS. Concepts in hypertension: the Croonian Lecture 1979. *J R Coll Phys* 1979;**14**:141–52.
3   Rose G. Hypertension in the community. In: Bulpitt CJ (ed). *Handbook of hypertension*. Vol 6: *Epidemiology of hypertension*. Elsevier, Amsterdam, 1985:1–14.
4   Intersalt Cooperative Research Group. Intersalt: an international study of electrolyte excretion and blood pressure. Results for 24 hour urinary sodium and potassium excretion. *Br Med J* 1988;**297**:319–28.

5   Elliott P, Stamler J, Nichols R, Dyer AR, Stamler R, Kesteloot H et al. Intersalt revisited: further analyses of 24 hour sodium excretion and blood pressure within and across populations. *Br Med J* 1996;**312**: 1249–53.

6   Smith WCS, Crombie IK, Tavendale RT et al. Urinary electrolyte excretion, alcohol consumption and blood pressure in the Scottish Heart Health Study. *Br Med J* 1988;**297**:329–30.

7   Klatsky AL, Friedman GD, Armstrong MA. The relationships between alcoholic beverage use and other traits to blood pressure: a new Kaiser Permanente study. *Circulation* 1986;**73**:628–36.

8   Law MR, Frost CD, Wald NJ. By how much does dietary salt reduction lower blood pressure? I—Analysis of observational data among populations. *Br Med J* 1991;**302**:811–5.

9   Frost CD, Law MR, Wald NJ. By how much does dietary salt reduction lower blood pressure? II—Analysis of observational data within populations. *Br Med J* 1991;**302**:815–8.

10   Law MR, Frost CD, Wald NJ. By how much does dietary salt reduction lower blood pressure? III—Analysis of data from trials of salt reduction. *Br Med J* 1991;**302**:819–24.

11   Fagard R, Bielen P, Hespel P, Lijnen P, Staessen J, Vanhees L et al. Physical exercise in hypertension. In: Laragh JH, Brenner BM, eds. *Hypertension: pathophysiology, diagnosis and management.* New York, Raven Press, 1990:1985–98.

12   Pickering TG. Psychosocial stress and hypertension: clinical and experimental studies. In: Swales JD (ed). *Textbook of hypertension.* Oxford, Blackwell Scientific, 1994:640–54.

13* Lever AF, Harrap SB. Essential hypertension: a disorder of growth with origins in childhood? *J Hypertens* 1992;**10**:101–20.

14* Barker DJP. *Mothers, babies and disease in adult life.* London, BMJ Publishing Group, 1994.

15   MacMahon S, Peto R, Cutler J et al. Blood pressure, stroke and coronary heart disease: part 1, prolonged differences in blood pressure: prospective observational studies corrected for the regression dilution bias. *Lancet* 1990;**335**:765–74.

16   Collins R, Peto R, MacMahon S et al. Blood pressure, stroke and coronary heart disease: part 2. Short-term reductions in blood pressure: overview of randomized drug trials in their epidemiological context. *Lancet* 1990;**335**:827–38.

17   MacMahon S. Blood pressure as a risk factor. In: Swales JD (ed). *Textbook of hypertension.* Oxford, Blackwell Scientific, 1994:46–57.

18   Mongeau J-G. Heredity and blood pressure. *Semin Nephrol* 1989;**9**: 208–16.

19 He J, Klag MJ, Whelton PK, Chen J-Y, Mo J-P, Qian M-C et al. Migration, blood pressure pattern and hypertension: the Yi Migrant Study. *Am J Epidemiol* 1991;**134**:1085–101.

20 Elford J, Phillips A, Thomson AG, Shaper AG. Migration and geographic variations in blood pressure in Britain. *Br Med J* 1990;**300**:291–5.

21 de Swiet M, Fayers P, Shinebourne EA. Blood pressure survey in a population of normal infants. *Br Med J* 1976;**ii**:9–11.

22 Rosner B, Hennekens CH, Kass EH, Miall WE. Age-specific correlational analysis of longitudinal blood pressure data. *Am J Epidemiol* 1977; **106**:306–13.

23 de Swiet M, Fayers P, Shinebourne EA. Value of repeated blood pressure measurements in children—the Brompton study. *Br Med J* 1980;**i**:1567–9.

24 Andre JL, Deschamps JP, Petit JC, Gueguen R. Change of blood pressure over five years in childhood and adolescence. *Clin Exp Hypertens* 1986;**8**:539–45.

25 Hofman A, Valkenburg HA. Determinants of change in blood pressure during childhood. *Am J Epidemiol* 1983;**117**:735–43.

26 Clarke WR, Woolson RF, Lauer RM. Changes in ponderosity and blood pressure in childhood; the Muscatine Study. *Am J Epidemiol* 1986;**124**: 195–206.

27 Marmot MG. Geography of blood pressure and hypertension. *Br Med Bull* 1984;**40**:380–6.

28 Knuiman JT, Hautvast JGAJ, Zwiauer KFM et al. Blood pressure and excretion of sodium, potassium, calcium and magnesium in 8 and 9 year-old boys from 19 European centres. *Eur J Clin Nutr* 1988;**42**: 847–55.

29 Brotons C, Singh P, Nishio T, Labarthe DR. Blood pressure by age in childhood and adolescence: a review of 129 surveys worldwide. *Int J Epidemiol* 1989;**18**:824–9.

30 Intersalt Cooperative Research Group. Appendix tables. Centre specific results by age and sex. *J Hum Hypertens* 1989;**3**:331–407.

31 Whincup PH. *A study of blood pressure in childen in nine British towns.* PhD thesis. London University, 1991.

32 Beaglehole R, Eyles E, Salmond C, Prior I. Blood pressure in Tokelaun children in two contrasting environments. *Am J Epidemiol* 1978;**108**: 283–8.

33 Beaglehole R, Eyles E, Prior IAM. Blood pressure and migration in children. *Int J Epidemiol* 1979:**8**:5–10.

34 Miller RA, Shekelle RB. Blood pressure in tenth-grade students. Results from the Chicago Heart Association Pediatric Heart Screening Project. *Circulation* 1976;**54**:993–1000.

35   Khaw KT, Marmot MG. Blood pressure in 15 to 16 year-old adolescents of different ethnic groups in two London schools. *Postgrad Med J* 1983;**59**:630–1.

36   Voors AW, Foster TA, Frerichs RR et al. Studies of blood pressure in children, ages 5-14 years, in a total biracial community. *Circulation* 1976;**54**:319–27.

37   Shaper AG. Communities without hypertension. In: Shaper AG, Hutt MSR, Fejfar Z, eds. *Cardiovascular disease in the tropics*. London, BMA, 1974:77–83.

38   Salmond CE, Prior IAM, Wessen AF. Blood pressure patterns and migration: a 14-year study of adult Tokelauans. *Am J Epidemiol* 1989: **130**:37–52.

39   Poulter NR, Khaw KT, Hopwood BE, Mugambi M, Peart WS, Rose G, Sever PS. The Kenyan Luo Study: observations on the initiation of a rise in blood pressure. *Br Med J* 1990;**300**:967–72.

40   Rosenthal T, Grossman E, Knecht A, Goldbourt U. Blood pressure in Ethiopian immigrants in Israel: comparison with resident Israelis. *J Hypertens* 1989;**7 (suppl 1)**:S53–5.

41   Goldbourt U, Khoury M, Landau E, Reisin LH, Rubinstein A. Blood pressure in Ethiopian immigrants: relationship to age and anthropometric factors, and changes during their first year in Israel. *Isr J Med Sci* 1991;**27**:264–7.

42   O'Dea K. Interpretation of genetic versus environmental factors—lessons from the Australian aborigines when westernized. In: Smith A (ed). *Hypertension as an insulin resistant disorder. Genetic factors and other mechanisms*. Amsterdam, Elsevier, 1991:69–87.

43   Cappuccio FP. Electrolyte intake and human hypertension: part B, calcium and magnesium. In Swales JD (ed). *Textbook of hypertension*. Oxford, Blackwell Scientific, 1994:551–66.

44   Arroll B, Beaglehole R. Does physical activity lower blood pressure: a critical review. *J Clin Epidemiol* 1992;**45**:439–47.

45   Williams PT, Fortmann SP, Terry RB, Garay SC, Vranizan KM, Ellsworth N et al. Associations of dietary fat, regional adiposity and blood pressure in men. *JAMA* 1987;**257**:3251–6.

46   Smoak CG, Burke GL, Webber LS, Harsha DW, Srinivasan SR, Berenson GS. Relation of obesity to clustering of cardiovascular disease risk factors in children and young adults. The Bogalusa Heart Study. *Am J Epidemiol* 1987;**125**:364–72.

47   Shaper AG. Origins and consequences of obesity. Ciba Foundation Symposium no. 201; Chichester, John Whiley, 1996:90–107.

48   Holland FJ, Stark O, Ades AE, Peckham CS. Birth weight and body mass index in childhood, adolescence, and adulthood as predictors

of blood pressure at age 36. *J Epidemiol Community Health* 1993;**47**: 432–5.

49 Havlik RJ, Hubert HB, Fabsitz RR et al. Weight and hypertension. *Ann Int Med* 1983;**98**:855–9.

50 Cutler JA. Randomized clinical trials of weight reduction in non-hypertensive persons. *Ann Epidemiol* 1991;**1**:363–70.

51 Ounsted MK, Cockburn JM, Moar VA, Redman CWG. Factors associated with the blood pressures of children born to women who were hypertensive during pregnancy. *Arch Dis Child* 1985;**60**:631–5.

52* Law CM, de Swiet M, Osmond, C, Fayers P, Barker DJP, Cruddas AM, Fall CHD. Initiation of hypertension in utero and its amplification throughout life. *Br Med J* 1993;**306**:24–7.

53 Wadsworth M, Kuh DJL. Childhood influences on adult health: a review of recent work in the 1946 national British birth cohort (the MRC National Study of Health and Development). *Paediat Perinat Epidemiol* 1997;**11**:2–20.

54 Bruce NG, Wannamethee G, Shaper AG. Life-style factors associated with geographic blood pressure variations among men and women in the UK. *J Hum Hypertens* 1993;**7**:229–38.

55 Maheswaran R, Gill JS, Davies P, Beevers DG. High blood pressure due to alcohol, a rapidly reversible effect. *Hypertension* 1991;**17**: 787–92.

56 Elliott P, Dyer A, Stamler R. The Intersalt Study: results for 24 hour sodium and potassium, by age and sex. *J Hum Hypertens* 1989;**3**: 323–30.

57 Cooper R, Soltero I, Liu K et al. The association between urinary sodium excretion and blood pressure in children. *Circulation* 1980;**62**:97–104.

58 Cooper R, Liu K, Trevisan M et al. Urinary sodium excretion and blood pressure in children: absence of a reproducible association. *Hypertension* 1983;**5**:135–9.

59 Cooper R, Van Horn L, Liu K et al. A randomized trial on the effect of decreased dietary sodium intake on blood pressure in adolescents. *J Hypertens* 1984;**2**:361–6.

60* Hofman A, Hazebroek A, Valkenburg HA. A randomized trial of sodium intake and blood pressure in newborn infants. *JAMA* 1983; **250**:370–3.

61 Hofman A. Sodium intake and blood pressure in newborns: evidence for a causal connection. In: *Children's blood pressure: report of the 88th Ross conference on paediatric research*. Ross Laboratories, Columbus, Ohio, 1989.

62 Geleijnse JM, Hofman A, Witteman JCM, Hazebroek AAJM, Valkenburg HA, Grobbee DE. Long term effects of neonatal sodium restriction on blood pressure (abstract). *J Hypertens* 1996;**14 (suppl 1)**: S210.

63   Lucas A, Morley R, Hudson GJ, Bamford MF, Boon A, Crowle P. Early sodium intake and later blood pressure in preterm infants. *Arch Dis Child* 1988;**63**:656–7.

64   Cappuccio FP, MacGregor GA. Does potassium supplementation lower blood pressure? A meta-analysis of published trials. *J Hypertens* 1991; **9**:465–73.

65   Whincup PH, Cook DG, Papacosta O, Jones SR. Relations between sodium:creatinine and potassium:creatinine ratios and blood pressure in childhood (abstract). *J Hypertens* 1992;**10**:1434.

66   Geleijnse JM, Grobbee DE, Hofman A. Sodium and potassium intake and blood pressure change in childhood. *Br Med J* 1990;**300**: 899–902.

67   Lever AF, Beretta-Piccoli C, Brown JJ, Davis DL, Frazer R, Robertson JIS. Sodium and potassium in essential hypertension. *Br Med J* 1981; **283**:463–7.

68   McGarvey ST, Zinner SH, Willett WC, Rosner B. Maternal prenatal dietary potassium, calcium, magnesium and infant blood pressure. *Hypertension* 1991;**17**:218–24.

69   Law CM, Shiell AW. Is blood pressure inversely related to birthweight: strength of evidence from a systematic review of the literature. *J Hypertens* 1996;**14**:935–41.

70   Barker DJP, Osmond C, Golding J, Kuh D, Wadsworth MEJ. Growth in utero, blood pressure in childhood and adult life, and mortality from cardiovascular disease. *Br Med J* 1989;**298**:564–7.

71*   Barker DJP, Bull AR, Osmond C, Simmonds SJ. Fetal and placental size and risk of hypertension in adult life. *Br Med J* 1990;**301**:259–62.

72   Martyn CN, Barker DJP, Jespersen S, Greenwald S, Osmond C, Berry C. Growth in utero, adult blood pressure and arterial compliance. *Br Heart J* 1995;**73**:116–21.

73*   Leon DA, Koupilova I, Lithell HO, Berglund L, Mohsen R, Vagero D et al. Failure to realise growth potential in utero and adult obesity in relation to blood pressure in 50 year-old Swedish men. *Br Med J* 1996; **312**:401–6.

74*   Elford J, Whincup PH, Shaper AG. Early life experience and adult cardiovascular disease. Longitudinal and case-control studies. *Int J Epidemiol* 1991;**20**:833–44.

75   Whincup PH, Cook DG, Shaper AG. Early influences on blood pressure: a study of children aged 5–7 years. *Br Med J* 1989;**299**:587–91.

76   Law CM, Barker DJP, Bull AR, Osmond C. Maternal and fetal influences on blood pressure. *Arch Dis Child* 1991;**66**:1291–5.

77   Whincup PH, Cook DG, Papacosta O. Do maternal and intrauterine factors influence blood pressure in childhood? *Arch Dis Child* 1992; **67**:1423–9.

78 Seidman DS, Laor A, Gale R et al. Birth weight, current body weight, and blood pressure in late adolescence. *Br Med J* 1991;**302**:1235–7.

79 Macintyre S, Watt G, West P et al. Correlates of blood pressure in 15 year olds in the West of Scotland. *J Epidemiol Community Health* 1991;**45**:143–7.

80 Taylor SJC, Whincup PH, Cook DG, Papacosta O, Walker M. Size at birth and blood pressure: cross sectional study in 8–11 year old children. *Br Med J* 1997;**314**:475–80.

81 Higgins MW, Keller J, Moore F et al. Studies of blood pressure in Tecumseh, Michigan. I. Blood pressure in young people and its relationship to personal and familial characteristics and complications of pregnancy in mothers. *Am J Epidemiol* 1980;**111**:142–55.

82 Thorne MC, Wing AL, Paffenbarger RS Jr. Chronic disease in former college students. VII. Early precursors in nonfatal coronary heart disease. *Am J Epidemiol 1968;***87**:520–9.

83 Trevisan M, Krogh V, Klimowski L et al. Absence of siblings—a risk factor for hypertension? *N Engl J Med* 1991;**324**:1285.

84* Lucas A. Programming by early nutrition in man. In: Bock GR, Whelan J, eds, *The childhood environment and adult disease*. Chichester: John Wiley and Sons, 1991:38–55.

85 Launer LJ, Hofman A, Grobbee DE. Relation between birthweight and blood pressure; longitudinal study of infants and children. *Br Med J* 1993;**307**:1451–4.

86 Hashimoto N, Kawasaki T, Kikuchi T, Takahashi H, Uchiyama M. The relationship between the intrauterine environment and blood pressure in 3 year-olds Japanese children. *Acta Paediatrica* 1996;**85**:132–8.

87* Whincup PH, Cook DG, Papacosta O. Birth weight and blood pressure; cross-sectional and longitudinal relationships in childhood. *Br Med J* 1995;**311**:773–6.

88 Barker DJP, Godfrey KM, Osmond C, Bull A. The relation of fetal length, ponderal index and head circumference to blood pressure and the risk of hypertension in adult life. *Paediatr Perinat Epidemiol* 1992;**6**:3544.

89 Moore VM, Miller AG, Boulton TJC, Cockington RA, Hamilton Craig I, Magarey AM, Robinson JS. Placental weight, birth measurements and blod pressure at age 8 years. *Arch Dis Child* 1996;**74**:538–41.

90 Williams S, St George IM, Silva P. Intrauterine growth retardation and blood pressure at age seven and eighteen. *J Clin Epidemiol* 1992;**45**:1257–63.

91 Carr-Hill R, Campbell DM, Hall MH, Meredith A. Is birthweight determined genetically? *Br Med J* 1987;**295**:687–9.

92 Robson EB. The genetics of birthweight. In: Falkner F, Tanner JM, eds. *Human growth*. Vol I: *Principles and prenatal growth*. New York: Plenum Press, 1978:285–97.

93 Langley SC, Jackson AA. Increased systolic blood pressure in adult rats induced by fetal exposure to maternal low protein diets. *Clin Sci* 1994; **86**:217–22.

94 Edwards CRW, Benediktsson R, Lindsay RS, Seckl JR. Dysfunction of placental glucocorticoid barrier: link between fetal environment and adult hypertension? *Lancet* 1993;**341**:355–7.

95 Stein ZA, Susser M. The Dutch famine 1944–45, and the reproductive process. I. Effect on six indices at birth. *Pediatr Res* 1975;**9**:70–6.

96 Rush D. Effects of changes in protein and calorie intake during pregnancy on growth of the human fetus. In: Chalmers I, Enkin M, Keirse MJNC, eds. *Effective care in pregnancy and childbirth*. Oxford, Oxford University Press, 1989:255–80.

97 Campbell DM, Hall MH, Barker DJP, Cross J, Shiell AW, Godfrey KM. Diet in pregnancy and the offspring's blood pressure 40 years later. *Br J Obs Gynae* 1996;**103**:273–80.

98 Godfrey KM, Redman CWG, Barker DJP, Osmond C. The effect of maternal anaemia and iron deficiency on the ratio of fetal weight to placental weight. *Br J Obstet Gynaecol* 1991;**98**:886–91.

99 Perry IJ, Beevers DG, Whincup PH, Bareford D. Predictors of ratio of placental weight to fetal weight in a multiethnic community. *Br Med J* 1995; **310**:436–9.

100 Whincup PH, Cook DG, Papacosta O, Walker M, Perry I. Maternal factors and development of cardiovascular risk: evidence from a study of children. *J Hum Hypertens* 1994;**8**:337–43.

101 Gibson HM. Plasma volume and glomerular filtration rate in pregnancy and their relationship to differences in fetal growth. *J Obstet Gynae Br Commonw* 1973, 80:1067–74.

102 Lucas A, Morley R. Does early nutrition in infants born before term programme later blood pressure? *Br Med J* 1994;**309**:304–8.

103 Ravelli G-P, Stein ZA, Susser MW. Obesity in young men after famine exposure in utero and early infancy. N Engl J Med 1976;**295**:349–53.

104 Law CM, Barker DJP, Osmond C, Fall CHD, Simmonds SJ. Early growth and abdominal fatness in adult life. *J Epidemiol Community Health* 1992;**46**:184–6.

105 World Health Organization. *Prevention in childhood and youth of adult cardiovascular diseases: time for action*. Technical Report Series No 792. WHO, Geneva, 1990.

C Biological and Social Processes

7 Fetal growth and development: the role of nutrition and other factors

Ivan J Perry

It is hypothesized that the risk of cardiovascular disease and diabetes in adult life is programmed in utero by specific patterns of abnormal fetal growth associated with maternal undernutrition. This hypothesis raises fundamental questions about patterns of fetal growth in utero and about the role of factors other than nutrition in fetal growth and development. An unambiguous concept of nutrition that relates to the mother's diet, growth, and development in childhood, and her diet during pregnancy, facilitates the testing of precisely formulated hypotheses in work on nutrition, fetal growth and adult disease. Different patterns of fetal growth retardation in pregnancy form a continuum that depends mainly on the severity and timing of thenutritional or other insult. Growth failure in the third trimester tends to be asymmetrical, with weight loss but a relative sparing of fetal length. The hypothesis that nutritional insults in early pregnancy set the fetus on a low growth trajectory leading tosymmetrical growth retardation is less securely based. The concept of nutritional programming is undoubtedly plausible in biological terms. However, a less discrete and deterministic model of programming is proposed, involving interactions between the maternal and fetal genotype, the mother's environment and life style (including diet), her prepregnancy nutritional status, metabolism and physiology, the hormonal, metabolic and circulatory milieu which sustains fetal growth and the infant's postnatal environment. The effects of prenatal nutrition on fetal growth in man depend on the timing of nutritional exposures in relation to critical periods of development and on interactions with the mother's prepregnancy nutritional status and aspects of the mother's metabolism and physiology such as glucose tolerance and blood pressure. Given an environment with adequate nutrition to sustain optimal growth in a girls childhood

145

and adolescence, dietary intake during pregnancy probably accounts for a relatively small amount of variation in fetal growth. Future studies need to examine, using reliable methods, the distribution and determinants of fetal growth rates and patterns within and between populations. Studies of prenatal diet, fetal growth, and pregnancy outcome that address problems of measurement error and explore interactions between diet and maternal physiology are also likely to prove rewarding.

7.1 Introduction

'As you sow, so shall you reap'

The health of mothers and infants is a central public health concern, and the notion that poor nutrition at critical periods of development in fetal life is a key determinant of health in childhood and adult life[1-2] has considerable resonance. Thus, the nutritional programming hypothesis has helped refocus interest in the role of maternal nutrition in fetal growth and development. This work, which has provided such a valuable millennial fillip for chronic adult disease epidemiology, also raises fundamental questions about patterns of fetal growth in utero and about the role of factors other than nutrition in fetal growth and development. It has become clear that nutrition needs to be placed in context within the broader framework of other maternal, fetal, and uterine/placental factors which are known to influence fetal growth.[3-6]

7.1.1 Fetal origins: a conceptual framework

It is now clear that various markers of fetal growth consistently predict cardiovascular disease risk.[1,2,7,8] It remains unclear however, as to whether these associations are primarily a manifestation of intrauterine 'programming' of cardiovascular disease risk due to poor maternal nutrition or 'programming' due to other influences in utero unrelated to maternal undernutrition, such as defective placentation, maternal glucose intolerance and hypertension or other aspects of the maternal hormonal, metabolic, or circulatory milieu. Alternatively, the link between low birthweight and later disease may be confounded by genetic factors related to both low birthweight and cardiovascular disease, or by postnatal environmental factors (notably poverty and social disadvantage) which link mother and infant.[9] In considering sources of variation in fetal growth, the focus of this review is on nutrition (and markers of maternal nutritional status including height, pregravid weight, and gestational weight gain) with particular reference to the nutritional programming hypothesis.[1-2] The focus of this work, to date, has been largely on the effects of maternal undernutrition at critical periods of development on fetal growth. There is a

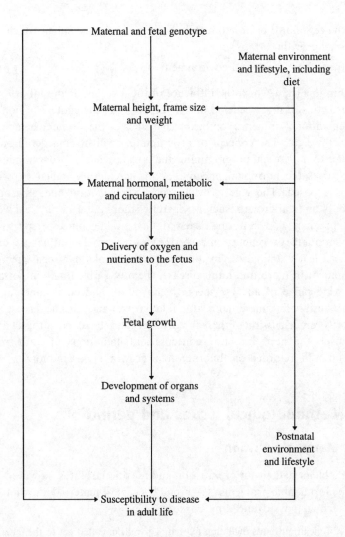

Figure 7.1 Fetal origins of adult disease: a conceptual framework.

need however to broaden the concept of programming, to consider a wider canvas, such as that in Fig. 7.1, which includes:

(i) the fetal genotype,

(ii) the maternal genotype,

(iii) the mother's social and physical environment,

(iv) the mother's prepregnancy nutritional status, her metabolism and physiology,

(v) her diet during pregnancy,

(vi) the resultant hormonal, metabolic and circulatory milieu which sustains fetal growth

(vii) the infant's postnatal environment.

Within this framework, the influence of the fetal and maternal genotype on fetal growth will be considered and it will be set in the context of non-genetic intergenerational influences on birthweight such as the mother's height and her own birthweight. The concept of programming will be considered both with reference to nutritional programming and a wider view of programming which encompasses the hormonal, metabolic, and circulatory milieu to which the fetus is exposed. The role of wider social, behavioural and environmental influences on fetal growth, such as cigarette smoking[10] and physical workload during pregnancy[11] will not be reviewed. Given a life course perspective, there is a continuum of genetic, intrauterine, and postnatal influences on adult disease. Clearly therefore, in the context of links between growth and development in utero and adult disease, there is a potentially important role for a wide range of adverse social, behavioural, and environmental factors which plausibly link maternal health, fetal growth and chronic disease in adult life. However, discussion of these factors is beyond the scope of this chapter. At the outset, the need for clear concepts and definitions of both 'maternal nutrition' and 'retarded or abnormal fetal growth' is paramount.

7.2 Methodological issues and definitions

7.2.1 Maternal nutrition

The reliable measurement of nutrition and nutritional status, however defined, presents formidable problems.[12] A broad concept of maternal nutrition may be used, such as that advanced by Barker,[13]

'. . . I mean nutrients including oxygen. The nutrients that get to the fetus are clearly related to the many aspects of the mother's physiology, her preconceptual stores, her competence to sustain fetal growth and maybe to a minor extent what she eats in pregnancy, and whether the mother exercises in pregnancy. Delivery of nutrients to the fetus is a very complicated agenda.' (p.238)

Although it is difficult to quibble with such a comprehensive and all embracing concept of maternal nutrition, there is potential for confusion between nutritional intake/nutritional status and other factors critical to the mother's competence to sustain fetal growth such as her level of blood pressure or glucose tolerance. Moreover, it is not clear that such a broad concept of nutrition facilitates the testing of precisely formulated hypotheses. Here, the term maternal nutrition refers to nutritional intake during pregnancy, i.e.

intake of calories and of macro and micronutrients, and nutritional status as measured by markers such as prepregnancy weight and height.

7.2.2 Fetal growth

The fertilised ovum faces three interrelated challenges in utero,

(i) implantation and survival,

(ii) differentiation or the development of new structures and

(iii) growth.

These challenges correspond approximately to the blastogenic, embryonic and fetal phases of development. Growth during the blastogenic and embryonic phases of development, which span the first 8 postovulatory weeks, consists of an increase in cell numbers (hyperplasia). By the end of this period, the embryo is only about 3 cm long and weighs approximately 6 g but has already developed several thousand structures.[14] The fetal phase of development, from the third through the ninth month, is characterized both by hyperplasia, an increase in the number of cells, and by hypertrophy, an increase in the size of existing cells, with the latter gradually becoming predominant.[15] In the first half of pregnancy the length of the fetus increases rapidly with peak length growth velocity before 20 weeks. By contrast, the rate of increase in fetal weight does not peak until the third trimester, at 30–32 weeks.[16–17]

The definition of normal and abnormal fetal growth has long been beset by confusion and controversy. For obvious reasons, work in this area has focused on the identification of a minority of infants at high risk of morbidity and mortality in the neonatal period. Birthweight is consistently and reliably recorded and is a good predictor of neonatal death and other adverse outcomes.[18] Early work focused on 'maturity' at birth and the concept of in utero growth failure did not emerge until the 1940s.[3] Infants weighing 2.5 kg or less are at substantially increased risk of adverse outcomes, and until the 1960s, such infants were described as 'premature'. Work in the early 1960s highlighted the fact that low birthweight infants are a mixture of those born too soon ('preterm') and those born too small ('small for dates'). The concept of 'small for dates' or 'growth retardation' which then emerged was based on the distribution of birthweight by gestational age in various reference populations[19] with an arbitrary cut-off point, usually at the 10th or 3rd percentile. Although theoretically attractive, adjustment of birthweight for gestational age was not a major advance in efforts to identify fetal growth retardation, as gestational age at birth is measured with low reliability relative to birthweight. Moreover, different populations have different fetal growth norms, depending on factors such as ethnic origin,[6] maternal height,[20] smoking prevalence[21] and altitude,[22] differences which highlight the important distinction between 'clinically normal' and 'biologically ideal' fetal growth. The distinction between being born 'too soon' and 'too small' is often blurred. Preterm and 'small for gestational age' births share many common antecedents, such as maternal short stature,[18] and in studies of placental morphology a number of similar histopathological abnormalities are documented in these syndromes.[23] Thus fetal growth norms based on infants born at 34 weeks gestation do not provide an unbiased reflection of normal fetal growth at this gestation. Similarly, studies of fetal growth retardation at 'term' probably exclude a severely affected subgroup of infants, those who are both preterm and growth retarded.

Much work in recent decades has addressed the need to further 'disaggregate' low birthweight with a view to elucidating specific aetiological factors. In a series of postmortem studies on infants with birthweight below two standard deviations for gestation, Gruenwald highlighted the extent to which the effects of growth retardation are uneven or 'asymmetrical' in the majority of such infants.[24] These infants tend to have relatively large heads, a modest reduction in length relative to the reduction in weight, and thinner skinfolds. The greatest reduction in weight occurs in organs such as the liver and thymus and the least in brain weight. It is suggested that such disproportionate fetal growth reflects an inadequate supply of oxygen or nutrients (failure of the supply line) at the time of rapid increase in fetal weight in middle to late gestation but after the peak in fetal length growth velocity.[3,16–17] By contrast, it is suggested that symmetrical growth retardation, with equal reduction in brain and body size and normal skinfold thickness, is either a normal variant, reflecting low genetic growth potential or is due to adverse influences acting in early pregnancy, during the phase of cellular hyperplasia[15] which set the fetus on a low growth trajectory.

This concept of early down regulation of fetal growth leading to either 'proportionate' or 'disproportionate' fetal growth retardation, has been central to the development of the nutritional programming (or fetal origins) hypothesis. It is suggested, for instance, that coronary heart disease is not associated with proportionate fetal growth arising from nutritional insults in early gestation but with disproportionate growth due to nutritional deprivation in mid and late gestation.[25] Thus the hypothesis is able to accommodate historical and geographical trends in coronary heart disease (CHD) rates that might otherwise seem inconsistent with a major aetiological role for fetal growth retardation. For example, in most western industrialized countries, CHD mortality was lower at the turn of the century than in the 1950s and it is difficult to reconcile these trends with changes in fetal nutrition and growth unless one proposes an association with a specific pattern of fetal growth retardation which has emerged during this period. Similarly, it is suggested that the current low rates of CHD in developing countries such as China, despite evidence of suboptimal maternal nutrition extending over a prolonged period, reflect 'proportionate' fetal growth retardation.[2] However, this model of fetal growth has attracted sceptical commentary.[26] Kramer has argued that fetal growth retardation is largely a third trimester phenomenon, as fetal growth in early pregnancy requires relatively little nutritional support, and therefore the notion of an early nutritional insult, which determines body proportions, is implausible.[26] Many populations in developing countries have mean birthweights which are similar to those in industrialized countries and growth failure in these environments is largely a postnatal phenomenon.[27]

The concept that an in utero insult in the third trimester produces disproportionate fetal growth is undoubtedly more plausible, although, in practice, reliable differentiation between symmetrical and asymmetrical growth retardation is often difficult.[4] In particular, the concept of brain sparing in asymmetrical growth retardation has proved difficult to document in all but the most extreme cases.[28] Ponderal index at birth (weight/length^3), is advanced as a continuous measure of fetal growth asymmetry. Ponderal index, essentially a measure of 'fatness/ thinness' at birth, is undoubtedly more sensitive to intrauterine adversity than birthweight[29] and is predictive of poor neonatal outcome.[30–32] Unfortunately, the usefulness of ponderal index and other indices such as the ratio of head circumference to length, is constrained by measurement error, in particular measurement of length at birth. Ponderal index is reported to be a poor predictor of skinfold thickness at birth[33] and in a study of high risk pregnancies it has been shown not to predict fetal growth velocity (based on serial ultrasound scans from 27 weeks) after adjustment for birthweight and gestational age.[34] Moreover, as ponderal index is highly correlated with birthweight, it needs to be evaluated in relation to birthweight rather than against a single absolute standard for the whole population.[35] Thus the lower end of the normal range of ponderal index for infants weighing 3500 g is higher than for infants weighing 2500 g. This highlights the difficulty of identifying infants with birthweight and length within the normal range but with fetal growth retardation relative to their genetic growth potential. The use of postnatal catch-up growth[36] represents an interesting approach to this problem which has yet to be fully exploited, although clearly this method raises concerns about variation in the rate of catch-up growth depending on the underlying cause and interactions with the level of nutritional and emotional support in the postnatal environment. In studies of the late effects of fetal growth retardation in adults, the use of birthweight relative to attained adult height[8] represents a similar approach to this problem, which although elegant is clearly imprecise. Thus, reliable measures of fetal growth retardation, that represent a substantial advance on birthweight combined with accurate gestational age, remain elusive. Ultimately, longitudinal studies from early pregnancy using advances in ultrasonographic biometry and fetal Doppler technology combined with relatively hard end-points such as postnatal catch-up growth under optimal conditions should allow more reliable definition and characterisation of fetal growth retardation.[37]

7.3 Sources of variation in fetal growth

Size at birth is clearly a complex outcome that depends on a host of different influences. Classification is arbitrary and difficult and inevitably incomplete (Table 7.1). Broadly, we need to consider:

(i) the fetal genotype,

(ii) the maternal genotype,

(iii) other stable maternal characteristics such as height, pelvic frame size and other indirect markers of lifelong nutritional status,

(iv) maternal characteristics that vary between pregnancies such as age, parity, prepregnancy weight, smoking, and diet,

(v) a range of specific influences related to placental function and the uterine environment such as defective placentation which is linked to both 'idiopathic' intrauterine growth retardation' and pre-eclampsia,

(vi) factors in the general environment, of which altitude is an obvious example, with a fall in mean birthweight of 100 g per 1000 metres above sea level.[22]

Quantitative estimates of the proportion of variation in birthweight explained by these different factors in a western industrialised setting[38] suggest that 10–15% is explained by the fetal genotype, approximately 25% by maternal genotype and other stable characteristics of the mother, some 20% by maternal factors that vary between pregnancies, with the remainder due to ill-defined factors related to placental function and the uterine environment.

7.3.1 Fetal and maternal genotype and familial clustering of birthweight

There is a strong tendency for consecutive births to the same mother to have similar birthweights. The birthweight correlation coefficient (r) between full siblings range from 0.36 to 0.62, with a median of approximately 0.5.[38] However, paternal half-siblings (i.e. having the same father but different mother) show a much lower correlation ($r = 0.1$) than maternal half-siblings ($r = 0.5$).[38] This suggests that the fetal genotype makes a relatively small contribution to variation in birthweight. Indeed it is clear that familial

Table 7.1 Factors known to influence fetal growth

Fetal and Maternal Genotype

Maternal factors

Age
Parity
Height/frame size, 'maternal constraint of fetal growth'
Maternal birth weight
Pre-pregnancy weight
Weight gain during pregnancy
Obstetric history (including previous still birth and birth weight of previous infants
Hypertension and pre-eclampsia
Glucose tolerance and diabetes
Other chronic maternal disease, e.g. renal impairment, anti-phospholipid syndrome
Maternal anaemia
Cigarette smoking
Ethnic origin
Socioeconomic status
Social support
Physical activity level
Physical work load during pregnancy
Alcohol consumption
Illicit drug use
Nutrition

Fetal factors

Sex
Multiple pregnancy
Chromosomal anomalies
Inborn errors of metabolism

Placental factors/Uterine environment

Reduced placental blood flow (Uteroplacental hypoperfusion)
Other placental and cord abnormalities
Intrauterine infections

General environment factors

Altitude
Environmental pollution e.g. lead

clustering of birthweight is largely determined by maternal factors, including the maternal genotype, but mainly by non-genetic factors, including maternal size and the mother's own birthweight.[39–40] The importance of maternal size was demonstrated by Walton and Hammond's classic cross-mating study of Shire horses and Shetland ponies.[41] The mares of these breeds differ fourfold in size. The hybrid foal from the Shetland mare was small, Shetland-sized, whereas the Shire mare's foal from the same hybridisation was three times larger. These observations, which have been replicated in other animals, including cattle and mice, suggest that 'maternal or uterine constraint' is an important determinant of fetal growth and is mainly a late gestation phenomenon.[3] There is considerable evidence that the mother's own birthweight contributes to non-genetic familial clustering of birthweight,[40] interacting with other maternal factors.[42] In the US 1988 National Maternal and Infant Health Survey, the risk of delivering a low birthweight infant (<2.5 kg) was increased over 14-fold (in multivariate analysis) among mother's who themselves were low birthweight and had a history of a previous low birthweight child relative to a baseline group of mother's of normal birthweight and with a previous child of normal birthweight. The relative risk (RR) of low birthweight was intermediate among mother's with low birthweight but with a previous infant of normal birthweight (RR = 2.6) and among those of normal birthweight but with a previous low birthweight infant (RR = 5.4). These effects were seen clearly in white and black mothers, in smokers and non-smokers and were independent of a wide range of covariates, including maternal height, prepregnancy weight, education, parity and pregnancy interval.[42] Wang and colleagues hypothesize that these intergenerational effects are due to in utero programming of postnatal reproductive function.[42] As with the general programming hypothesis, this is arguably a speculative leap from birth to childbearing across a considerable expanse of potential confounders. It also raises the question of what is meant by programming and whether the concept of programming is biologically plausible.

7.3.2 Programming

Programming is said to occur 'when an early stimulus or insult, operating at a critical or sensitive period, results in a permanent or long term change in the structure or function of the organism'.[43] Nature is replete with examples of programming.[2] A clear example of the phenomenon is the lifelong effect of early exposure to sex hormones on sexual physiology. For example, a female rat injected with testosterone on the fifth day after birth will develop normally until puberty but will fail to ovulate or show normal patterns of female sexual behaviour thereafter. The release of gonadotropin by the hypothalamus has been irreversibly altered from the cyclical female pattern to the tonic male pattern. The same injection of testosterone given a few days later has little effect on reproductive function.[44] In the American alligator, the temperature at which eggs are hatched determines not only the sex of the offspring but also postnatal growth rate, skin pigmentation, and the animals' preferred temperature in adult life, with alligators gravitating towards an environment which has the same temperature as the one in which they were hatched.[45]

7.3.2.1 Programming and nutrition

Closer to the current discussion, Winick and colleagues in the late 1960s studied rats severely deprived of protein at different stages of early brain development and subsequently rehabilitated. In early gestation, when the cells were rapidly multiplying (hyperplastic growth) there was evidence from biochemical measures of DNA and RNA that the number of cells was irreversibly depleted and the effects of dietary restriction were permanent, whereas in later gestation, when the cells were enlarging but were no longer hyperplastic, the effects of diet were reversible.[15] On the basis of similar experiments in the 1960s, McCance and Widdowson postulated a critical period early in development when 'the regulating centres of the hypothalamus are being coordinated with rate of growth'.[46] They showed, for instance, that rats undernourished from 3 to 6 weeks after birth remained permanently small whereas similar deprivation between 9 and 12 weeks was followed by catch-up growth.[47] Apart from effects on growth, there is evidence from animal models of programming effects of maternal nutrition on specific aspects of the offspring's physiology. For instance, pregnant rats starved in early pregnancy and then nutritionally rehabilitated produce obese offspring[48] and rats born to mothers given a low protein diet before and during pregnancy have been shown to have persistently raised blood pressure.[49] Overnutrition at critical periods can also have long term consequences. McGill and colleagues, in a series of experiments over 20 years, have demonstrated long term deferred, adverse effects of infant nutrition, particularly breast as compared with formula feeding, and over feeding as compared with normal or underfeeding, on serum HDL-cholesterol concentrations, adiposity and atherosclerosis in the baboon, a large primate with cholesterol metabolism similar to that of humans.[50]

7.3.2.2 Programming and the maternal-uterine milieu

Diet during pregnancy influences the maternal uterine milieu, interacting with the mother's prepregnancy nutritional status, metabolism, and physiology. There is evidence from animal experiments and in man that the hormonal, metabolic, and circulatory milieu in which the fetus finds itself can exert long term effects on physiology and risk of disease in adult life. In the rat, it has been shown that changes in the glucose concentrations to which the fetus is exposed produce effects on glucose tolerance in the offspring which persist through several generations, mimicking genetic transmission.[51]

In the Pima Indian community, the children of mothers with diabetes during pregnancy were found to have a substantially higher prevalence of diabetes (45%) at age 20–24 years than the children of women who developed diabetes after pregnancy (8.4%).[52] Freinkel suggests that various factors associated with the diabetic intrauterine environment, such as elevated concentrations of glucose, ketones, amino acids, and lipids, exert direct effects on the developing fetus ('fuel mediated teratogenesis') which confer a higher risk of obesity, insulin resistance, and abnormal glucose tolerance in childhood and early adult life.[53]

These observations extend the notion of programming from a narrow focus on the effects of nutritional deprivation in pregnancy alone or on the effects of other well-circumscribed insults[54] to a broader concept that includes wide ranging but often more subtle perturbations of the uterine environment. This broader concept, however, raises questions about the feasibility of isolating specific programming effects, particularly 'nutritional programming' effects from the wider canvas of potential modulators of the uterine environment in which the pregnancy is sustained, as summarized in Fig. 7.1. This point is well illustrated when we consider the effects of the mother's blood pressure on fetal growth and interrelations between pre-eclampsia, maternal hypertension, and idiopathic fetal growth retardation.

7.3.2.3 Hypertension and idiopathic fetal growth retardation

Pre-eclampsia is a syndrome peculiar to human pregnancy, characterized clinically by hypertension and proteinuria. Pre-eclampsia, especially if severe, poses a significant threat to the health and wellbeing of the mother and is associated with marked derangement of uteroplacental blood flow (utero-placental ischaemia) with high risk of fetal growth retardation.[55] Women with established essential hypertension at the outset of pregnancy are at increased risk of developing pre-eclampsia[55–56] and they are at substantially increased risk of giving birth to a growth retarded infant regardless of whether they develop pre-eclampsia. It has been assumed that, aside from these specific hypertensive syndromes, maternal blood pressure levels do not influence fetal growth. Recent work based on measurements of 24 h ambulatory blood pressure in pregnancy provide evidence of a continuous inverse association between maternal blood pressure across the normal range and fetal growth as reflected by birthweight, ponderal index, and infant's head circumference.[57] Thus there is evidence that both pathological and 'high normal' blood pressure are associated with reduced fetal growth. These observations raise the possibility that the reported associations between retarded fetal growth and adult hypertension are confounded by maternal blood pressure which is associated both with fetal growth retardation via placental vascular insufficiency and with hypertension in the offspring via the shared genes and environment which link a mother and her child. In this particular case it is not clear that one needs to invoke a specific hypothesis involving maternal nutrition and intrauterine programming.

In a significant minority of cases of fetal growth retardation no predisposing maternal or fetal factors are identified. Although this is a heterogenous group, there is considerable evidence that abnormal or defective placentation is an important element in the pathogenesis of idiopathic fetal growth retardation.[58-59] The key placental changes are failure of placental trophoblastic invasion of the uterine spiral arteries with failure to convert these arteries into low resistance uteroplacental vessels and 'acute atherosis' of the spiral arteries supplying the placenta. This latter term refers to fibrinoid necrosis of the arterial wall with an intramural accumulation of fat-laden macrophages and a perivascular mononuclear cell infiltrate.[58] The pathogenesis of acute atherosis is unknown but an immunological basis is suspected. These placental changes however are not specific to idiopathic intrauterine growth retardation but are also observed in cases of pre-eclampsia,[58-59] and to a lesser extent with cases of preterm birth.[23] Idiopathic intrauterine growth retardation and pre-eclampsia share similar haemodynamic abnormalities in pregnancy, including a relative failure of the early pregnancy expansion of the maternal vascular compartment which normally leads to a fall in blood pressure and increased cardiac output in anticipation of the higher demands for flow, nutrients, and oxygen in late pregnancy.[60] This suggests that some cases of idiopathic intrauterine growth retardation form part of a broader syndrome or spectrum of disorders which are characterized by failure of maternal circulatory adaptation to the presence of trophoblastic tissue .[60-61] The ultimate causes of this syndrome are unknown but a failure of maternal–fetal immunological tolerance is likely to emerge as an important factor.[62]

7.3.2.4 Programming: mechanisms and caveats

It is clear that in biological terms the concept that an insult or stimulus at a critical period of development can produce (or programme) lasting effects on the organism is plausible. Different mechanisms have been proposed to explain the durability of programming effects including, at the cellular level, permanent effects of nutritional deprivation on cell numbers (as suggested by the work of Winick and colleagues[15]), alteration of gene expression and selective survival or 'natural selection' of particular clones of cells.[43] As discussed above, higher level effects are also plausible, including effects on the structure and function of particular organs,[63] up or down regulation of hormone receptors and Freinkel's concept of 'fuel mediated teratogenesis'.[53] Unfortunately in the context of work on the aetiology of chronic disease in adult life such as CHD, the term 'programming' has mechanistic and deterministic connotations which sit uneasily with a multifactorial, component cause model of aetiology.[64] Moreover, a degree of scepticism about the permanence or irreversibility of many 'programming' effects on the function of the organism and the expression of disease is warranted. There is clearly a broad spectrum of programming scripts ranging from those apparently written in stone by a single author, such as that of the American alligator, to those written in less durable material by a committee, such as the child of a mother with gestational diabetes whose risk of developing non-insulin dependent diabetes will depend on additional genetic and postnatal life style factors such as obesity and lack of exercise. Despite these caveats, the notion of critical periods of development has undoubtedly been helpful in work on maternal nutrition and fetal growth.

7.4 Maternal nutrition and fetal growth

Interest in prenatal nutrition has waxed and waned over the last 100 years, as succinctly reviewed by Susser and Stein.[65] The late 19th century movement to promote improvement in the diet of pregnant women, led by Budin in France and Ballantyne in Britain, faltered when animal experimentalists failed to detect important effects of diet on pregnancy outcome. Interest was restored during the Great Depression in the 1930s by the efforts of nutritionists such as Boyd-Orr, and in the early 1940s a number of studies reporting positive effects of food or vitamins on pregnancy outcomes were reported.[66-67] The effects of wartime starvation and privation on fetal growth and mortality, such as that associated with the 18-month Leningrad siege[68] and the 6 month Dutch famine[65] further emphasized the importance of diet in pregnancy. However, two major observational studies published in the 1950s again cast doubt on the importance of nutrition during pregnancy, (above a critical threshold), for fetal growth.[69-70] Thomson measured the food intake of 479 Aberdeen primigravidae during the seventh month of pregnancy using weighed food intakes and food diaries and found no significant associations between birthweight and either calorie intake or the intake of specific nutrients after adjustment for maternal height and weight. He concluded that 'within the range of diets in this survey, the influence of diet on birthweight must be small, indeed negligible'.[70]

Although the effects of starvation, severe and moderate malnutrition on fetal growth are not seriously disputed,[68,71-72] the contribution of lesser degrees of malnutrition to fetal growth retardation remains contentious.[73] Much of the earlier and current controversy in this area reflects the fact that the effects of prenatal nutrition on human fetal growth are critically dependent on both the timing of nutritional exposures in relation to critical periods of development (as suggested by the programming model) and on interactions with the mother's prepregnancy nutritional status, metabolism, and physiology. As indicated earlier, nutritional status is generally inferred indirectly from measures such as maternal height, pregravid weight and skinfold thickness.

7.4.1 The timing of the nutritional insult

The importance of the timing of the nutritional exposure in man is clearly illustrated by the data from the Dutch famine.[65] This famine, which was due to a Nazi-imposed transport embargo in western Holland, lasted 6 months from November 1944 to May 1945, when Holland was liberated from the Occupation. Clear effects of third trimester famine exposure were seen on birthweight and placental weight, and to a lesser extent on length and head circumference. Recovery of birthweight and other indices of fetal growth after the famine ended was rapid, indicating that exposure to severe malnutrition in early pregnancy had little evidence on fetal growth. Although these data provide unequivocal evidence of the importance of nutritional deprivation at a critical period of gestation, there was no evidence in these data of the setting of fetal growth on a low trajectory by early exposure to severe malnutrition.[65] In this context it is noteworthy that although famine exposure produced long term effects on obesity among survivors (with more obesity among those exposed in early gestation and less in those exposed in late gestation[74]), no permanent effect of famine exposure at any stage of gestation were detectable on height at age 19 years in this economically developed country.[65] It is often assumed that short stature in adult life, such as that commonly seen in economically underdeveloped countries, largely reflects the growth trajectory set in utero.[2] However it is clear that there are substantial postnatal influences on both adult height and (surprisingly) body shape, principally the levels of nutrition and the incidence of infectious disease in childhood. Even minor illness in childhood is associated with slowing of growth, and the nutritional requirements to sustain catch-up growth are high. Thus, the large secular trend in height in Japan between 1950 and 1980 was almost entirely due to increases in leg length, related to improved social conditions in childhood rather than improved diet in pregnancy.[27] These observations emphasize the need for caution in extrapolating data from programming experiments in animals to human.

7.4.2 Interactions with prepregnancy nutritional status

A short interval between pregnancies has been linked with low birthweight, via effects on both fetal growth[75] and risk of preterm birth, and there is some evidence that this may reflect, at least partially, the need for the mother to restore nutrient reserves depleted in the course of the previous pregnancy. Maternal height and 'frame size', regarded as a marker of lifelong nutritional status, has already been shown to be a determinant of fetal growth, especially in the third trimester. Data from a large number of studies indicate a strong relation between maternal pregravid weight, gestational weight gain (which mainly reflects calorie intake during pregnancy) and infant birthweight. [76–77] Essentially, birthweight increases steadily with increasing pregravid weight and with increasing gestational weight gain. As shown in Table 7.2[14,78] these effects are independent of each other but are additive in their combined effects and are seen in smokers and non-smokers. As one would expect, the effect of gestational weight gain on birthweight is most marked in underweight women, an observation consistent with findings from intervention studies.[79]

There is evidence that the distribution of body fat also influences fetal growth independently of pregravid weight and gestational weight gain. Brown and colleagues have described independent associations between the mother's waist–hip ratio measured before conception or in early pregnancy and the infant's birthweight, length, and head circumference.[80] Central obesity is associated with a number of metabolic changes that may influence fetal growth, including elevated circulating levels of triglycerides[81] and free fatty acids,[82] insulin resistance, hyperinsulinaemia, and higher fasting glucose levels.[83] Insulin and insulin-like growth factors, which are also influenced by maternal nutrient intake, are particularly important regulators of fetal growth.[84] Pregnancy itself induces insulin resistance and hyperinsulinaemia in the mother,[85] which facilitates the transfer of nutrients from mother to fetus. This phenomenon (and other adverse maternal sequelae of pregnancy such as

Table 7.2 Mean birth weight (g) of term live births by maternal pregravid weight, gestational weight gain and smoking status. Adapted from Luke[14] and Taffel.[78]

Pregravid weight and smoking	Weight gain (lbs)					% change (<16 lb vs ≥36 lb gain)
	<16	16–20	21–25	26–35	≥36	
Underweight						
Non-smoker	2927	3100	3276	3374	3483	19.0
Smoker	2631	2821	3069	3174	3314	26.0
Normal weight						
Non-smoker	3097	3231	3428	3471	3606	16.4
Smoker	2918	3065	3135	3292	3398	16.4
Overweight						
Non-smoker	3330	3458	3526	3581	3665	10.0
Smoker	3258	3365	3379	3384	3519	8.0

pre-eclampsia) has been interpreted in terms of 'maternal-fetal genetic conflict', i.e. meeting the fetal requirements to maximise delivery of nutrients and oxygen at the expense of the mother's interest in maintaining her health and well-being.[86] Further discussion of the range of maternal and placental hormonal and metabolic influences on fetal growth is clearly beyond the scope of this review.[87] However, the associations between maternal waist–hip ratio and fetal growth emphasize the extent to which maternal nutrition (however defined) and the maternal hormonal–metabolic milieu are mutually interdependent and again they suggest a broader, less rigidly deterministic programming model.

7.4.3 Nutritional deficits and fetal/placental growth in economically developed countries

Inadequate folic acid intake has been clearly linked with malformations of the developing embryo in early pregnancy.[88] However, the importance of other common nutritional deficits on fetal growth in developed countries is uncertain. Dietary restriction in previously well nourished pregnant sheep is associated with placental hypertrophy[72] which is interpreted as a compensatory phenomenon.[89] Barker and colleagues have suggested that in humans, placental hypertrophy, which results in discordance between birth and placental weight with an elevated placental ratio, is a relatively sensitive marker of inadequate nutrition such as that associated with iron deficiency anaemia.[89] This group have reported a striking association between an elevated placental ratio at birth and essential hypertension in middle age.[90] Using data from the Oxford record linkage system, Godfrey *et al.* have described a specific association between low maternal haemoglobin combined with a fall in mean cell volume during pregnancy and elevated placental ratio.[91] By contrast, Perry *et al.* found that maternal obesity was the dominant predictor of an elevated placental ratio, in a study of European, Asian and Afro-Caribbean women from a relatively deprived UK inner city community.[92] No associations with indices of iron deficiency anaemia, including serum ferritin, were detected. Similarly, Whincup and colleagues detected no consistent relation between indices of iron deficiency anaemia and placental ratio in a study of over 600 children, nor was there evidence in this study of an association between maternal anaemia during pregnancy and blood pressure at age 9–11 years.[93]

Godfrey *et al.* examined the effects of diet on fetal and placental growth in a prospective study involving a group of over 500 mothers who delivered at term in Southampton.[94] Diet was assessed using a food frequency questionnaire administered in early and late pregnancy. A complex pattern of associations and interactions emerged. High carbohydrate intakes in early pregnancy were associated with reduced birth and placental weight, and lower protein intakes in late pregnancy were also associated with reduced birth and placental weight. Although data from experimental studies in sheep are advanced to support the biological plausibility of these findings,[72] there is a clear need for replication in other studies in humans. There is observational evidence of an inverse association between dietary protein intake and birthweight[95] but this is inconsistent with the data from intervention studies when protein supplementation alone is used[96] (see section 12.3 in Chapter 12 for more details). In data from Campbell and colleagues in Aberdeen, intriguing associations were detected between the mother's intakes of animal protein and carbohydrate during pregnancy and blood pressure in the offspring at age 40 years.[95] At relatively low protein intakes (below 50 g/day) there was a positive association between carbohydrate intake and blood pressure whereas above 50 g/day an inverse association was found. Again, replication of these findings will be required. It is noteworthy that in neither of these studies was there evidence of placental hypertrophy in response to suboptimal nutrition. In summary, fetal growth depends on the mother's nutritional status before conception, her diet during pregnancy and interactions between these factors and aspects of the mother's metabolism and physiology such as glucose tolerance and blood pressure. In communities which provide adequate nutrition to sustain optimal growth in childhood and adolescence, dietary intake during pregnancy probably accounts for a relatively small amount of variation in fetal growth.

7.5 Conclusions

The fetal origins hypothesis has opened up an important and exciting agenda on the patterns and determinants of fetal growth and development. Barker and colleagues have set work in this area on a high growth trajectory and progress will be limited only by our collective imagination and our ability to develop narrowly focused hypotheses which make specific and testable predictions. The latter will depend critically on improvements in methods used to both measure fetal growth rates from early gestation and to derive quantitative, in utero indices of asymmetry and other abnormal patterns of fetal growth. Work on the distribution and determinants of fetal growth rates and patterns within and between populations using robust and reliable methods should then attract high priority. Further observational studies are needed of prenatal diet, fetal growth, and pregnancy outcome which address problems of measurement error with adequate sample size and repeated measures and which explore interactions between diet and the mother's metabolism and physiology. Ultimately, detailed and long term follow-up of the offspring from such studies and their parents will help place nutritional programming within a broader life course canvas, which includes genetic, intrauterine and postnatal determinants of adult morbidity and premature mortality.

References

Those marked with an asterisk are especially recommended for further reading

1   *Barker DJP, ed. *Fetal and infant origins of adult disease*. London: BMJ Publishing Group, 1992.
2   *Barker DJB. *Mothers, babies, and disease in later life*. London: BMJ Publishing Group, 1994.
3   Trudinger B. Fetal growth disorders. In: Moore TR, *et al.*, eds, *Gynecology and obstetrics: a longitudinal approach*. Edinburgh: Churchill Livingstone, 1993:487–98.
4   Cunningham FG, MacDonald PC, Gant NF, eds.. Preterm and post-term pregnancy and inappropriate fetal growth. In: Williams JW, ed. *Williams obstetrics*. 19th edition. East Norwalk (Conneticut): Appleton & Lange, 1989:741–77.
5   Robinson JS. Fetal growth. In: Turnbull A, Chamberlain G, eds, *Obstetrics*. Edinburgh: Churchill Livingstone, 1989:141–50.
6   McFadyen IR. Fetal growth. In: Studd J, ed, *Progress in obstetrics and gynaecology*. Vol. 5. Edinburgh: Churchill Livingstone, 1985:58–77.
7   Lithell HO, McKeigue PM, Berglund L, Mohsen R, Lithell UB, Leon DA. Relation of size at birth to non-insulin dependent diabetes and insulin concentrations in men aged 50–60 years. *Br Med J* 1996;**312**: 406-10.
8   Leon DA, Kupilova I, Lithell HO, Berglund L, Mohsen-R,; Vagero-D, Lithell UB, McKeigue-PM. Failure to realise growth potential in utero and adult obesity in relation to blood pressure in 50 year old Swedish men. *Br Med J* 1996; **312**:401–6.
9   Ben-Shlomo Y, Davey Smith G. Deprivation in infancy or in adult life: which is more important for mortality risk. *Lancet* 1991;**337**:530–34.
10 Brooke OG, Anderson HR, Bland JM, Peacock JL, Stewart CM. Effects on birthweight of smoking, alcohol, caffeine, socioeconomic factors, and psychosocial stress. *Br Med J* 1989;**298**:795–801.
11 Launer LJ, Villar J, Kestler E, deOnis M. The effect of maternal work on fetal growth and duration of pregnancy: a prospective study. *Br J Obstet Gynaecol*. 1990;**97**:62–70.
12 Caggiula AW, Orchard TJ, Kuller LH. Epidemiologic studies of nutrition and heart disease. In: Feldmad EB, ed, *Nutrition and heart disease*. Edinburgh: Churchill Livingstone, 1983:1–27.
13 Barker DJ. The placenta in intrauterine growth retardation. Discussion. In: Ward RHT, Smith SK, Donnai D, eds, *Early fetal growth and development*. London: RCOG Press, 1994:238.
14 Luke B. Nutritional influences on fetal growth. *Clin Obstet Gynecol* 1994;**36**:538–49.

15   Winick M, Noble A. Cellular response in rats during malnutrition at various ages. *J Nutr* 1966;**89**:300–6.

16   Tanner JM. *Fetus into man.* Boston: Harvard University Press, 1978:40.

17   Falkner F, Holzgreve W, Schloo RH. Prenatal influences on postnatal growth. *Eur J Clin Nutr* 1994;**46(Suppl 1)**:S15–24.

18   Lumley J. Epidemiology of prematurity. In: Yu VYH, Wood EC, eds. *Prematurity.* Churchill Livinstone. Edinburgh 1987;1–24.

19   Battaglia FC, Lubchenco LO. A practical classification of newborn infants by weight and gestational age. *J Pediatr* 1967;**71**:159–63.

20   Thomson AM, Billewicz WZ, Hytten FE. The assessment of fetal growth. *J Obstet Gynaecol Br Commonw* 1968;**75**:903–16.

21   Anderson GD, Blidner IN, McClemont S, Sinclair JC. Determinants of size at birth in a Canadian population. *Am J Obstet Gynecol* 1984;**150**:236–44.

22   McCullough RE, Reeves JT, Liljegren RL. Fetal growth retardation and increased infant mortality at high altitude. *Arch Environ Health* 1977; **32**:36–9.

23   Salafia CM, Vogel CA, Vintzileos AM, Bantham KF, Pezzullo J, Silberman L. Placental pathologic findings in preterm birth. *Am J Obstet Gynecol* 1991;**165**:934–8.

24   Gruenwald P. Pathology of the deprived fetus and its supply line. In: Elliott K, Knight J, eds, *Size at Birth.* Ciba Foundation Symposium No 27. Amsterdam: Associated Scientific Publishers, 1974:3–9.

25   Barker DJP. Fetal origins of coronary heart disease. *Br Med J* 1995;**311**: 171–4.

26   Kramer M. In: Early nutrition and lifelong health. Sixteenth Marabou Symposium. Discussion. *Nutrition Reviews* 1996;**54(II)**:S56–73.

27   Eveleth PB, Tanner JM. Environmental influences on growth. In: Eveleth PB, Tanner JM. *Worldwide variation in human growth.* Cambridge: 2nd edition. Cambridge University Press, 1991,191–207.

28   Crane JP, Kopta MM. Comparative newborn anthropometric data in symmetric versus asymmetric intrauterine growth retardation. *Am J Obstet Gynecol* 1980;**138**:518–22.

29   Perry IJ, Beevers DG. The definition of pre-eclampsia. *Br J Obstet & Gynaecol* 1994;**101**:587–91.

30   Colley NV, Tremble JM, Henson GL, Cole TJ. Head circumference/ abdominal circumference ratio, ponderal index and fetal malnutrition. Should head circumference/abdominal circumference ratio be abandoned? *Br J Obstet Gynaecol* 1991;**98**:524–7.

31   Patterson RM, Pouliot MR. Neonatal morphometrics and perinatal outcome: who is growth retarded? *Am J Obstet Gynecol* 1987;**157**:691–3.

32   Fay RA, Dey PL, Saadie CMJ, Buhl JA, Gebski VJ. Ponderal index: a better definition of the at risk group with intrauterine growth problems

than birth-weight for gestational age in term infants. *Aust NZ Obstet Gynecol* 1991;**31**:17–9.

33 Frisancho AR, Compton A, Matos J. Ineffectiveness of body mass indices for the evaluation of neonate nutritional status. *J Pediatr* 1986; **108**:993–5.

34 *Peterson S, Larsen T, Greisen G. Judging fetal growth from body proportions at birth. *Early Hum Dev* 1992;**30**:139–46.

35 *Chard T, Costeloe K, Leaf A. Evidence of growth retardation in neonates of apparently normal weight. *Eur J Obstet & Gynecol Reprod Biol* 1992;**45**:59–62.

36 Bates JA, Evans JA, Mason G. Differentiation of growth retarded from normally grown fetuses and prediction of intrauterine growth retardation using Doppler ultrasound. *Br J Obstet & Gynecol* 1996; **103**:670–5.

37 Craigo SD. The role of ultrasound in the diagnosis and management of intrauterine growth retardation. *Semin Perinatol* 1994;**18**:292–304.

38 Robson EB. The genetics of birthweight. In: Falkner F, Tanner JM, eds. *Human Growth. Vol 1: Principles and prenatal growth.* New York: Plenum Press, 1978:285–97.

39 Ounsted M, Ounsted C. Maternal regulation of intrauterine growth. *Nature* 1966;**212**:995–7.

40 Klebanoff MA, Graubard BI, Kessel SS, Berendes HW. Low birthweight across generations. *JAMA* 1984;**252**:2423–7.

41 Walton A, Hammond J. The maternal effects on growth and conformation in Shire-horse-Shetland-pony crosses. *Proc R Soc Lond [Biol]* 1938; **125**:311–35.

42 *Wang X, Zuckerman B, Coffman GA, Corwin MJ. Familial aggregation of low birthweight among whites and blacks in the United States. *N Engl J Med* 1996;**333**:1744–9.

43 Lucas A. Programming by early nutrition in man. In: Bock GR, Whelan J, eds, *The childhood environment and adult disease.* Chichester: John Wiley & Sons, 1991:38–55.

44 Barraclough CA. Production of anovulatory, sterile rats by a single injection of testosterone propionate. *Endocrinology* 1961;**68**:62–7.

45 Ferguson MWJ. Overview of mechanisms in embryogenesis. In: Ward RHT, Smith SK, Donnai D, eds, *Early fetal growth and development.* London: RCOG Press, 1994:1–19.

46 McCance RA, Widdowson EM. Review lecture: the determinants of growth and form. *Proc R Soc Lond [Biol]* 1974;**185**:1–17.

47 Widdowson EM, McCance RA. The effect of finite periods of undernutrition at different ages on the composition and subsequent development of the rat. *Proc R Soc Lond [Biol]* 1963;**158**:329–42.

48 Anguita RM, Sigulem DM, Sawaya AL. Intrauterine food restriction is associated with obesity in young rats. *J Nutr* 1993;**123**:1421–8.

49   Langley SC, Jackson AA. Increased systolic blood pressure in adult rats induced by fetal exposure to maternal low protein diets. *Clin Sci* 1994;**86**:217–22.

50   McGill HC, Mott GE, Lewis DS, McMahon CA Jackson EM. Early determinants of adult metabolic regulation: effects of infant nutrition on adult lipid and lipoprotein metabolism. *Nutr Rev* 1996;**54(II)**: S31–40.

51   van Assche FA, Aerts L. Long-term effects of diabetes and pregnancy in the rat. *Diabetes* 1985;**34 (Suppl 2)**:S116–8.

52   Pettitt DJ, Bennett PH, Saad MF, Charles MA, Nelson RG, Knowler WC. Abnormal glucose tolerance during pregnancy in Pima Indian women. *Diabetes* 1991;**40 (Suppl 2)**:S126–30.

53   *Freinkel N. Of pregnancy and progeny. Banting Lecture 1980. *Diabetes* 1980;**29**:1023–35.

54   Gilbert T, Lelievre-Pegorier M, Merlet-Benichou C. Immediate and long-term renal effects of fetal exposure to gentamycin. *Pediatr Nephrol* 1990; **4**:445–50.

55   Taylor DJ. The epidemiology of hypertension during pregnancy. In: Rubin PC, ed. *Handbook of Hypertension Vol. 10; Hypertension in pregnancy*. Amsterdam, Elsevier, 1988;223–240.

56   Eskenazi B, Fenster L, Sidney S. A multivariate analysis of risk factors for pre-eclampsia. *JAMA* 1991;**226**:237–41.

57   Churchill D, Perry IJ, Beevers DG. Aambulatory blood pressure in pregnancy and fetal growth. *Lancet* 1997;**349**:7–10.

58   Fox H. The placenta in pregnancy hypertension. In: Rubin PC, ed. *Handbook of Hypertension Vol. 10; Hypertension in pregnancy*. Elsevier, Amsterdam, 1988;16–37.

59   *Fox H. The placenta in intrauterine growth retardation. In: Ward RHT, Smith SK, Donnai D, eds, *Early fetal growth and development*. London: RCOG Press, 1994:223–35.

60   *Peeters LLH. The effect of early maternal maladaption on fetal, growth. *J Perinat Med* 19994;**22 (Suppl 1)**:S9–16.

61   Khong TY, De Wolf F, Robertson WB, Brosens I. Inadequate maternal vascular response to placentation in pregnancies complicated by pre-eclampsia and by small for gestational-age infants. *Br J Obstet Gynaecol* 1986;**93**:1049–59.

62   Robillard PY, Hulsey TC, Perianin J, Janky E, Miri EH, Papiernik E. Association of pregnancy-induced hypertension with duration of sexual cohabitation before conception. *Lancet* 1994;**344**:973–5.

63   Mackenzie HS, Lawler EV Brenner BM. Congenital oligonephropathy: the fetal flaw in essential hypertension. *Kidney Int* 1996;**49 (Suppl 55)**: S30–4.

64   Rothman KJ. Causes. *Am J Epidemiol* 1976;**104**:587–92.

65   *Susser M, Stein Z. Timing in prenatal nutrition: a reprise of the Dutch famine study. *Nutr Rev* 1994;**52**:84–94.

66   Ebbs JH, Tisdall FF, Scott WA. The influence of prenatal diet on the mother and child. *J Nutr* 1941;**22**:515–26.

67   Cameron CS, Graham S. Antenatal diet and its influence on stillbirths and prematurity. *Glasgow Med J* 1944;**142**:1–7.

68   Antonov AN. Children born during the siege of Leningrad in 1942. *J Pediatr* 1947;**30**:250–9.

69   McGanity WJ, Cannon RO, Bridgfort EB, *et al.*. The Vanderbilt cooperative study of maternal and infant nutrition. V. Description and outcome of obstetrics sample. *Am J Obstet Gynecol* 1954;**67**:491–500.

70   Thomson AM. Diet in relation to the course and outcome of pregnancy. *Br J Nutr* 1959;**13**:509–25.

71   Treasure JL, Russell GFM. Intrauterine growth and neonatal weight in babies of women with anorexia nervosa. *Br Med J* 1988;**296**:1038.

72   *Robinson JS, Owens JA, De Barro T, lok F, Chidzanja S. Maternal nutrition and fetal growth. In: Ward RHT, Smith SK, Donnai D, eds, *Early fetal growth and development*. London: RCOG Press, 1994: 317–34.

73   Maternal nutrition and low birthweight. *Lancet* 1975;**ii**:445.

74   Ravelli GP, Stein ZA, Susser MW. Obesity in young men after famine exposure in utero and early infancy. *N Engl J Med* 1976;**295**:349–53.

75   Rawlings JS, Rawling VB, Read JA. Prevalence of low birthweight and preterm delivery in relation to the interval between pregnancies among white and black women. *N Engl J Med* 1995;**332**:69–74.

76   Eastman NJ, Jackson E. Weight relationships in pregnancy. I The bearing of maternal weight gain and prepregnancy weight on birthweight in full term pregnancies. *Obstet Gynecol Surv* 1968;**23**:1003–24.

77   Thomson AM. Fetal growth and size at birth. In: Barron SL, Thomson AM, eds, *Obstetrical Epidemiology*. London: Academic Press, 1983: 89–142.

78   Taffel S. *Maternal weight gain and the outcome of pregnancy, United States, 1980*. Washington, DC:US Govt. printing office, 1986. US Dept of Health and Human Services publication PHS 86–1922. Vital and Health Statistics, series 21, No. 44.

79   Viegas OAC, Scott PH, Cole TJ, Eaton P, Needham PG, Wharton BA. Dietary protein energy supplementation of pregnant Asian mothers at Sorrento, Birmingham. II: Selective during third trimester only. *Br Med J* 1982;**285**:592–5.

80   Brown JE, Potter JD, Jacobs DR, Kopher RA, Rourke MJ, Barosso GM, Hannan PJ, Schmid L A. Maternal waist-to-hip ratio as a predictor of newborn size: results of the Diana Project. *Epidemiology* 1996; **7**:62–66.

81   McKeigue PM, Pierpoint T, Ferrie JE, Marmot MG. Relationship of glucose intolerance and hyperinsulinaemia to body fat pattern in South Asians and Europeans. *Diabetologia* 1992;**35**:785–91.

82   Campaigne BN. Body fat distribution in females: metabolic consequences and implications for weight loss. *Med Sci Sports Exer* 1990;**22**:291–97.

83   McKeigue PM, Shah B, Marmot MG. Relationship of central obesity and insulin resistance with high diabetes prevalence and cardiovascular risk in South Asians. *Lancet* 1991;**337**:382–6.

84   Fowden AL. The role of insulin in prenatal growth. *J Dev Physiol* 1989;**12**:173–82.

85   Cousins L. Insulin sensitivity in pregnancy. *Diabetes* 1991;**40 (Suppl 2)**:S39–43.

86   Haig D. Genetic conflicts in human pregnancy. *Q Rev Biol* 1993;**68**: 495–525.

87   Evain-Brion D. Hormonal regulation of fetal growth. *Horm Res* 1994;**42**:207–14.

88   Daly LE, Kirke PN, Molloy A, Weir DG, Scott JM. Folate levels and neural tube defects. Implications for prevention. *JAMA* 1995;**274**: 1698–702.

89   Godfrey KM, Barker DJP. Maternal nutrition in relation to fetal and placental growth. *Eur J Obstet & Gynecol Reprod Biol* 1995;**61**:15–22.

90   Barker DJP, Bull AR, Osmond C, Simmonds SJ, Fetal and placental size and the risk of hypertension in adult life. *Br Med J* 1990;**301**:259–62.

91   Godfrey KM, Redman CWG, Barker DJP, Osmond C. The effect of maternal anaemia on the ratio of fetal weight to placental weight. *Br J Obstet & Gynaecol* 1991;**98**:886–91.

92   Perry IJ, Beevers DG, Whincup PH, Bearford D. Predictors of ratio of placental weight to foetal weight in multiethnic community. *Br Med J* 1995;**310**:436–9.

93   Whincup P, Cook D, Papacosta O, Walker M, Perry IJ. Maternal factors and development of cardiovascular risk: evidence from a study of blood pressure in children. *J Hum Hypertens* 1994;**8**:337–43.

94   Godfrey K, Robinson S, Barker DJP, Osmond C, Cox V. Maternal nutrition in early and late pregnancy in relation to placental and fetal growth. *Br Med J* 1996;**312**:410–4.

95   Campbell DM, Hall MH, Barker DJP, Cross J Shiell AW, Godfrey KM. Diet in pregnancy and the offspring's blood pressure 40 years later. *Br J Obstet & Gynaecol* 1996;**103**:273–80.

96   Kramer MS. Effects of energy and protein intakes on pregnancy outcome: an overview of the research evidence from controlled clinical trials. *Am J Clin Nutr* 1993;**58**:627–35.

8 Social pathways between childhood and adult health

Diana Kuh, Chris Power, David Blane, and Mel Bartley

There are two main ways that socioeconomic factors throughout the life course affect adult health and disease risk. First, they affect exposures to known or suspected causal factors during gestation, infancy, childhood, adolescence, or young adulthood which are part of long term *biological* chains of risk. Second, they form part of *social* chains of risk that begin with a socially compromised start to life, operate throughout the life course partly via educational and other learning experiences, and lead to adult socioeconomic circumstances which affect disease risk through exposures to causal factors in later life. Causal factors at each life stage include physical hazards and behaviours with known or suspected biological pathways, but may also include stressful life conditions which affect biological resources through psychosocial processes which are only beginning to be understood. Thus evidence from two types of studies are reviewed in this chapter: (1) aetiological studies which have examined how variations in adult disease are related to social factors at different stages of the life course in order to understand biological chains of risk, and; (2) studies of social chains of risk, which have investigated either the extent to which individuals experience continuity in their socioeconomic environment or how they interact with their environment in ways that lead to socially patterned exposures which may damage or protect health capital.

8.1 Introduction

Previous chapters have focused on biological risk factors at different stages of the life course and their independent and combined effects on adult disease. This chapter develops the idea that socioeconomic factors throughout the life course affect adult health and disease risk. This is because health-damaging exposures or health-enhancing opportunities are socially patterned, and because an individual's response, which may modify their impact or alter the risk of future exposures will be powerfully affected by their social and economic experience. Unlike biological progamming which is hypothesized to occur during critical periods of development, the positive or adverse effects of the socioeconomic environment are hypothesized to be due to cumulative exposure over the life course, although some developmental stages may be more sensitive.

The term 'socially patterned' implies that resources and opportunities are constrained by the various forms of social stratification (such as socio-economic class, race and gender) and by the nature of the roles associated with social institutions such as the family, educational institutions, or occupational groups. These, in turn, change over time and differ between societies. Using a simple life course framework we first discuss how the constraints and opportunities afforded by socioeconomic position link childhood to adult health. This framework is then extended to emphasize the interactions that occur between an individual and the environment (particularly the family and the school) through which behavioural and psychosocial processes operate which may have long term implications for adult health. The effects of race or gender are not addressed.

8.2 Pathways between childhood and adult health: a simplified framework

Figure 8.1 provides a simplified framework which shows the hypothesized major pathways via which childhood socioeconomic factors affect later life health. Longitudinal studies with prospective social and biological information collected in childhood and adulthood, such as the Medical

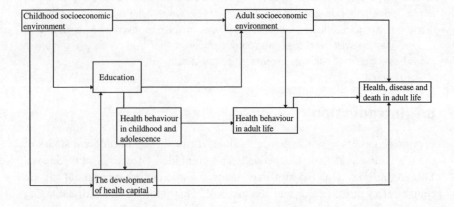

Figure 8.1 Pathways between childhood and adult health:a simplified framework

Research Council National Survey of Health and Development (the 1946 birth cohort)[1-3] and the National Child Development Study (the 1958 birth cohort),[4-6] provide particularly valuable sources of data for reviewing the evidence for these pathways. This chapter emphasizes the earlier stages of the life course. It only briefly discusses the adult factors underlying the well documented strong and graded associations between adult socio-economic status (measured by adult social class or education) and mortal-ity, morbidity, and other health outcomes and behaviours which occur in Britain,[7-11] the US,[12-19] and other developed countries,[20] as these are dis-cussed in Chapter 11 and reviewed elsewhere. Nor does it address how adult health behaviours and other risk factors increase chronic disease risk, as this has been discussed in previous chapters.

8.2.1 Continuity in the socioeconomic environment over the life course

There is plenty of evidence from intergenerational studies that those from more favoured family backgrounds have a much better chance of achieving high socioeconomic positions or earnings in adult life.[21-31] In the 1958 cohort, a man whose father was in social class I or II was twice as likely to be in the same class position himself at 33 years than one whose father had been a skilled manual worker, and nearly three times more likely than one whose father had been in social class IV or V.[30] These results are almost identical for the 1946 cohort.[2,32] Conversely, the risk of unemployment in the 1958 cohort was greatest for those whose fathers suffered unemployment. Whereas almost 10% of men were unemployed, this was true of over 19% of those whose fathers had themselves been unemployed in 1974 (when the cohort member was 16), and fully 50% of those whose fathers had also been unemployed when they were 7 and 11 years of age in 1965 and 1969. The risk of unemployment for a year or more, and of low income, was also higher for those with fathers in lower quintiles of the income distribution.[30]

How much of the continuity between child and adult socioeconomic circumstances is mediated by educational experience (see Fig. 8.1)? There is substantial evidence from cohort studies of a powerful effect of family background (in terms of parental education, father's social class and other parental or household characteristics) on educational opportunity and attainment.[1,2,4,25,33,34] In turn, educational attainment is a powerful predictor of adult income and occupation.[23,24,28,30,31] Some studies show no independent effect of childhood socioeconomic status on adult earnings once education has been accounted for.[23] In contrast, findings from the 1946 birth cohort show that father's social class was still an independent predictor of male midlife earnings,[28] and maternal education was still an independent predictor of women's earnings,[31] even after allowing for own educational experience. It is likely that besides the powerful influence that well educated middle class parents have on their children's educational achievement, they also develop social and personal skills in their offspring (such as motivation and self direction, manners of speech and peer identification), and provide financial backing and social contacts which help prepare their child for a similar class position and capacity for earning.[35,36]

8.2.2 Importance of socioeconomic career for adult health

Although it is well documented that adults in the poorest socioeconomic circumstances have the worst health, only a few studies have looked at the effect of length and timing of exposure. A Scottish cohort study with data on social class in adulthood and retrospective data on father's occupation and own occupation at labour market entry found that those who remained in less favoured circumstances throughout life experienced the highest mortality risk,[37] suggesting that risk accumulates over the life course. Most,[37-44] but not all[45,46] of the studies which have looked at the timing of exposure have found that childhood socioeoconomic circumstances have an inverse relationship with cardiovascular morbidity or mortality independent of subsequent adult social position, suggesting that some underlying causes may have their effect in early life. These studies, and the relationships between conventional cardiovascular risk factors and socioeconomic position at different life stages are discussed in more detail in section 11.3 of Chapter 11.

Analyses using information from the birth cohort studies have examined a wider set of health experiences. In the 1958 cohort, socioeconomic circumstances prevailing at each stage of childhood and adolescence were found to be relevant to health differences among young adults.[6] In the 1946 cohort, adult socioeconomic factors were better predictors than father's social class of those in the poorest health at 36 years[47] or physically disabled at age 43 years,[48] but father's social class and level of education were better predictors of those in the best of health at 36 years, regardless of the later social environment.[47] In this study, the risks for those who remained in less favoured circumstances throughout life were not compared with the risks for those who were only in such circumstances in adulthood.

Generally, intergenerational upward social mobility has been linked to better adult health[49] and increased life expectancy[37,50,51] through its association with improved life conditions or health behaviours. However, for some health outcomes, such social mobility may carry adverse health consequences (this is also the case for geographical migration, see Chapter 10). For example, Forsdahl[52] suggested that deprivation in childhood followed by relative affluence in adulthood would increase coronary disease risk (see chapter 3, section 3.2). There is some evidence that successful men who surmount a childhood of disadvantage have more health problems.[53] Blood pressure seems to be particularly vulnerable to social mobility. For example, in the 1946 birth cohort it was found that of the men from manual social classes who did not receive any educational qualifications, those who rose within the manual classes in comparison with their fathers had significantly higher mean systolic blood pressures than those who had remained in the same class.[54] This is similar to Dressler's work on life style incongruity[55] which found that in African-American communities in the US, those who demonstrated material success which was not supported with other credentials, such as higher education, were more likely to be hypertensive. Whether in these examples the processes involved are primarily biological or psychosocial (see section 8.3) remains to be seen.

8.2.3 Childhood socioeconomic circumstances, the acquisition of health capital and adult health

We have used the term 'health capital' to mean the accumulation of biological resources, inherited and acquired during earlier stages of life which determine current health and future health potential, including resilience to future environmental insults. This concept of health capital is analogous to the notion of constitution used in the interwar years (see Chapter 2).

How do the independent or cumulative socioeconomic experiences of the previous generation and of the individual in infancy, childhood and adolescence affect the acquisition of health capital, as shown in Fig. 8.1? Recently Wadsworth[56,57] reviewed some of the evidence, showing that poverty, unemployment, poor home circumstances, and parental education are associated with many aspects of health in early life which, as the previous chapters have discussed, may raise adult disease risk. These include poor prenatal and postnatal growth, respiratory infection, and poor maternal and child nutrition. Socioeconomic factors in childhood predict adult stature[58] through their association with early nutrition and exercise which are essential for skeletal development;[59] those who attain high levels of peak bone mass are less likely to reach the critical threshold for osteoporosis in later life even if there is no difference in the rate of bone loss during ageing. Intergenerational links, although not shown in Fig. 8.1, are suggested by research which has shown that poor social circumstances during gestation or childhood affect a young women's subsequent reproductive performance and pregnancy outcome.[60–64]

The associations between early physical growth and development and later health may be due to social as well as biological pathways. For example, it is not clear whether the poorer subsequent physical and mental development of low birth weight babies represent biological sequelae or social influences.[65] This is because low birth weight babies are more likely to be born into poor families and to remain in disadvantaged circumstances during childhood.[65,66]

But even if the adverse sequelae are primarily biological in origin, it is evident that they may be be modified by social influences[67,68]

Another example is the well documented relationship between adult height and cardiovascular morbidity and mortality.[41,69–73] Height is both a marker of child health and development[74] and of childhood socioeconomic conditions.[75] Although this evidence has been used to support the idea that the early environment influences adult health, an alternative interpretation is that height influences adult health through its effect on adult socioeconomic position. This is because social mobility, in terms of occupation and marriage, is selective with respect to height.[71,76–79] Another interpretation is that the relationship between height and mortality is due to differential rates of shrinkage according to health.[80]

Similarly, overweight and obesity are risk factors for adult health (see Chapters 4 and 6) but they also predict an individual's social and economic trajectory, particularly for women.[81–83] For example, one study found that fatter women were less likely to marry and had poorer job opportunities and lower incomes than other women.[81] Could these findings be explained by the fact that those from lower socioeconomic groups are more likely to be fat?[78,84,85] As the findings were independent of baseline socioeconomic status they appear to reflect the socioeconomic consequences of overweight. Thus both biological and social pathways over the life course may explain the relationship between overweight and adult health.

Biological and social pathways also operate for those with serious or chronic childhood illnesses. Social class differences exist in the incidence of serious illness, particularly in the first 5 years of life.[78] Childhood illness and disability have long term consequences for adult health,[47,86] disability[48] and handicap.[87] This may be due to the biological sequelae associated with a specific disorder or because individual and societal expectations and opportunities are lowered (for example through educational disruption and underachievement, poor self esteem, or stigmatization). For example, children with chronic illness in the 1946 birth cohort study compared with other cohort members were at increased risk of unemployment in adult life (possibly because the disruption of education reduced their chances of educational attainment), were less likely to be homeowners and had reduced social support due to higher parental death rates.[88]

8.3 Extending the framework: individual social capital and chains of risk

The framework in Fig. 8.1 is a simple representation of the social and economic constraints and opportunities which may link the socioeconomic environment in childhood to adult health. Once psychosocial[89] or behavioural[90] explanations are invoked, the framework has to be extended to allow for interactions between the individual and the environment.

Within any given material and social-structural context, an individual's behaviour will help to shape both their current circumstances and future life trajectory. One of the important influences on behaviour is the individual's social capital, by which we mean the accumulation of social and cognitive skills, self esteem, coping strategies, attitudes, and values. The development of social capital is a major function of childhood and adolescence. This process is thought to be shaped primarily by characteristics of the family and the school, influenced in turn by the socioeconomic and cultural characteristics of the time and the place (Fig. 8.2).

The idea of a 'chain of risk' offers a dynamic framework for studying the interplay over time between intrinsic (i.e. individual social capital and

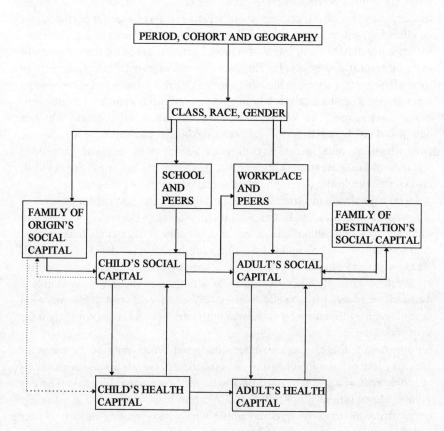

Figure 8.2 The development of individual social capital* over the life course and its relationship with individual health capital.

*Comprises cognitive and social skills, coping strategies, self esteem, attitudes and values. A family's social capital also includes relationships between family members.

behaviour) and extrinsic (i.e. material and cultural) influences on individual life trajectories and associated health risks. This concept was developed by Rutter in his seminal discussion of the pathways between childhood and adult life.[91] He argued that 'the impact of some factor in childhood may lie less in the immediate behavioural change it brings about than the fact it sets into motion a chain reaction in which one 'bad' thing leads to another, or, conversely, that a good experience makes it more likely that another one will be encountered' (p.27).[91] Rutter's interest was in psychopathological continuities and disconti-nuities over the life span, but his conceptual framework is also relevant in understanding the psychosocial and behavioural processes underlying path-ways between the early social environment and adult health. Individual characteristics, such as self esteem, coping strategies, and cognitive and social skills act as mediators along these pathways. Adolescence and young adult-hood are critical periods because many important 'life transitions' are nego-tiated during this time (decisions about training, careers, marital partners, and childbearing) which may act as key links in chains of advantage and adversity. In this more dynamic and interactive model, parents are more than the sum of material resources they supply. The social capital of parents affects the care of their offspring in very early life which may influence growth and development through psychoendocrine mechanisms, with implications for later health. For example, Hertzman and Wiens[68] report a study which showed that that rats handled daily between birth and weaning had lower basal corticosterone concentrations and faster physiological recovery in stressful situations throughout life. Parenting skills, and the quality of the role models provided, also contribute to the development of social capital in offspring.

Social capital will, in turn, affect educational progess, and the negotiation of important life transitions. In this way, it contributes to the social position and the level of social support achieved in adult life. It also contributes to the maintenance of health capital by influencing health related behaviours and, perhaps, psychoendocrine responses[89,92–94] to environmental stressors in adult life, such as unemployment. Educational attainment, beyond being simply a mediator between, or a good marker of, childhood and adult material advantage, may therefore be associated with later health because of these links with social capital.[95]

Poor family functioning or other childhood stress may set a chain of adversity into motion by inhibiting the aquisition of social capital such as skills or self esteem which may lead to poor school performance (Fig. 8.3). There is some evidence (see section 8.3.3) that adolescent behaviours, such as smoking, heavy drinking or early experimentation in sexual activity, which cluster together and are seen as problem behaviours in the wider society, are associated with poor school performance and low self esteem. Early sexual activity carries a risk of teenage pregnancy and this may act as a key link in a chain of risk.

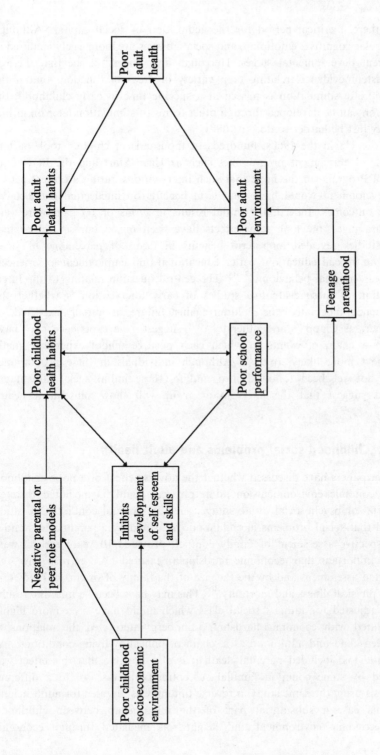

Figure 8.3 Examples of chains of risk

Is there a critical period for the acquisition of social capital? Although particular cognitive, emotional, and social abilities are more easily acquired at different developmental stages, Hertzman and Wiens[68] argue that there is 'consistent evidence, relating to a variety of areas of function, that if the appropriate stimulation is missed at a specific time in early childhood, the function can be developed through other forms of stimulation later on in life. It may just be harder to do.' (p.1088)

In the US in the 1960s, hundreds of thousands of children took part in preschool enrichment programmes such as Head Start and the Perry Preschool Program, in the hope that such interventions during a critical period of development would have long term benefits on intellectual and behavioural outcomes. Indeed, the initial results in terms of IQ gain were very encouraging;[96] the long term effects have been mixed but several evaluative studies revealed long term benefits in terms of percentage of years spent in special education, better educational and employment experiences, and less criminal behaviour.[97–100] The central question relating to the interpretation of these evaluative studies of early intervention is whether the experience 'inoculated' the children against failure, as initially expected, or whether, as Clapp[101] and others[1,102–104] suggest, 'the experience may have begun a chain of events in which each positive school experience made the next more likely' (p.5).[101] Although individuals in these programmes have not yet been followed into midlife, these initial social advantages would suggest that the intervention group will show subsequent health gains.

8.3.2 Childhood social problems and adult health

Recent papers have discussed whether the adverse effect of a poor childhood socioeconomic environment on adult physical health is mediated through material or psychosocial disadvantage, such as parental conflict. One study found that social problems in childhood (measured by a parental loss and a retrospective assessment of family conflict, provided 10 years earlier) were more important than economic hardship (measured by a retrospective self reported assessment and by the the size of the family of origin) in predicting adult physical illness and mortality.[105] This may have been because the results were adjusted for father's social class which might have been more highly correlated with economic hardship. Lundberg interpreted the relationship between child and adulthood as a 'chain of unhealthy living conditions'. As parental loss included parental death it is also possible that this effect was caused by some common familial susceptibility to disease. In a different analysis using the same study, a reverse finding was revealed for adult height. In this case a substantial part of the relationship between childhood socioeconomic environment and height was mediated through economic conditions in the family of origin rather than through family conflict or parental loss.[106]

There is a substantial body of evidence to show that children of divorced parents have more short term health and behavioural problems, less successsful educational, occupational and marital careers, and poorer mental health and health habits in adult life.[107–117] Parental conflict rather than divorce as such appear to increase the risk of poor psychosocial adjustment.[111,114] These findings suggest that both psychosocial and socioeconomic chains of risk may be operating, both of which could impact on physical health. Parental divorce but not parental death in childhood has been found to predict adult mortality in the US Terman sample, reducing life expectancy by at least 4 years.[118] Other measures of the childhood socioeconomic environment did not raise mortality risk, but this sample is highly selected in terms of sociodemographic factors because the original sample of children were selected on the basis of high IQ scores. This will have reduced the ability to detect such effects. Furthermore, divorce amongst the parents of this sample was a relatively rare event and may have had a different meaning compared with divorce among parents of later generations. Information was not given on the future career trajectories of this sample, and whether these differed between those who experienced parental divorce and those who did not.

Despite some methodological problems these studies raise the intriguing possibility that psychosocial processes may be important in explaining the link between the childhood environment and adult physical health. In the 1946 cohort, survey members with parents who provided low levels of care and high levels of control (based on retrospective assessments by adult offspring) had significantly less social support in adult life.[119] Another study showed that having a warm or affectionate parent was associated with adult social accomplishment in terms of having a long, happy marriage, children and relationships with close friends in midlife.[120] In this study, parental harmony or a difficult childhood were not so important. These two studies[119,120] which link parenting style with adult interpersonal competence support a psycho-social interpretation and suggest possible mediating factors, as social support and marriage have been linked to adult health and mortality.[121–124]

Studies that have looked at earlier stages of the life course also provide support for psychosocial processes. For example, in a US study[125] high levels of reported family conflict were associated with prospective increases in physical symptoms among adolescents. In a cohort study of Scottish young people, measures of family functioning were more powerful than measures of material deprivation in predicting health 3 years later,[126] and stressful life events in mid adolescence influenced future career trajectories.[127] The 1958 birth cohort provides several examples of possible psychosocial processes: social adjustment (as measured by the Rutter Behaviour score) accounted for some of the class inequalities in self reported health at 23 years and affected future social mobility.[6] It also showed that shortness in childhood was associated with reports of psychosocial problems, such as bedwetting.[128] Furthermore, height in childhood had a stronger association with unemployment than adult height.[129] This suggested that indirect health selection (through psychosocial processes) rather than direct selection of shorter men out of the labour market was operating, thus adding a fourth explanation for the link between height and health besides the three others discussed in section 8.2.3. For example, family conflict might temporarily retard child growth and also raise the risk of later unemployment. In such a case the development of both social and health capital would have been impeded by the same childhood adversity.

8.3.3 The development of health behaviours

Conceptualizing the development of health behaviours as a 'chain of risk' encourages researchers to study whether habits established in childhood carry over to adult life, and to examine hypothesized links between the attributes of the child or adolescent and the characteristics of their socioeconomic environment (in particular family, school and peer influences) which predict take up and subsequent maintenance or cessation of behaviour. The difficulty of changing established health behaviours is well documented[130,131] and emphasizes the need to study these early influences on their development.[132] This is not to deny that these influences on adult behaviour will be modified by the social and economic constraints and opportunities encountered later (see section 8.4).

So far most studies have concentrated on a single behaviour and usually examined only some of the links in any chain of risk, often lacking any theoretical framework with which to understand the processes involved.[32,133] An exception was the study by Jessor and Jessor[134,135] into the personal and environmental factors that predict onset, continuity, and change in problem adolescent behaviours because it offered a conceptual framework, looked for common influences on several behaviours, and elicited some of the underlying psychosocial processes.

Least attention has been paid to the establishment of food preferences or dietary patterns, although family influences are likely to operate from infancy. In the 1946 cohort certain nutrient intakes at 36 years were associated with social class of origin[136] but surprisingly little is known either about cultural factors or psychosocial processes influencing food selection.[137,138] Studies since the 1930s have repeatedly pointed out that low income families cannot afford a healthy diet (see for example[139–141]) and healthy food is often less available and more expensive in poorer than in richer neighbourhoods.[142] Besides any nutritional impact on health, a poor diet may have a long term influence on food preferences.

Most attention has been paid to the uptake of cigarette smoking and alcohol drinking in adolescence. This is a time when when decisions about ways of living become increasingly the responsibility of the young person and health damaging behaviours tend to cluster.[135,143–149] The healthiness or otherwise of behaviourial choices in adolescence may be of less importance compared with other functions they serve: as markers of transition into the adult world; for gaining admission to peer groups or making oneself attractive to the opposite sex; as a sign of personal identity, independence, and autonomy; as a coping mechanism for adolescent anxiety, failure, and stress; or simply because certain activities are fun. Thus, there may be greater similarities in early life influences on adolescent behaviours than on long term continuity and change in these behaviours.

Generally, studies on the uptake of smoking and drinking and participation in physically active leisure pursuits point to the importance of parents, siblings and peers.[138,150–160] Whether the effects are mediated through role modelling, attitudes, or parental skills in developing autonomy in the offspring[161] is unclear. The influence of parents on their children's drinking habits appears to be complex, in that parents who are heavy drinkers or who abstain are less likely to be imitated by their children[162] and children whose parents disapprove of drinking are more likely to drink away from home where they may be affected by peer relationships.[163] Parental divorce and other indications of poor functioning in the family of origin are predictive of smoking[110] and problem drinking in midlife[109,164] although not always among young adults.[165] In general, Lau et al.[166] speculated that parental influences on health behaviours and beliefs would persist throughout life unless the child was exposed, during certain sensitive periods, to important social models whose behaviour and beliefs differed from those of the parent. This idea of sensitive periods or events (adolescence, leaving home, going on to higher education, or setting up home with a partner) is similar to Rutter's point that the negotiation of life transitions during adolescence acts as a key link in chains of risk.

Educational characteristics, such as low aspirations, earlier school leaving, and poor educational performance are associated with the uptake of smoking and drinking.[151,167–171] Smoking and excess drinking may act as a defence against a derogated self image,[168] whereas participation in sports may enhance self esteem.[172]

Using 1946 birth cohort data on personality collected at 16 years and smoking habit up to 25 years, smokers were both more neurotic and more extrovert than non-smokers, neurotic extroverts were most likely to take up smoking and stable extroverts were most likely (at least among men) to have given up by the age of 25 years.[173] Those who initiate smoking at younger ages are less likely to give up.[174–176] Those who drink heavily in adolescence are likely to continue to do so in early adulthood.[134,177] There is evidence from retrospective studies[178–183] and a prospective study[184] that those who participated in active leisure pursuits during childhood were more likely than their peers to continue to do so in adult life.

In late adolescence or early adult life key life transitions provide an opportunity to discontinue adolescent behaviour patterns. For example, the acquisition of educational qualifications is associated with healthier diets, less smoking and more exercise in adult life,[136,184–186] and the formation of stable partnerships and families moderates heavy drinking.[187]

8.4 Adult factors

According to the argument presented so far in this chapter, individuals entering adult life may bring with them a number of sources of risk for later health, such as a poor growth and development, a greater risk of exposure and vulnerability to psychosocial stress, and behaviours, such as cigarette smoking; all these have been influenced by the early social environment. The extent to which these sources of risk in early life account for variations in individual risk or social class gradients in health is as yet unknown. The individual then incurs additional sources of risk due to the constraints and opportunities afforded by adult socioeconomic position, which, as has been shown, is itself the outcome of earlier socioeconomic processes. The impact of these risks is exacerbated because they affect those who are already most vulnerable. The question of whether a good start to life protects against the impact of poor adult circumstances has been little studied.

Adults in the lower socioeconomic groups have less healthy diets,[185] are more likely to smoke[175] and are less likely to engage frequently in sports activities[188] compared with those in the upper groups. Although some of these relationships may be accounted for by early life influences, in particular by education, a Scottish cohort study previously decribed[37] found that such behavioural risk factors were more strongly associated with socioeconomic position in adulthood rather than childhood.[189] For example, current financial constraints and living in poor neighbourhoods are likely to restrict diet[142] and reduce social participation, including such things as membership of sports clubs. Similarly, smoking may be an effective coping strategy in low income households.[190]

The impact of these behaviours on health should not be overstated. They only explain some of the social inequalities in adult health[185] and coronary heart disease mortality (see Chapter 11),[191,192] and even when people are successful at changing their behaviour, the effect has often been less than expected.[193–195] Evidence from the Health and Lifestyle Survey[185] suggests that health related behaviours may have more impact on health in the non-manual classes, perhaps because other factors play a greater role in the manual classes.

Exposure to physical hazards and stressful life conditions are socially stratified.[196,197] Manual socioeconomic groups are at higher risk of exposure to a range of physical hazards in their residential and occupational environments.[198] Adverse social circumstances often involve both these material disadvantages and the social exclusion associated with experiences such as low income and unemployment.[89] The low status attached to occupying a position at or near the bottom of a social hierarchy is in itself a source of stress, particularly in times of rising social expectations and growing social inequality, as witnessed in Britain and the US and many other developed countries in the last 20 years.[89,114] During the economic recessions of the 1970s and 1980s, adults in the lower socioeconomic groups were more likely to experience unemployment than those in the upper socioeconomic groups.[199] Unemployment carries significant risks to health.[200–204] Manual workers with health problems were more likely to lose their jobs and withdraw permanently from the labour market where their health may deteriorate more rapidly because of a lower standard of living.[199] In the 1946 cohort, the socioeconomic consequences of disability were shown to be more severe for manual compared with nonmanual workers.[48]

Labour market experience in adult life, particularly in respect of income from occupational pensions has a powerful affect on the standard of living after retirement, with implications for health in old age.[205,206] This is likely to increase with the erosion of state pensions and a greater reliance on occupational pensions. As the birth cohort studies mature it will be possible to study how socioeconomic factors in childhood, adolescence, and adult life accumulate and impact on the ageing process.

In adult life, the individual's social capital will influence their response to the socioeconomic environment, moderating its effects on disease risk and the ageing process generally, and modifying the risk of further exposure to adversity. Although this chapter has focused on the ways in which social capital is influenced by early life experiences, midlife is thought to be a developmental stage in its own right[207,208] with opportunities to acquire new social and personal skills and coping strategies.

8.5 Social change

The twentieth century has witnessed radical changes in living conditions and family patterns in Britain, the US, and other developed countries.[114,209,210] These have affected each birth cohort at a different stage of the life course, providing a unique generational experience with different implications for health and other life chances. For example, studies have shown how growing up in during the Great Depression affected the development of boys and girls in different ways[211] or how the experience of US military service allowed some men to break the chain of risk associated with early disadvantage by reshaping their life course.[212] Career opportunities expanded for many young people in the postwar period with the growth of non-manual occupations and the associated expansion in secondary and further education. In contrast, young people entering the labour market during the 1970s and 1980s were at a greatly increased risk of unemployment, and more restricted career opportunities.[114] Growing inequality in the distribution of income and the experience of unemployment in the developed countries over the last 20 years have increased the proportion of the population living in relative poverty.[89,114] Children have been particularly affected by this increase in relative poverty, particularly those living with single parents or whose parents have divorced.[56,213–215] These trends have worrying implications for the development of social and health capital in these younger generations and for their health in later life.

8.6 Conclusions

This chapter has shown that to understand the influence of the life course on health and the prevalent adult chronic diseases, the biological processes of development, growth, and ageing need to be examined in relation to living standards and stressful life conditions, which vary across the life course and by position in the social hierarchy. The example of chronic obstructive airways disease summarizes the main points and illustrates the accumulation of biological and social risk over the life course.[216] During early life, crowded living conditions, poor housing and air quality, financial constraints, and poor parental behaviour may adversely affect nutrition during pregnancy or the intensity and frequency of respiratory infections during early childhood, damaging or restricting lung development and growth. During adolescence, parents and peers and educational experience influence the uptake of cigarette smoking. In adulthood, cultural influences, exposure to stress, and individual characteristics affect the chance of giving up smoking, and the type of occupation affects exposure to fumes and dust. The progressive loss of respiratory function eventually begins to limit the level of physical activity the individual can sustain. Although this may not interfere with the performance of a sedentary white collar occupation, it may force retirement from a physically arduous manual job.[217] Occupational pension provisions will influence living standards once out of the workforce and will continue to influence the course of the disease. Thus, even though the clinically overt stages of this disease do not become manifest until later life, its development involves the interaction of both biological and social chains of risk throughout life.[218] Epidemiologists who view social factors only as potential confounders limit their understanding of the natural history of the disease.

In this cumulative life course model, biological chains of risk emphasize the development of health capital in fetal and early childhood whereas social chains of risk emphasize the whole of childhood when the acquisition of social capital is rapid, and late adolescence and young adulthood when key life life transitions are made. The use of more sophisticated statistical models will permit the testing of hypothesized chains of risk, incorporating biological, social, and psychosocial factors. Data will be available from the maturing of the birth cohort studies and from follow ups of historical cohort studies. In this way the accumulation of risks to health over the life course may be further elucidated.

References

Those marked with an asterisk are especially recommended for further reading.

1   Douglas JWB, Ross JM, Simpson HR. *All Our Future*. London: Peter Davis, 1968.
2* Wadsworth MEJ. *The imprint of time: childhood, history and adult life*. Oxford: Oxford University Press, 1991.
3   Wadsworth MEJ, Kuh DJL. Childhood influences on adult health: a review of recent work in the British 1946 national birth cohort study, the MRC National Survey of Health and Development. *Paediat Perinat Epidemiol* 1997;**11**:2–20.
4   Fogelman K, ed. *Growing up in Great Britain. Papers from the National Child Development Study*. London: The MacMillan Press Ltd, 1983.
5   Ferri E, ed. *Life at 33. The fifth follow-up of the National Child Development Study*. London: National Children's Bureau, 1993.
6* Power C, Manor O, Fox AJ. *Health and class: the early years*. London: Chapman Hall, 1991.
7   Black D, Morris JN, Smith C, Townsend P. *Inequalities in health: report of a Research Working Group*. London: Department of Health and Social Security, 1980.
8   Townsend PN, Davidson N, Whitehead M. *Inequalities in health*. London: Penguin, 1988.
9* Department of Health. *Variations in Health: what can the Department of Health and the NHS do?* London: Department of Health, 1995.
10 Davey Smith G, Bartley M, Blane D. The Black Report on socio-economic inequalities in health 10 years on. *Br Med J* 1990;**301**:373-7.
11 Marmot MG, Bobak M, Davey Smith G. Explanations for social inequalities in health. In: Amick III BC, Levine S, Tarlov AR, Chapman Walsh D, eds. *Society and health*. London: Oxford University Press, 1995:172–210.

12   Antonovsky A. Social class, life expectancy and overall mortality. *Milbank Mem Fund Q* 1967;**45**:31–73.

13   Antonovsky A. Social class and the major cardiovascular diseases. *J Chron Dis* 1968;**21**:65–106.

14   Kitagawa EM, Hauser PM. *Differential mortality in the United States: a study in socioeconomic epidemiology.* Cambridge, M.A.: Harvard University Press, 1973.

15   Feldman JJ, Makuc DM, Kleinman JC, Cornoni-Huntley J. National trends in educational differentials in mortality. *Am J Epidemiol* 1989; **129**:919–33.

16   Elo IT, Preston SH. Educational differentials in mortality: United States, 1979–85. *Soc Sci Med* 1996;**42**:47–57.

17   Davey Smith G, Neaton JD, Wentworth D, Stamler R, Stamler J. Socioeconomic differentials in mortality risk among men screened for the multiple risk factor intervention trial: I. White men. *Am J Public Health* 1996;**86**:486–96.

18   Davey Smith G, Wentworth D, Neaton JD, Stamler R, Stamler J. Socioeconomic differentials in mortality risk among men screened for the multiple risk factor intervention trial: II. Black men. *Am J Public Health* 1996;**86**:497–504.

19   Diez-Roux AV, Nieto FJ, Tyroler HA, Crum LD, Szklo M. Social inequalities and atherosclerosis. *Am J Epidemiol* 1995;**141**:960–72.

20   Kunst AE, Mackenbach HP. The size of mortality differences associated with educational level in nine industrialized countries. *Am J Public Health* 1994;**84**:932–7.

21   Glass DV(ed). *Social mobility in Britain.* London: Routledge and Kegan Paul, 1954.

22   Sewell WH, Hauser RM. *Education,occupation, and earnings: achievement in the early career.* London: Academic Press, 1975.

23   Fagerlind I. *Formal Education and Adult Earnings: a longitudinal study on the economic benefits of education. Stockholm Studies in Educational Psychology 21.* Stockholm, Sweden: Wiksell International, 1975.

24   Goldthorpe JH. *Social mobility and class structure in modern Britain.* Oxford: Clarendon Press, 1980.

25   Halsey AH, Heath AF, Ridge JM. *Origins and destinations: family, class and education in modern Britain.* Oxford: Clarendon Press, 1980.

26   Britten N. Models of intergenerational class mobility: findings from the National Survey of Health and Development. *Br J Sociol* 1981;**32**: 224–38.

27   Atkinson AB, Maynard AK, Trinder GG. *Parents and children: incomes in two generations.* London: Heinemann Educational Books, 1983.

28   Kuh D, Wadsworth M. Childhood influences on adult male earnings in a longitudinal study. *Br J Sociol* 1991;**42**:537–55.

29   Connolly S, Micklewright J, Nickell S. *The occupational success of young men who left school at sixteen.* EUI Working Paper ECO No. 92.61. Florence: European University Institute, 1992.

30   Johnson P, Reed H. Two Nations? *The Inheritance of Poverty and Affluence.* Institute for Fiscal Studies Commentary No 53. London: IFS, 1996.

31   Kuh D, Head J, Hardy R, Wadsworth M. The influence of education and family background on women's earnings in midlife: evidence from a British national birth cohort study. *Br J Sociol Education* **(in press):**

32   Kuh DJL. *Assessing the influence of early life on adult health.* PhD thesis. London University, 1993.

33   Floud JE, Halsey AH, Martin FM. *Social class and educational opportunity.* London: Heinemann, 1950.

34   Douglas JWB. *The home and the school.* London: MacGibbon & Kee, 1964.

35   Bowles S. Understanding unequal economic opportunity. In: Atkinson AB, ed. *Wealth, income and inequality.* 1980: Oxford University Press, 1996;173–85.

36   Kohn ML. *Class and conformity: a study in values.* Chicago: University of Chicago Press, 1977.

37   Davey Smith G, Hart C, Blane D, Gillis C, Hawthorne V. Lifetime socioeconomic position and mortality: prospective observational study. *Br Med J* 1997;**314**:547–52.

38   Gliksman MD, Kawachi I, Hunter D, Colditz GA, Manson JE, Stampfer MJ, Speizer FE, Willett WC, Hennekens CH. Childhood socioeconomic status and risk of cardiovascular disease in middle aged US women: a prospective study. *J Epidemiol Community Health* 1995;**49**:10–5.

39   Burr ML, Sweetnam PM. Family size and paternal unemployment in relation to myocardial infarction. *J Epidemiol Community Health* 1980; **34**:93–5.

40   Kaplan GA, Salonen JT. Socioeconomic conditions in childhood and ischaemic heart disease during middle age. *Br Med J* 1990;**301**:1121–3.

41   Notkola V, Punsar S, Karvonen MJ, Haapokoski J. Socio-economic conditions in childhood and mortality and morbidity caused by coronary heart disease in adulthood in rural Finland. *Soc Sci Med* 1985;**21**:517–23.

42   Vågerö D, Leon D. Effect of social class in childhood and adulthood on adult mortality. *Lancet* 1994;**343**:1224–5.

43   Gillum RF, Paffenbarger RS. Chronic disease in former college students. XVII Socio-cultural mobility as a precursor of coronary heart disease and hypertension. *Am J Epidemiol* 1978;**108**:289–98.

44   Wannamethee SG, Whincup PH, Shaper G, Walker M. Influence of fathers' social class on cardiovascular disease in middle-aged men. *Lancet* 1996;**348**1259–63.

45 Lynch JW, Kaplan GA, Cohen RD, Kauhanen J, Wilson TW, Smith NL, Salonen JT. Childhood and adult socioeconomic status a predictors of mortality in Finland. *Lancet* 1994;**343**:524–7.

46 Hasle H. Association between living conditions in childhood and myocardial infarction. *Br Med J* 1990;**300**:512–3.

47 Kuh DJL, Wadsworth MEJ. Physical health status at 36 years in a British national birth cohort. *Soc Sci Med* 1993;**37**:905–16.

48 Kuh DJL, Wadsworth MEJ, Yusuf EJ. Burden of disability in a post war birth cohort. *J Epidemiol Community Health* 1994;**48**:262–9.

49 Power C, Matthews S, Manor O. Inequalities in self rated health in the 1958 birth cohort: lifetime social circumstances or social mobility? *Br Med J* 1996;**313**:449–53.

50 Mare RD. Socio-economic careers and differential mortality among older men in the United States. In: Vallin J, D'Souza S, Palloni A, eds. *Measurement and analysis of mortality*. Oxford: Clarendon Press, 1990; 362–387.

51 Dahl E, Kjaersgaard P. Social mobility and inequality in mortality. *Eur J Public Health* 1993;**31**:24–32.

52 Forsdahl A. Are poor living conditions in childhood and adolescence an important risk factor for arteriosclerotic heart disease? *Br J Prev Soc Med* 1977;**31**:91–5.

53 Caspi A. Prolegomena to a model of continuity and change in behavioural development. In: Bock GR, Whelan J, eds. *The childhood environment and adult disease*. Chichester (Ciba Foundation Symposium 156): Wiley, 1991;209–23.

54 Wadsworth MEJ, Cripps HA, Midwinter RA, Colley JRT. Blood pressure at age 36 years and social and familial factors, cigarette smoking and body mass in a national birth cohort. *Br Med J* 1985; **291**:1534–8.

55 Dressler WW. Education, lifestyle and arterial blood pressure. *J Psychosom Res* 1990;**34**:515–23.

56 Wadsworth MEJ. Family and education as determinants of health. In: Blane D, Brunner E, Wilkinson RJ, eds. *Social organisation and health*. London: Routledge, 1996;152–70.

57 Wadsworth MEJ. Health inequalities in the life course perspective. *Soc Sci Med* 1997;**44**:859–70.

58 Kuh D, Wadsworth MEJ. Parental height, childhood environment and subsequent adult height in a national birth cohort. *Int J Epidemiol* 1989;**18**:663–8.

59 Cooper C, Cawley M, Bhalla A, Egger P, Ring F, Morton L, Barker D. Childhood growth, physical activity and peak bone mass in women. *J Bone Miner Res* 1995;**10**:940–7.

60 Drillien CM. The social and economic factors affecting the incidence of premature birth. *J Obstet Gynaecol Br Emp* 1957;**64**:161–84.

61 Baird D. The epidemiology of low birth weight: changes in incidence in Aberdeen 1948–72. *J Biosoc Sci* 1974;**6**:323–41.

62 Lumey LH, Van Poppel FWA. The Dutch famine of 1944–5: mortality and morbidity in past and present generations. *Social History of Medicine* 1994;229–46.

63 Hart N. Famine, maternal nutrition and infant mortality: a re-examination of the Dutch Hunger Winter. *Popul Stud* 1993;**47**:27–46.

64 Emanuel I. Intergenerational studies of human birth weight from the 1958 birth cohort. I. Evidence for a multigenerational effect. *Br J Obstet Gynaecol* 1992;**99**:67–74.

65 Russell M, Carr-Hill R, Illsley R. The sociological study: differences relevant to the childhood environment. In: Illsley R, Mitchell RG, eds. *Low birth weight: a medical, psychological and social study*. Chichester: John Wiley & Sons, 1984;51–90.

66 Bartley M, Power C, Blane D, Davey Smith G. Birthweight and later socio-economic disadvantage: evidence from the 1958 British cohort study. *Br Med J* 1994;**309**:1475–9.

67* Illsley R, Mitchell RG, eds. *Low birth weight: a medical, psychological and social study*. Chichester: John Wiley & Sons, 1984.

68 Hertzman C, Wiens M. Child development and long-term outcomes: a population health perspective and summary of successful interventions. *Soc Sci Med* 1996;**43**:1083–95.

69 Waaler HTH. Height, weight and mortality. The Norwegian experience. *Acta Med Scand* 1984; **(Suppl 679)**:1–56.

70 Marmot MG, Rose GA, Shipley MJ, Hamilton PJS. Employment grade and coronary heart disease in British civil servants. *J Epidemiol Community Health* 1978;**32**:244–9.

71 Nystrom Peck AM. Childhood environment, intergenerational mobility, and adult health - evidence from Swedish data. *J Epidemiol Community Health* 1992;**46**:71–4.

72 Yarnell JWG, Limb ES, Layzell JM, Baker IA. Height: a risk marker for ischaemic heart disease: prospective results from the Caerphilly and Speedwell heart disease studies. *Eur Heart J* 1992;**13**:1602–5.

73 Rich EJW, Manson JE, Stampfer MJ, et al. Height and the risk of cardiovascular disease in women. *Am J Epidemiol* 1995;**142**:909–17.

74 Floud R, Wachter K, Gregory A. *Height, health and history. Nutritional status in the United Kingdom 1750–1980*. Cambridge: Cambridge University Press, 1990.

75 Fogel RW. Physical growth as a measure of the economic well-being of populations: the eighteenth and nineteenth centuries. In: Falkner F,

Tanner JM, eds. *Human growth: a comprehensive treatise, Volume 3. Methodology: ecological, genetic and nutritional effects on growth.* New York: Plenum Press, 1986;263–305.

76   Illsley R. Social class selection and class differences in relation to stillbirths and infant deaths. *Br Med J* 1955;**2**:1520–4.

77   Illsley R, Kincaid JC. Social correlations of perinatal mortality. In: Butler NR, Bonham DG, eds. *Perinatal mortality.* Edinburgh: Churchill Livingstone, 1963;270–86.

78   Wadsworth MEJ. Serious illness in childhood and its association with later life achievements. In: Wilkinson RG, ed. *Class and health.* London: Tavistock Publications, 1986;50–74.

79   Power C, Fogelman K, Fox AJ. Health and social mobility during the early years of life. *Q J Soc Affairs* 1986;**2**:397–413.

80   Leon D, Davey Smith G, Shipley M, Strachan D. Height and mortality in London: early life influences, socio-economic confounding or shrinkage? *J Epidemiol Community Health* 1995;**49**:5–9.

81   Gortmaker SL, Must A, Perrin JM, Arthur MS, Dietz WH. Social and economic consequences of overweight in adolescence and young adulthood. *N Engl J Med* 1993;**329**:1008–12.

82   Sonne-Holm S, Sorenson TIA. Prospective study of attainment of social class of severely obese subjects in relation to parental social class, intelligence, and education. *Br Med J* 1986;**292**:586–9.

83   Sargent ID, Blanchflower DG. Obesity and stature in adolescence and earnings in young adulthood. *Arch Pediatr Adolesc Med* 1994;**148**:681–7.

84   Braddon FEM, Rodgers B, Wadsworth MEJ, Davies JMC. Onset of obesity in a 36 year birth cohort study. *Br Med J* 1986;**293**:299–303.

85   Power C, Moynihan C. Social class and changes in weight for height between childhood and early adulthood. *Int J of Obes* 1988;**12**: 445–53.

86   Power C, Peckham C. Childhood morbidity and adulthood ill health. *J Epidemiol Community Health* 1990;**44**:69–74.

87   Kuh D, Lawrence C, Tripp J, Creber G. Work and work alternatives for disabled young people. *Disability, Handicap and Society* 1988;**3**:3–26.

88   Pless IB, Cripps HA, Davies JMC, Wadsworth MEJ. Chronic physical illness in childhood and psychological and social circumstances in adolescence and early adult life. *Dev Med Child Neurol* 1989;**31**:746–55.

89* Wilkinson RG. Unhealthy Societies. *The affliction of inequality.* London: Routledge, 1996.

90   Pincus T, Callahan LF. Associations of low formal education level and poor health status: behavioral, in addition to demographic and medical, explanations? *J Clin Epidemiol* 1994;**47**:355–61.

91* Rutter M. Pathways from childhood to adult life. *J Child Psychol Psychiatry* 1989;**1**:23–51.

92 Kiecolt-Glaser JK, Glaser R. Psychoneuroimmunology and health consequences:data and shared mechanisms. *Psychosom Med* 1995;**57**: 269–74.

93 Sapolsky RM. *Stress, the ageing brain and the mechanism of neuron death.* Cambridge,Massachusetts: MIT Press, 1992.

94 Brunner E. The social and biological basis in cardiovascular disease in the workers. In: Blane D, Brunner E, Wilkinson R, eds. *Health and Social Organization: towards a health policy in the 21st Century.* London: Routledge, 1996;272–99.

95 Winkleby MA, Jatulis DE, Frank E, Fortmann SP. Socioeconomic status and health: how education, income, and occupation contribute to risk factors for cardiovascular disease. *Am J Public Health* 1992;**82**: 816–20.

96 Bronfenbrenner V. Is early intervention effective? Facts and principles of early intervention: a summary. In: Clarke AM, Clarke ADB, eds. *Early experience: myth and evidence.* New York: The Free Press, 1976.

97 Brown B. *Found: Long-term gains from early intervention.* American Association for the Advancement of Science. Selected Symposia Series. Boulder Colorado: Westview Press, 1978.

98 Berrueta-Clement JR, Schweinhart LJ, Barnett WS, Epstein AS, Weikart DP. *Changed lives: the effects of the Perry Preschool Program through age 19.* Ypsilanti, Michigan: The High/Scope Press, 1984.

99 Washington V, Oyemade OJ. *Project Head Start. Past, present, and future trends in the context of family needs.* New York and London: Garland Publishing Inc, 1987.

100 Schweinhart LJ, Barnes HV, Weikart DP. *Significant benefits. The High/ Scope Perry Preschool Study through age 27.* Monographs of the High/ Scope Educational Research Foundation 10., 1993.

101 Clapp G. *Child Study Research: Current perspectives and applications.* Lexington, Mass: Lexington Books, Heath and Company, 1988.

102 Clarke-Stewart KA, Fein GG. Early childhood programs. In: Mussen PH, ed. *Handbook of child psychology.* Vol. II. 4th ed. New York: John Wiley & Sons, 1983;917–99.

103 Scarr S, Weinberg RA. The early childhood enterprise. Care and education of the young. *Am Psychol* 1986;**41**:1140–5.

104 Clarke AM, Clarke ADB. Thirty years of child psychology: a selective review. *J Child Psychol Psychiatry* 1986;**27**:719–59.

105 Lundberg O. The impact of childhood living conditions on illness and mortality in adulthood. *Soc Sci Med* 1993;**36**:1047–52.

106 Nystrom Peck M, Lundberg O. Short stature as an effect of economic and social conditions in childhood. *Soc Sci Med* 1995;**41**:733–8.

107 Wadsworth MEJ, Maclean M. Parents' divorce and children's life chances. *Children and Youth Services Review* 1986;**8**:145–59.

108 Wallerstein JS, Corbin SB. Daughters of divorce: report from a ten-year follow-up. *Am J Orthopsychiatry* 1989;**59**:593–604.

109 Kuh D, Maclean M. Women's childhood experience of parental separation and their subsequent health and socio-economic status in adulthood. *J Biosoc Sci* 1990;**22**:121–35.

110 Wadsworth MEJ, Maclean M, Kuh D, Rodgers B. Children of divorced parents: a summary and review of findings from a national long-term follow-up study. *Fam Pract* 1990;**7**:104–9.

111 Amato PR, Keith B. Parental divorce and adult well–being: a meta-analysis. *J Mar Fam* 1991;**53**:43–58.

112 Pope H, Mueller CW. The intergenerational transmission of marital instability: comparisons by race and sex. *J Soc Issues* 1976; **32**:49–66.

113 Rodgers B, Power C, Hope S. Parental divorce and adult psychological distress. Evidence from a national birth cohort. *J Child Psychol Psychiatry* **(in press):**

114* Hess LE. Changing family patterns in Western Europe: opportunity and risk factors for adolescent development. In: Rutter M, Smith DJ, eds. *Psychosocial disorders in young people: time trends and their causes.* Chichester: John Wiley & Sons Ltd, 1995;104–93.

115 McLanahan SS, Bumpass L. Intergenerational consequences of family disruption. *Am J Sociol* 1988;**94**:130–52.

116 Wallerstein JS. The long term effects of divorce on children. *J Am Acad Child Adolesc Psychiatry* 1991;**30**:344–60.

117 Kiernan KE. The impact of family disruption in childhood on transitions made in young adult life. *Popul Stud* 1992;**46**:213–34.

118 Schwartz JE, Friedman HS, Tucker JS, Tomlinson-Keasey C, Wingard DL, Criqui MH. Sociodemographic and psychosocial factors in childhood as predictors of adult mortality. *Am J Public Health* 1995;**85**: 1237–45.

119 Rodgers B. Reported parental behaviour and adult affective symptoms 2: mediating factors. *Psychol Med* 1996;**26**:63–77.

120 Franz CE, McClelland DC, Weinberger J. Childhood antecedents of conventional social accomplishment in midlife adults: a 36-year prospective study. *J Pers Soc Psychol* 1991;**60**:586–95.

121 Berkman LF, Syme L. Social networks, host resistance, and mortality: a nine-year follow-up study of Alameda county residents. *Am J Epidemiol* 1979;**109**:186–204.

122 Ben-Shlomo Y, Davey Smith G, Shipley M, Marmot MG. Magnitude and causes of mortality differences between married and unmarried men. *J Epidemiol Community Health* 1993;**47**:200–5.

123 Wyke S, Ford G. Competing explanations for associations between marital status and health. *Soc Sci Med* 1992;**34**:523–32.

124 MacIntyre S. The patterning of health by social position in contemporary Britain: directions for sociological research. *Soc Sci Med* 1986;**23**: 393–415.

125 Mechanic D, Hansell S. Divorce, family conflict, and adolescents' wellbeing. *J Health Soc Behav* 1989;**30**:105–16.

126 Sweeting H, West P. Family life and health in adolescence: a role for culture in the health inequalities debate? *Soc Sci Med* 1995;**40**:163–75.

127 Sweeting H, West P. The patterning of life events in mid- to late adolescence: markers for the future? *J Adolesc* 1994;**17**:283–304.

128 Power C, Manor O. Asthma, enuresis and chronic illness: long term impact on height. *Arch Dis Child* 1995;**73**:298–304.

129 Montgomery SM, Bartley MJ, Cook DG, Wadsworth MEJ. Health and social precursors of unemployment in young men in Great Britain. *J Epidemiol Community Health* 1996;**50**:415–22.

130 McCormick J, Skrabanek P. Coronary heart disease is not preventable by population interventions. *Lancet* 1988;**1**:839–41.

131 Oliver MF. Doubts about preventing coronary heart disease. *Br Med J* 1992;**304**:393–4.

132 Falkner F. *Prevention in childhood of health problems in adult life.* Geneva: WHO, 1980.

133 Nutbeam D, Aar L, Catford J. Understanding children's health behaviour: the implications for health promotion for young people. *Soc Sci Med* 1989;**29**:317–25.

134 Jessor R, Jessor S. *Problem behaviour and psychosocial development. A longitudinal study of youth.* New York: Academic Press, 1977.

135 Jessor R. Adolescent development and behavioral health. In: Matarazzo J, ed. *Behavioral health.* New York: Wiley, 1984:69–90.

136 Braddon FEM, Wadsworth MEJ, Davies JMC, Cripps HA. Social and regional differences in food and alcohol consumption and their measurement in a national birth cohort. *J Epidemiol Community Health* 1988;**42**: 341–9.

137 Rozin P. The acquisition of food habits and preferences. In: Matarazzo J, ed. *Behavioral health.* New York: Wiley, 1984:590–607.

138 Sallis JF, Nader PR. Family determinants of health behaviors. In: Gochman DS, ed. *Health bhavior.* New York: Plenum, 1988:107–24.

139 Boyd Orr J. *Food, health and income.* London: Macmillan, 1937.

140 Durward L. *Poverty in pregnancy: the cost of an adequate diet for expectant mothers.* London: Maternity Alliance, 1988.

141 *National Children's Home Poverty and Nutrition Survey.* London: National Children's Homes, 1992.

142 Soonan A, MacIntyre S, Anderson A. Scotland's health—a more difficult challenge for some? The price and availability of healthy foods in socially

contrasting localities in the West of Scotland. *Health Bull* 1993;**51**: 276–84.

143 Plant MA, Peck DF, Samuel E. *Alcohol, drugs and school-leavers.* London: Tavistock Publications, 1985.

144 Welte JW, Barnes GM. Youthful smoking patterns and relationships to alcohol and other drug use. *J Adolesc* 1987;**10**:327–40.

145 Battjes RJ. Smoking is an issue in alcohol and drug abuse treatment. *Addict Behav* 1988;**13**:225–30.

146 Burke GL, Hunter SM, Croft JB, Cresanta JL, Berenson GS. The interaction of alcohol and tobacco use in adolescents and young adults: Bogalusa Heart Study. *Addict Behav* 1988;**13**:387–93.

147 Townsend J, Wilkes H, Haines A, Jarvis M. Adolescent smokers seen in general practice: health, lifestyle, physical measurements, and response to antismoking advice. *Br Med J* 1991;**303**:947–50.

148 Lader D, Matheson J. *Smoking among secondary school children in 1990.* London: OPCS HMSO, 1991.

149 Health Education Authority. *Tomorrow's young adults.* London: Health Education Authority, 1992.

150 Charlton A, Blair V. Predicting the onset of smoking in boys and girls. *Soc Sci Med* 1989;**29**:813–8.

151 Goddard D. *Why children start smoking.* London: HMSO, 1990.

152 Swan AV, Murray M, Jarrett L. *Smoking behaviour from pre-adolescence to young adulthood.* Aldershot: Avebury, 1991.

153 Maddox GL. *The domesticated drug: drinking among collegians.* New Haven: College and University Press, 1970.

154 Murray M, Kiryluk S, Swan AV. Relation between parents' and children's smoking behaviour and attitudes. *J Epidemiol Community Health* 1985;**39**:169–74.

155 Gordon NP, McAlister AL. Adolescent drinking: issues and research. In: Coates T, Peterson AC, Perry C, eds. *Promoting adolescent health: A dialog on research and practice.* London: Academic Press Inc, 1982: 201–24.

156 Greendorfer SL, Lewko JH. Role of family members in sport socialization of children. *Res Q* 1978;**49**:146–52.

157 Snyder EE, Spreitzer EA. Correlation of sport participation among adolescent girls. *Res Q* 1976;**47**:804–9.

158 Rossow I, Rise J. Concordance of parental and adolescent health behaviors. *Soc Sci Med* 1994;**38**:1299–305.

159 Royal College of Physicians. *Smoking and the young.* London: Royal College of Physicians, 1992.

160 Marsh A, McKay S. Poor smokers. London: Policy Studies Institute, 1994 161 Pratt L. Child rearing methods and children's health behavior. *J Health Soc Behav* 1973;**14**:61–9.

162 Harburg E, Davis DR, Caplan R. Parent and offspring alcohol use: imitative and aversive transmission. *J Stud Alcohol* 1982; **43**:497–516.

163 McKechnie RJ, Cameron D, Cameron IA, Drewery J. Teenage drinking in South-West Scotland. *Br J of Addict* 1977;**72**:287–95.

164 Tennant C, Bernardi E. Childhood loss in alcoholics and narcotic addicts. *Br J of Addict* 1988;**83**:695–703.

165 Estaugh V, Power C. Family disruption in early life and drinking in young adulthood. *Alcohol and Alcoholism* 1991;**26**:639–44.

166 Lau RR, Quadrel MJ, Hartman KA. Development and change of young adults' preventive health beliefs and behavior: influence from parents and peers. *J Health Soc Behav* 1990;**31**:240–59.

167 Green G, MacIntyre S, West P, Ecob R. Like parent like child? Associations between drinking and smoking behaviour of parents and their children. *J Addict* 1991;**86**:745–58.

168 Borland BL, Rudolph JP. Relative effects of low socio-economic status, parental smoking and poor scholastic performance on smoking among high school students. *Soc Sci Med* 1975;**9**:27–30.

169 Margulies RZ, Kessler RC, Kandel DB. A longitudinal study of onset of drinking among high-school students. *J Stud Alcohol* 1977;**38**:897–912.

170 Jessor R, Jessor SL. Adolescent development and the onset of drinking: a longitudinal study. *J Stud Alcohol* 1975;**36**:27–51.

171 Wilks J, Callan VJ, Austin DA. Parent, peer and personal determinants of adolescent drinking. *Br J of Addict* 1989;**84**:619–30.

172 Biddle S, Armstrong . Children's physical activity: an exploratory study of psychological correlates. *Soc Sci Med* 1992;**34**:325–31.

173 Cherry N, Kiernan K. Personality scores and smoking behaviour. *Br J Prev Soc Med* 1976;**30**:123–31.

174 Catford JC, Nutbeam D, Woolaway M. Effectiveness and cost benefits of smoking education. *Community Med* 1984;**6**:264–72.

175 Wald N, Kiryluk S, Barby S, Doll R, Pike M, Peto R. *U.K. Smoking statistics.* Oxford: Oxford University Press, 1988.

176 Breslau N, Peterson EL. Smoking cessation in young adults: age at initiation of cigarette smoking and other suspected influences. *Am J Public Health* 1996;**86**:214–20.

177 Ghodsian M, Power C. Alcohol consumption between the ages of 16 and 23 in Britain: a longitudinal study. *Br J of Addict* 1987;**82**:175–80.

178 Patrick C. Relation of childhood and adult leisure activities. *J Soc Psychol* 1945;**21**:65–79.

179 Sofranko AJ, Nolan MF. Early life experiences and adult sports participation. *Res Q* 1976;**47**:804–9.

180 Yoesting DK, Burkhead DL. Significance of childhood recreation experience on adult leisure behaviour: an exploratory analysis. *J Leisure Res* 1973;**5**:25–36.

181 Clark CHH. *National Adult Physical Fitness Survey. President's Council on Physical Fitness and Sports Newsletter.* Washington D.C.: Special Edition, 1973.

182 Dishman RK, Sallis JF, Orenstein DR. The determinants of physical activity and exercise. *Public Health Rep* 1985;**100**:2:158–71.

183 Sports Council and Health Education Authority. *Allied Dunbar National Fitness Survey. A report on activity patterns and fitness levels.* London: Sports Council, 1992.

184 Kuh DJL, Cooper C. Physical activity at 36 years: patterns and childhood predictors in a longitudinal study. *J Epidemiol Community Health* 1992;**46**:114–9.

185 Blaxter M. *Health and Lifestyles.* London: Routledge, 1990.

186 Fenner N. Leisure, exercise and work. In: Cox BD, Blaxter M, Buckle ALJ, Fenner NP, Golding JF, Gore M, Huppert FA, Nickson J, Roth M, Stark J, Wadsworth MEJ, Whichelow M, eds. *The Health and Lifestyle Survey.* London: Health Promotion Trust, 1987;85–95.

187 Power C, Estaugh V. The role of family formation and dissolution in shaping drinking behaviour in early adulthood. *Br J Addict* 1990;**85**: 521–30.

188 Office of Population Censuses and Surveys. *General Household Survey 1986. Series GHS. No.16.* London: HMSO, 1989.

189 Blane D, Hart CL, Davey Smith G, Gillis CR, Hole DJ, Hawthorne VM. The association of cardiovascular disease risk factors with socioeconomic position during childhood and during adulthood. *Br Med J* 1996;**313**: 1434–8.

190 Graham H. Women and smoking in the United Kingdom: the implications for health promotion. *Health Promotion* 1988;**3**:371–82.

191 Rose G, Marmot MG. Social class and coronary disease. *Br Heart J* 1981;**45**:13–9.

192 Davey Smith G, Shipley MJ, Rose G. The magnitude and causes of socioeconomic differentials in mortality: further evidence from the Whitehall Study. *J Epidemiol Community Health* 1990;**44**:265–70.

193 Ockene JK, Kuller LH, Svendsen KH, Meilahn E. The relationship of smoking cessation to coronary heart disease and lung cancer in the multiple risk factor intervention trial (MRFIT). *Am J Public Health* 1990;**80**:954–8.

194 Rose G, Colwell L. Randomised controlled trial of anti-smoking advice: final (20 year) results. *J Epidemiol Community Health* 1992;**46**:75–7.

195 Holme I, Hjermann I, Helgeland A, Leren P. The Oslo Study: diet and anti-smoking advice. Additional results from a 5 year primary preventive trial in middle-aged men. *J Prevent Med* 1985;**14**:279–92.

196 Blane D. An assessment of the Black Report's explanations of health inequalities. *Sociol Health Illness* 1985;**7**:423–45.

197 Pearlin LI. The sociological study of stress. *J Health Soc Behav* 1989;**30**:241–56.

198 Blane D, Bartley M, Davey Smith G. Disease aetiology and materialist explanations of socioeconomic mortality differentials. *Eur J Public Health* **(in press):**

199 Bartley M, Owen C. Relation between socioeconomic status, employment, and health during economic change, 1973–93. *Br Med J* 1996;**313**: 445–59.

200 Cook DG, Cummins RO, Bartley MJ, Shaper AG. Health of unemployed middle aged men in Great Britain. *Lancet* 1982;**i**:1290–4.

201 Moylan S, Millar J, Davies R. *For richer, for poorer—DHSS Cohort study of unemployed men.* London: HMSO, 1984.

202 Moser KA, Fox AJ, Jones DR. Unemployment and mortality in the OPCS Longitudinal Study. *Lancet* 1984;**ii**:1324–8.

203 Moser KA, Goldblatt PO, Fox AJ, Jones DR. Unemployment and mortality: comparison of the 1971 and 1981 Longitudinal Study samples. *Br Med J* 1987;**294**:86–90.

204 Morris JK, Cook DG, Shaper AG. Loss of employment and mortality. *Br Med J* 1994;**308**:1135–9.

205 Evandrou M, Falkingham J. Social security and the life course: developing sensitive policy alternative. In: Arber S, Evandrou M, eds. *Ageing, independence and the life course.* London: Jessica Kingsley Publishers, 1993;201–23.

206 Hancock R, Weir P. *More ways than means: a guide to pensioners' incomes in Great Britain during the 1980s.* London: Age Concern Institute of Gerontology, Kings College, London, 1994.

207 Baltes PB, Baltes NM. *Succesful aging: perspectives from the behavioural sciences.* Oxford: Oxford University Press, 1990.

208 Lachman M, James JB. *Multiple paths of midlife development.* Chicago: University of Chigaco Press, 1997.

209* Smith DJ. Living conditions in the twentieth century. In: *Psychosocial disorders in young people: time trends and their causes.* Chichester: John Wiley & Sons Ltd, 1995.

210 Halsey AH. *British social trends since 1900. A guide to the changing social structure of Britain.* Basingstoke: The Macmillan Press Ltd, 1988.

211 Elder GHJr, Caspi A. Economic stress in lives: developmental perspectives. *J Soc Issues* 1988;**44**:25–45.

212 Elder GH Jr. Military times and turning points in men's lives. *Dev Psychol* 1986;**22**:233–45.

213 Fuchs VR, Reklis DM. America's children: economic perspectives and policy options. *Science* 1992;**255**:41–6.

214 Wadsworth MEJ, Kuh DJL. Are gains in child health being undermined? *Dev Medi Child Neurol* 1993;**35**:742–5.

215 Cornia GA. *Child poverty and deprivation in industrialised countries: recent trends and policy options.* Florence: UNICEF International Child Development Centre: Innocenti Occasional Papers, No.2., 1990.

216 Mann SL, Wadsworth MEJ, Colley JRT. Accumulation of factors influencing respiratory illness in members of a national birth cohort and their offspring. *J Epidemiol Community Health* 1992;**46**:286–92.

217 Blane D, Davey Smith G, Bartley M. Social selection: what does it contribute to social class differences in health? *Sociol Health Illness* 1993;**15**:1–15.

218 Blane D. Social determinants of health: socioeconomic status, social class and ethnicity. *Am J Public Health* 1995;**85**:903–4.

D Explaining disease patterns

Evidence based practice patterns

9 Time trends

David P Strachan and Ivan J Perry

Analyses of time trends offer intriguing but inconclusive evidence relating to life course influences on adult disease. There appears to be a combination of linear and non-linear components which are not readily combined and quantified in terms of period and cohort effects. Furthermore, the major identifiable cohort effect, the effect of cigarette smoking on respiratory mortality, cannot be attributed to programming effects in early life. Age–period–cohort analyses thus provide a limited basis for inference regarding the relative importance of factors acting in childhood or adult life. Attempts to explain trends in mortality and morbidity from ischaemic heart disease, stroke and chronic obstructive pulmonary diseases have focused on recent documented changes in established risk factors related to adult life style. These explain some but not all of the observed trends, suggesting that a life course approach embracing factors acting in early as well as later life may be appropriate. Predictions of future mortality rates and disease burden need to acknowledge our uncertainties about the nature of many of the underlying cohort influences, the unpredictability of future changes in environment and life style, and the potential for changes in case-fatality resulting from advances in medical care.

9.1 Introduction

Mortality attributed to stroke among white males in the United States declined by more than 50% between 1960 and 1987.[1] Temporal variations such as this remind us that the occurrence of many diseases is not fixed and, with fuller understanding of underlying causes, may be amenable to public health intervention. Even where the disease burden is not preventable, exploration of time trends may allow a cautious prediction of future patterns and thus assist in the planning of health and social services. In this chapter, we discuss some of the methodological problems inherent in analysis of time trends and their relevance to the life course approach.

Interpretation of temporal variation in disease incidence, prevalence, mortality or health service utilisation should consider possible changes in:

- The information system which generated the data, including its coverage, completeness and certification or coding rules
- Clinical diagnosis, or the recognition and labelling of symptoms by patients.
- The natural history of disease, including effects of medical care on prognosis
- The incidence of disease

Because it is often difficult to disentangle true changes from possible artifacts, time trends rarely provide definitive evidence for or against a causal hypothesis. However, suggestive evidence relevant to the life course approach may emerge if there is evidence of either a *period* or *cohort* influence on incidence, prevalence, or mortality rates.

A period effect is evident when a similar (approximately parallel) shift in rates for each age group occurs during a particular calendar period. Period effects are commonly due to artifacts of the information system, but may represent real variations in incidence or natural history. In the context of a life course approach, they are of importance in that they must reflect the impact of factors operating in adult life, affecting a number of age groups simultaneously. For example, an epidemic of fatal asthma in Britain during the 1960s (Fig. 9.1) has been widely attributed to a change in case-fatality related to the introduction of high dose isoprenaline inhalers; it subsided when the Committee on Safety of Medicines issued a warning about their potential cardiotoxicity in acute life-threatening asthma.[2]

A cohort (or generation) effect is evident when age-specific rates rise and fall in parallel when plotted, not against year of occurrence (period), but against year of birth (cohort). Such variation may reflect the delayed consequences of programming influences early in life, although this is not necessarily the case. Cohort-related variations in lung cancer, for example, correspond closely to estimations of lifetime cigarette consumption (adjusted for changing tar composition) in different cohorts (Fig. 9.2). This aspect of adult life style displays such a clear cohort-related variation because smoking was widely adopted by men in active service during World War I, but did not become popular among women until World War II.

It is often difficult to disentangle period and cohort influences on disease occurrence, because *linear* trends (or 'drift') cannot reliably be assigned either to a cohort or a period effect.[4] It is only the *non-linear* variations which can be interpreted with confidence as a cohort or a period phenomenon. Multiple regression models summarising the multiplicative effects of age, period and cohort on mortality rates can be misleading unless the above limitations are acknowledged.[3,4]

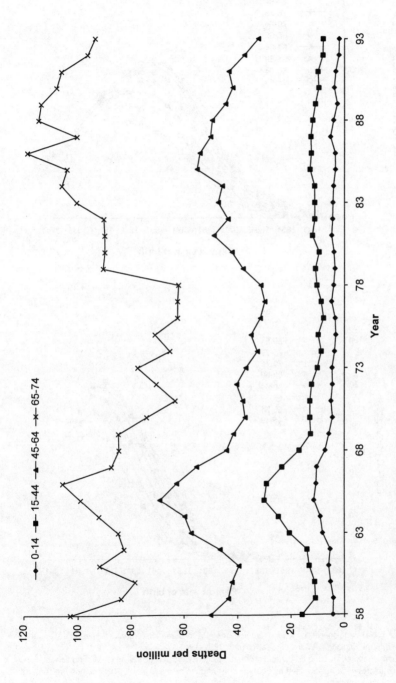

Figure 9.1 Age-specific asthma mortality rates for England & Wales, 1958-1993
Footnote: Prepared by Lung & Asthma Information Agency, St George's Hospital Medical School, London, from data published by the Office of Population Censuses and Surveys, London.

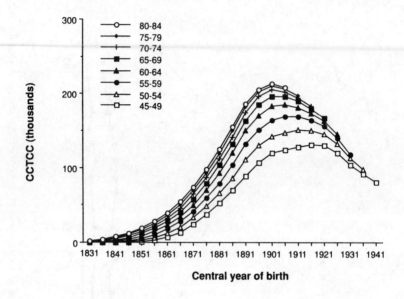

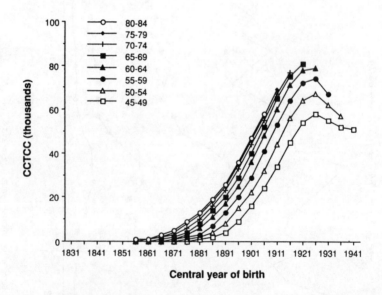

Figure 9.2(a) Age-specific cumulative lifetime cigarette consumption for males (upper figure) and females (lower figure), England & Wales, by year of birth 1831–1941
Footnote: Prepared by Lung & Asthma Information Agency, St George's Hospital Medical School, London, from estimates of cumulative lifetime cigarette consumption by Lee et al.[56] CCTCC: cumulative constant tar cigarette consumption

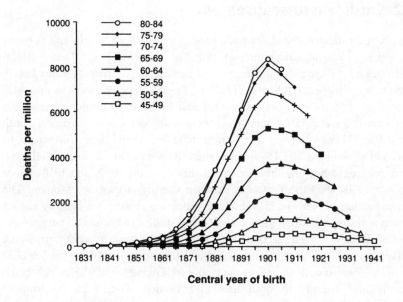

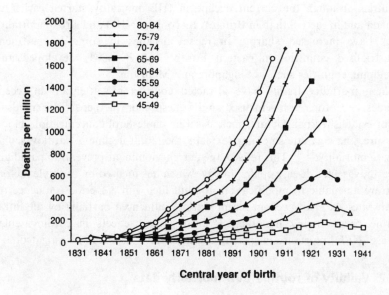

Figure 9.2(b) Age-specific lung cancer mortality rates for males (upper figure) and females (lower figure), England and Wales, by year of birth 1831–1941
Footnote: Prepared by Lung & Asthma Information Agency, St George's Hospital Medical School, London from mortality data published by the Office of Population Censuses and Surveys, London.

9.2 Cardiovascular diseases

This century has witnessed dramatic secular trends, both within and between countries, in age adjusted mortality rates for ischaemic heart disease (IHD) and stroke.[5-7] Figure 9.3 shows the age standardised mortality rates for all circulatory diseases, IHD, and stroke in England and Wales, for men and women aged 35–64 years, between 1901 and 1992.[7] In men and women there was a marked rise in IHD mortality from the early decades of the century until the 1940s. This was followed in men by a short decline and then a further rise to a second peak in the late 1970s. In women the post 1940s decline in IHD was more prolonged but rates also increased sharply in the 1960s and 1970s. Since the late 1970s IHD mortality has declined sharply in men and women. The stroke mortality trends in England and Wales this century are broadly similar in men and women, with a more or less steady decline in both sexes between the turn of the century and the late 1930s. This was followed by an upturn which peaked around 1940, coinciding with the change from the 4th to the 5th ICD revision. Since the 1950s stroke mortality in England and Wales has fallen sharply and steadily in both men and women. Trends in the broader 'circulatory disease' cause of death category are consistent with those for IHD and stroke (Fig. 9.3).

Broadly similar patterns have been observed in most western industrialized countries although the current decline in IHD mortality started earlier in Canada and in the US than in Britain.[6] By contrast, IHD and stroke mortality rates have increased sharply in recent decades in some less affluent industrialised countries in eastern Europe and in newly developed and developing countries such as Singapore and Mauritius.[5,8]

These mortality trends have attracted considerable attention in recent decades.[5,6,9,10] Interest has focused on the question of whether secular trends in major established risk factors, such as serum cholesterol concentration, blood pressure, and cigarette smoking, 'explain' the recent decline in cardiovascular disease mortality.[11-13] This reflects the current dominant prevention paradigm in cardiovascular disease epidemiology, which has focused on life style factors that are amenable to modification in adult life, with a 'period' influence on death rates.[14,15] However, in recent work,[16] influenced partially by the intra-uterine programming hypothesis,[17] birth cohort effects in cardiovascular disease (CVD) mortality in specific countries have also been investigated.

9.2.2 Validity of routine CVD mortality data

It is generally accepted that in most countries the trends in CVD mortality observed this century reflect real changes in mortality and that only a small proportion of the overall variation can be attributed to changes in diagnosis, classification, or coding procedures.[5] The validity of these trends is supported

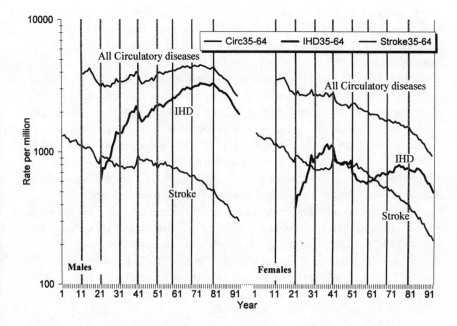

Figure 9.3 Mortality trends 1901–1992, for the circulatory system (all circulatory diseases, IHD, and stroke) in males and females aged 35–64 years, age standardized to the European population. Reproduced with permission from *The Health of Adult Britain 1841–1994* (1997). Copyright of the Crown 1997. With kind permission of the Controller of HMSO and of the Office for National Statistics.

by data from bridge coding exercises across ICD revision periods within countries such as the US,[18] the finding of consistent trends in broad and specific cause of death categories such as circulatory disease and IHD in most countries, the evident impact of the decline in IHD and stroke on all cause mortality in western industrialised countries, and the striking similarity in trends observed in a wide range of different developed countries.[6] Comparisons between countries are probably less secure than those within countries, particularly with regard to stroke mortality.[19] However, IHD mortality data from the World Health Organization MONICA study, which has monitored trends in incidence and mortality from cardiovascular disease in 26 countries during the past decade, are broadly consistent with the routine mortality data.[20]

9.2.3 Changes in incidence or case fatality?

There is considerable evidence that the decline in IHD mortality seen in developed countries in recent decades reflects a variable combination of trends in both incidence and case fatality.[21–24] For instance, in recent US data from the twin cities of Minneapolis and St Paul, there is clear evidence of declining in-hospital mortality, out-of-hospital mortality, and rates of hospitalization for first myocardial infarction in men and women between 1985 and 1990.[24] The contribution of falling in-hospital mortality to the overall decline in IHD mortality in this population has increased in this short period relative to the period between 1960 to 1986.[21] Similarly, the decline in stroke mortality can almost certainly be attributed to favourable trends in both incidence and case fatality,[25,26] although data on recent trends in stroke incidence rates are contradictory. There is evidence from the Framingham Study,[27] Olmsted County Minnesota,[28] Canada,[29] and New Zealand[30] which suggests minimal change or an increase in stroke incidence during the last decade. Declining trends in stroke incidence are documented in the Honolulu Heart Program,[31] in Japan[32] and more recently in the FINMONICA stroke study.[25] In the latter study however the trends in incidence, an average fall of 1.7% per year in men aged 25–74 years between 1983 and 1982 are dwarfed by the trends in mortality, with an average fall of 5.2% per year.

9.2.4 Trends in risk factors and cardiovascular disease mortality

For over four decades investigators have linked national food consumption data with trends in IHD mortality.[33] For instance, positive associations are described between the slope of the decline in consumption of saturated fat and dietary cholesterol in the mid 1960s and the rate of decline in IHD mortality between 1969–75 in 20 countries.[33] Similarly, falling tobacco consumption and increased consumption of grains, legumes, fruit, and vegetable intakes were associated with higher rates of decline in IHD mortality in these analyses. Despite the well rehearsed limitations of ecological data,[34] it is noteworthy that these findings have been largely sustained in observational studies based on individuals.[35]

Vartiainen and colleagues[11] have estimated the extent to which secular trends in IHD risk factors explain the sharp decline in IHD mortality seen in Finland in recent decades. Using data on trends in risk factors from five large population based surveys between 1972 and 1992, they have estimated that 80% of the observed decline in IHD mortality in men and 72% of the decline in IHD mortality in women, could be attributed to changes in serum cholesterol concentration, blood pressure, and smoking. Almost half of the decline was apparently attributable to falling serum cholesterol concentration, a trend which almost certainly reflects substantial dietary change in Finland during this period with falling consumption of saturated fat and a marked increase in vegetable consumption.[36] Broadly similar findings on trends in risk factors and changes in IHD mortality are described in other countries.[13,37] Clearly, estimates of the percentage change in mortality 'explained' in these analyses merit cautious interpretation given the limited number of risk factors studied, methodological concerns related to measurement error in serial risk factor surveys, and the choice of appropriate lag periods between changes in exposures and outcomes at the population level. It is noteworthy that in Finland, as in other industrialized countries, IHD mortality has fallen despite increasing obesity.

Using the same risk factor data, it has been estimated that almost half of the decline in stroke mortality in Finland between 1972 and 1992 could be attributed to a fall in diastolic blood pressure.[12] Although anti-hypertensive drug therapy undoubtedly contributed to this trend it should be emphasized that the entire blood pressure distribution in Finland was shifted downwards during this period, reflecting perhaps dietary change such as decreased salt intake.[36] Although stroke shares common risk factors with IHD, notably blood pressure and cigarette smoking, there are marked differences in mortality trends for these conditions within and between countries.[6] For instance in Japan, which has low and falling IHD mortality rates, stroke mortality has fallen since the early 1960s from the highest rate in the world (approximately 1700/100 000 per annum) to less than 500/100 000 per annum, a level below that found in some countries in eastern Europe such as Hungary and Bulgaria. Although the different trends for stroke and IHD mortality may partially reflect discordant trends for thrombotic, embolic and haemorrhagic stroke, there may be important specific determinants of stroke mortality (and by extension incidence) which have not yet been identified. There has been a sharp fall in dietary salt intake in Japan in recent decades, which may have contributed to the decline in stroke mortality via effects on the population blood pressure distribution.[38] It has also been suggested, on the basis of ecological data and experiments in animals, that salt may exert direct effects on stroke risk, independent of effects on blood pressure.[39–41] Salt is also likely to act as a marker for other nutrients relevant to stroke risk, notably fruit and vegetables.[42,43]

9.2.5 Birth cohort effects

Despite the importance of period of death effects such as adult diet and life style, there is clear evidence of important birth cohort effects in IHD mortality in Britain[16] and other countries.[44] Osmond[16] has reviewed IHD mortality rates in England and Wales between 1952 and 1991 using log-linear models to assess the separate effects of period and birth cohort on variation in the rates. While the peak in IHD mortality rates observed towards the end of the 1970s was largely attributable to period effects, there was evidence of a fall in IHD risk in each successive year of birth during the period of observation. Baker et al.,[45] reviewing similar data, have highlighted the extent to which IHD mortality rates fell in all age groups, from the youngest to the over-75s, and in all regions of the country at the same time, in the 1970s. Although this is consistent with strong period effects, it is not clear that one can discount coexisting birth cohort effects without modelling the data.

Sverre,[44] reviewing Norwegian IHD mortality trends between 1966 and 1986, describes strong birth cohort effects in men (but not in women), with a sharp rise in risk in successive birth cohorts between 1870 and 1900 and a steady decline thereafter during the period of observation to 1930. Osmond[16] has suggested that the favourable birth cohort trends detected in his analysis of British IHD mortality data may be attributed to improvements in maternal health, physique, and nutrition during the course of this century. It should be noted, however, that these factors have not necessarily improved steadily since the turn of the century.[46] Moreover, the programming hypothesis, as currently formulated, does not make clear predictions about the effects of historical changes in maternal nutrition on CVD event rates. Associations are described between a range of markers of fetal growth and different disease end-points in adult life which depend on the timing and severity of the nutritional insult in utero and on interactions with risk factors related to adult life style.[47]

As with IHD, there is evidence in the data for stroke mortality for England and Wales of both period and cohort effects. It is noteworthy however that after a fall in stroke risk in successive cohorts born between 1880 and 1910, there is evidence of increasing risk in cohorts born between 1910 and 1940.[48] However, these cohort effects did not produce a clear and prolonged upturn in mortality as they were offset by stronger period effects from 1951–54 onwards. Explanations for this adverse birth cohort trend are elusive, although the possibility that cigarette smoking was a factor (as with respiratory disease) must be considered.

9.2.6 Projections of future disease burden

The current decline in IHD incidence and mortality in developed countries seems likely to continue given the evidence of favourable birth cohort trends in at least some developed countries,[16,44] broadly favourable trends in risk factors[13] and evidence of an accelerating decline in case fatality.[24] The recent sharp decline in case fatality seen in US data[24] probably reflects the widespread use of thrombolytic therapy combined with greater emphasis on secondary prevention measures such as smoking cessation and lipid lowering therapy.[49] As the rate of decline to-date has varied in different socioeconomic groups in developed countries,[5] inequalities in IHD morbidity and mortality are likely to assume greater importance. The prospects for eastern Europe and for developing countries are less clear as we lack key data on trends in risk factor. Additional data from the WHO MONICA Project, which will soon be available, will greatly facilitate projections on the course of the IHD epidemic into the next century.[13]

The prospects for continuing decline in stroke mortality even in developed countries seem less secure, given the recent fall off in the rate of decline in some countries,[1] the evidence in Britain of unfavourable birth cohort trends between 1910 and 1940[48] and the lack (as yet) of specific therapeutic interventions of proven effectiveness in acute stroke. Blood pressure levels are key determinant of stroke risk.[50] Although there is evidence of favourable trends in blood pressure in a number of developed countries[13] it is difficult to see how these trends can be sustained into the next century, given the rising prevalence of obesity and physical inactivity in children and adults in most developed countries.[51]

9.2.7 Summary

The striking secular trends in IHD and stroke mortality observed in Britain and in most westernised industrialized countries during the course of this century reflect real changes in incidence and mortality. Secular trends in major risk factors, which are amenable to modification in adult life (such as serum cholesterol concentration, blood pressure, and cigarette smoking) appear to explain a substantial proportion of the decline in CVD mortality observed in recent decades. However, in analyses of routine mortality data, clear birth cohort effects are detectable. Given that aspects of adult life style, such as cigarette smoking, can be associated with birth cohort-related variation in mortality rates (Fig. 9.2), it is clear that age–period–cohort analyses provide a limited basis for inference regarding the relative importance of factors acting in early versus adult life.

9.3 Respiratory diseases

9.3.1 Chronic obstructive pulmonary diseases

Recent trends in mortality from chronic obstructive pulmonary diseases (COPD: chronic bronchitis, emphysema, asthma and chronic airflow obstruction) vary substantially by country and by gender.[52] Rates are generally stable or falling in men, and stable or rising in women, although male death rates have continued to rise in some west European countries, the US, and Canada during the 1980s.[53–56] Neither current nor past trends in cigarette smoking adequately explain the international variation in the direction of trends, although within countries smoking is universally a powerful risk factor for COPD mortality.[52] This paradox may reflect inadequacy of national smoking data or may be evidence of influential factors other than smoking.

Longer-term COPD mortality trends in England and Wales are well described by a cohort-related rise and fall superimposed on a downward linear drift.[55,56] The peak of the cohort effect corresponds to generations of men born around 1900 and women born some 20–30 years later. A similar cohort pattern emerges in Canadian death rates.[57] This non-linearity is clearly related to uptake of cigarette smoking (Fig. 9.2), but published age–period–cohort analyses have drawn different conclusions about whether the linear drift represents a cohort or period phenomenon.[55,56] Possible explanations considered in Chapter 5 include improved prenatal or postnatal growth, a decline in childhood respiratory infection, air pollution control, dietary changes, or introduction of antibiotics. The downward drift started in the late nineteenth century in all age-groups simultaneously[58] and therefore is more likely to be a period of death effect, at least at the start. Mortality from bronchitis and pneumonia among infants and young children did not start to decline until the early years of the twentieth century, so it is unlikely that this was the key influence on adult mortality.

There is clearer evidence that trends in morbidity have been influenced by changes in smoking behaviour. Reviews of British prevalence studies during the period 1950-1990[59,60] suggest a modest reduction in prevalence of persistent cough and phlegm in middle aged men. The decline (from about 25% in the 1950s and 1960s to about 15% in 1990) parallels a decline in current smoking (from 75% to 30%). There was no change among middle aged women (9–10% in the 1950s and 1960s, compared with 8–9% in the 1980s), reflecting more stable smoking habits (about 25% currently smoking in both periods). These patterns are similar to those for general practitioner contacts for chronic respiratory disease over a similar period.[60]

Marked reductions in urban smoke and sulphur dioxide air pollution over the past thirty years have reduced the daily and seasonal fluctuations in morbidity experienced by chronic bronchitic patients,[61] although the long term effect of air pollution control on respiratory mortality remains poorly evaluated. Previously marked geographical correlations between air pollution levels and respiratory mortality[62] became weaker as air pollution levels fell during the 1960s,[63] but it is too early to assess a possible cohort-related benefit from reduced pollution exposure in childhood.

9.3.2 Asthma and allergy

The prevalence of wheeze did not fall in line with the prevalence of cough and phlegm as British men gave up smoking during the 1960s and 1970s.[59] Since smoking is strongly related to reports of wheeze in middle age, this suggests that another factor may have been operating to increase the prevalence of wheeze. There is consistent evidence from Britain,[64] Australia,[65] and many other countries[66] of an increase in the prevalence of asthma and wheeze among children of school age, by about 50% in relative terms over the period 1965–1990.[64,65] Two studies of children[67,68] have also shown an increase in non-specific bronchial hyperresponsiveness, suggesting that these changes are not entirely explained by changes in parental reporting or labelling of symptoms.

Much less is known about trends in asthma in adults. Hospital admission rates are currently rising in all adult age groups in England and Wales and general practitioner contacts are also becoming more common.[69] These trends are not entirely explained by diagnostic transfer from chronic bronchitis and related diagnoses, but they could reflect changes in the use of health services rather than a true increase in morbidity. It is salutary to note that despite widespread use of effective therapies, and a decline from levels experienced in the 1960s and 1980s (Fig. 9.1), asthma mortality in England and Wales is currently at a similar level to that prevailing in the 1930s.[70]

Consistent evidence of an increase in asthma prevalence in younger adults emerges from three studies of military recruits, in Sweden,[71] Finland,[72] and Israel.[73] The 20-fold increase among Finnish conscripts from 1966 to 1989 is the most remarkable—this change is too large to be plausibly explained by changes in symptom reporting or disease labelling. There is also suggestive evidence of a rising prevalence of allergic rhinitis among American college students[74] and Swedish army conscripts.[71] Two studies of adult populations report an increasing prevalence of positive skin prick tests to common aeroallergens.[75,76] In contrast, no change in skin prick positivity and a *decrease* in prevalence of non-specific bronchial hyperresponsiveness was found in Busselton between 1981 and 1990.[77] Although not entirely consistent, these findings suggest that the prevalence of allergic sensitization may be rising and this would be a plausible explanation for an increase in the prevalence of asthma, particularly in young adults.

The skin prick results from the longitudinal study in Tucson, Arizona[76] are particularly interesting because age-specific prevalence data are available from two examinations 8 years apart. At each survey, the proportion of adults with positive skin prick reactions declined with age from about 40 onwards, yet on follow up, an increasing proportion of subjects in each age group were prick positive. Two explanations could be advanced for this. Skin prick reagents and test methods are notoriously difficult to standardize and this may have resulted in a systematic difference between the two surveys (an artifactual period effect). Alternatively, the decline in prevalence with age in the first survey could be a manifestation of a cohort effect, with earlier born generations carrying a reduced risk of allergic sensitization throughout life.

9.3.3 Projections of future disease burden

Apart from cigarette smoking, the reasons underlying the trends in respiratory mortality and morbidity are poorly understood. Because the influence of smoking appears in mortality trends as a cohort effect, it is possible to predict with some confidence its impact on future death rates. Thus, female death rates from COPD will tend to rise while those among men (apart from the oldest age groups) will tend to fall. Changes in the tar composition of cigarettes, inhalation behaviour and other factors may modulate these effects, and the impact of future tobacco control strategies are unknown. Superimposed on these trends is the downward drift in COPD mortality and a suspected rise in prevalence of asthma. The former is welcome but unexplained and therefore unpredictable. It is at least arguable that the increase in adult asthma is part of a more general increase in allergic diseases which may be attributable to developmental changes in the immune system related to living conditions early in life,[78] as discussed further in Chapter 5. Thus, the rising prevalence of asthma and allergy among children and adolescents may be a worrying foresight of future trends among adults.

References

Those marked with an asterisk are especially recommended for further reading

1* McGovern PG, Burke GL, Sprafka JM, Xue S, Folsom AR, Blackburn H. Trends in mortality, morbidity, and risk factor levels for stroke from 1960 through 1990. The Minnesota Heart Survey. *JAMA* 1992; **268**:753–9.

2 Inman WHW, Adelstein AM. Rise and fall of asthma mortality in England and Wales in relation to use of pressurised aerosols. *Lancet* 1969;**2**:279–83.

3 Clayton DG, Schifflers E. Models for temporal variation on cancer rates. II: Age–period–cohort models. *Stat Med* 1987;**6**:469–81.

4 Tarone RE, Chu KC. Evaluation of birth cohort patterns in population disease rates. *Am J Epidemiol* 1996;**143**:85–91.

5* Beaglehole R. International trends in coronary heart disease mortality, morbidity, and risk factor. *Epidemiolog Rev* 1990;**12**:1–15.

6* Thom TJ, Epstein FH. Heart disease, cancer, and stroke mortality trends and their interrelations. An international perspective. *Circulation* 1994;**90**:574–82.

7 Khaw K-T, Davey-Smith G, Ebrahim S, Murphy M, Charlton J. In: Charlton J, Murphy M, eds. *The health of adult Britain 1841–1994*. Office for National Statistics, London, HMSO, 1997.

8 Tuomilehto J, Li N, Dowse G, Gareeboo H, Chitson P, Fareed D, Min Z, Alberti KG, Zimmet P. The prevalence of coronary heart disease in the multiethnic and high diabetes prevalence population of Mauritius. *J Intern Med* 1993;**233**:187–94.

9   Gordon T, Thom T. The recent decrease in CHD mortality. *Prev Med* 1975;**4**:115–25.

10*   Higgins MW, Luepker RV, eds. Trends and determinants of coronary heart disease mortality: international comparisons. *Int J Epidemiol* 1989;**18 (suppl 1)**:S1–232.

11*   Vartiainen E, Puska P, Pekkanen J, Tuomilehto J, Jouilahti P. Changes in risk factors explain changes in mortality from ischaemic heart disease in Finland? *Br Med J* 1994;**309**:23–7.

12*   Vartiainen E, Cinzia S, Tuomilehto J, Kuulasmaa K. Do changes in cardiovascular risk factor explain changes in mortality from stroke in Finland? *Br Med J* 1995;**310**:901–4.

13   Dobson A, Bired git F, Kuulasmaa K *et al.* Relations of changes in coronary disease rates and changes in risk factor levels: methodological issues and a practical example. *Am J Epidemiol* 1996;**143**:1025–34.

14   Blackburn H. Trends and determinants of CHD mortality: changes in risk factors and their effects. Int J Epidemiol 1989;**18 (suppl 1)**:S210–5.

15   Shaper AG. Reflections on the Seven Countries Study. *Lancet* 1996; **347**:208.

16   Osmond C. Coronary heart disease mortality trends in England and Wales, 1952–1991. *J Public Health Med* 1995;**17**:404–10.

17   Barker DJP, ed. *Fetal and infant origins of adult disease*. London: BMJ Publishing Group, 1992.

18   Whelton SK, Klag MJ. Recent trends in the epidemiology of stroke. What accounts for the persistent decline in stroke mortality in western nations? *Curr Opin Cardiol* 1987;**2**:741–7.

19   Asplund K, Bonita R, Kuulasmaa K, Rajakangas AM, Schaedlich H, Suzuki K, Thorvaldsen P, Tuomilehto J. Multinational comparisons of stroke epidemiology. Evaluation of case ascertainment in the WHO MONICA Stroke Study. *Stroke* 1995;**26**:355–60.

20   Tunstall-Pedoe H, Kuulasmaa K, Amouyel P, Arveiler D, Rajakangas AM, Pajak A. Myocardial infarction and coronary deaths in the WHO Monica Project. Registration procedures, event rates and case-fatality rates in 38 populations from 21 countries in four continents. *Circulation* 1994;**90**:583–612.

21   Burke GL, Sprafka JM, Folsom AR, Luepker RV, Norsted SW, Blackburn H. Trends in CHD mortality, morbidity and risk factor levels from 1960 to 1986: the Minnesota Heart Survey. *Int J Epidemiol* 1989; **18 (suppl 1)**:S73–81.

22   Gillum RF. Trends in acute myocardial infarction and coronary heart disease death in the United States. *J Am Coll Cardiol* 1994;**23**:1273–7.

23   Traven ND, Kuller LH, Ives DG, Rutan GH, Perper JA. Coronary heart disease mortality and sudden death: trends and patterns in 35–44 year old white males, 1970–1990. *Am J Epidemiol* 1995;**142**:45–52.

24* McGovern PG, Pankow JS, Shahar E, Doliszny KM, Folsom AR, Blackburn H, Luepker RV. Recent trends in acute coronary heart disease—mortality, morbidity, medical care, and risk factors. The Minnesota Heart Survey Investigators. *N Engl J Med* 1996;**334**:884–90.

25 Tuomilehto J, Rastenyte D, Sivenius J et al. Ten-year trends in stroke incidence and mortality in the FINMONICA stroke study. *Stroke* 1996; **27**:825–32.

26 Shahar E, McGovern PG, Sprafka JM, Pankow JS, Doliszny KM, Luepker RV, Blackburn H. Improved survival of stroke patients during the 1980s. The Minnesota Stroke Survey. *Stroke* 1995;**26**:16.

27 Wolf PA, D'Agostino RB, O'Neal MA, Sytkowski P, Kase CS, Belanger AJ, Kannel WB. Secular trends in stroke incidence and mortality. The Framingham Study. *Stroke* 1992; **11**:1551–5.

28 Broderick JP, Phillips SJ, Whisnant JP, O'Fallon WM, Bergstrahl EJ. Incidence rates of stroke in the eighties: the end of the decline in stroke? *Stroke* 1989;**20**:577–82.

29 Mayo NE, Goldberg MS, Levy AR, Danys I, Korner-Bitensky N. Changing rates of stroke in the province of Quebec, Canada: 1981–1988. *Stroke* 1991;**22**:590–5.

30 Bonita R, Broad JB, Beaglehole R. Changes in stroke incidence and case fatality in Auckland, New Zealand, 1981–91. *Lancet* 1993;**342**:1470–3.

31 Kagan A, Popper J, Reed DM, MacClean CJ, Grove JS. Trends in stroke incidence and mortality in Hawaiian Japanese men. *Stroke* 1994;**25**: 1170–5.

32 Kodama K. Stroke trends in Japan. *Ann Epidemiol* 1993;**3**:524–8.

33 Stamler J. Opportunities and pitfalls in international comparisons related to patterns, trends and determinants of CHD mortality. *Int J Epidemiol* 1989;**18 (suppl 1)**:S3–18.

34 Morgenstern H. Uses of ecologic analysis in epidemiologic research. *Am J Public Health* 1982;**72**:1336–44.

35 Ascherio A, Rimm EB, Giovannucci EL, Spiegelman D, Stampfer M, Willett WC. Dietary fat and risk of coronary heart disease in men: cohort follow up study in the United States. *Br Med J* 1996;**313**:84–90.

36 Pietinen P. Changing dietary habits in the population: the Finnish experience. In: Ziant G, ed. *Lipids and health*. Amsterdam: Elsevier Science, 1990.

37 Sigfusson N, Sigvaldason H, Steingrimsdottir L et al. Decline in ischaemic heart disease in Iceland and change in risk factor levels. *Br Med J* 1991;**302**:1371–5.

38 Elliott P, Stamler J, Nichols R, et al. for the Intersalt cooperative research group. Intersalt revisited: further analyses of 24 hour sodium excretion and blood pressure within and across populations. *Br Med J* 1996;**312**:1249–53.

39   Perry IJ, Beevers DG. Salt intake and stroke, a possible direct effect. *J Hum Hypertens* 1992;**6**:23–5.

40   Tobian L, Hanlon S. High sodium chloride diets injure arteries and raise mortality with changing blood pressure. *Hypertens* 1990;**15**:900–3.

41   Antonios TFT, MacGregor GA. Salt—more adverse effects? *Lancet* 1996;**348**:250–1.

42   Gale CR, Martyn CN, Winter PD, Cooper C. Vitamin C and risk of death from stroke and coronary heart disease in a cohort of elderly people. *Br Med J* 1995;**310**:1563–6.

43   Gillman MW, Cupples LA, Gagnon D, Posner BM, Ellison RC, Castelli WP, Wolf PA. Protective effect of fruits and vegetables on development of stroke in men. *JAMA* 1995;**273**:1113–7.

44   Sverre JM. Secular trends in coronary heart disease mortality in Norway, 19661986. *Am J Epidemiol* 1993;**137**:301–10.

45   Baker D, Illsey R, Vagero D. Today or in the past? The origins of ischaemic heart disease. *J Public Health Med* 1993;**15**:243–8.

46   Webster C. Healthy or hungry thirties? *History Workshop Journal* 1982; **13**:110–29.

47   Barker DJP. Foetal origins of coronary heart disease. *Br Med J* 1995; **311**:171–4.

48   Wolfe CDA, Burney PGJ. Is stroke mortality on the decline in England? *Am J Epidemiol* 1992;**136**:558–65.

49   Scandinavian Simvastatin Survival Study Group. Randomised trial of cholesterol lowering in 4444 patients with coronary heart disease: The Scandinavian Simvastatin Survival Study (4S). *Lancet* 1994;**344**: 1383–9.

50   Collins R, Peto R, MacMahon S, et al. Blood pressure, stroke and coronary heart disease: Part 2, short term reductions in blood pressure: overview of randomised drug trials in their epidemiologic context. *Lancet* 1992;**335**:827–38.

51   Prentice AM, Jebb SA. Obesity in Britain: gluttony or sloth? *Br Med J* 1995;**311**:437–9.

52   Brown CA, Crombie IK, Tunstall-Pedoe H. Failure of cigarette smoking to explain international differences in mortality from chronic obstructive pulmonary disease. *J Epidemiol Community Health* 1994;**48**:134–9.

53   Thom TJ. International comparisons in COPD mortality. *Am Rev Respir Dis* 1989;**140 (suppl)**:S27–34.

54   Feinleib M, Rosenberg HM, Collins JG, Delozier JE, Pokras R, Chevarley FM. Trends in COPD morbidity and mortality in the United States. *Am Rev Respir Dis* 1989;**140 (suppl)**:S9–18.

55   Barker DJP, Osmond C. Childhood respiratory infection and adult chronic bronchitis in England and Wales. *Br Med J* 1986;**293**: 1271–5.

56*   Lee PN, Fry JS, Forey BA. Trends in lung cancer, chronic obstructive lung disease, and emphysema death rates for England and Wales 1941–85 and their relation to trends in cigarette smoking. *Thorax* 1990;**45**: 657–65.

57   Manfreda J, Mao Y, Litven W. Morbidity and mortality from chronic obstructive pulmonary disease. *Am Rev Respir Dis* 1989;**140 (suppl)**: S19–26.

58   Strachan DP. Trends in respiratory mortality in England and Wales. *Thorax* 1991;**46**:149.

59   Cook DG, Kussick SJ, Shaper AG. The respiratory benefits of stopping smoking. *J Smoking Relat Dis* 1990;**1**:45–58

60*   Strachan DP. Epidemiology: a British perspective. In: Calverley P, Pride N, eds. *Chronic obstructive pulmonary disease*. London: Chapman & Hall, 1995:47–68.

61   Waller RE. Control of air pollution: present success and future prospect. In: Bennett AE, ed. *Recent advances in community medicine I*. Edinburgh: Churchill Livingstone, 1978:59–72.

62   Gardner MJ, Crawford MD, Morris JN. Patterns of mortality in middle and old age in the county boroughs of England and Wales. *Br J Prev Soc Med* 1969;**23**:133–40.

63   Chinn S, Florey CDV, Baldwin IG, Gorgol M. The relationship of mortality in England and Wales 1969–73 to measurements of air pollution. *J Epidemiol Community Health* 1981;**35**:174–9.

64   Anderson HR. Is asthma really increasing? *Paed Resp Med* 1993;**1**:6–10.

65   Bauman A. Has the prevalence of asthma symptoms increased in Australian children? *J Paediatr Child Health* 1993;**29**:424–8.

66   Burr ML. Epidemiology of asthma. In: Burr ML, ed. *Epidemiology of clinical allergy*. Basel: Karger, 1993:80–102.

67   Burr ML, Butland BK, King S, Vaughan-Williams E. Changes in asthma prevalence: two surveys 15 years apart. *Arch Dis Child* 1989; **64**:1118–25.

68   Peat JK, van den Berg RH, Green WF, Mellis CM, Leeder SR, Woolcock AJ. Changing prevalence of asthma in Australian children. *Br Med J* 1994;**308**:1591–6.

69*   Department of Health Committee on the medical effects of air pollutants. *Asthma and outdoor air pollution. London:* HMSO, 1995. 85–100.

70   Burney PGJ. Asthma deaths in England and Wales 1931–85: evidence for a true increase in asthma mortality. *J Epidemiol Community Health* 1988;**42**:316–20.

71   Åberg N. Asthma and allergic rhinitis in Swedish conscripts. *Clin Exp Allergy* 1989;**19**:59–63.

72   Haahtela T, Lindholm H, Bjorkstein F, Koskenvuo K, Laitenen LA. Prevalence of asthma in Finnish young men. *Br Med J* 1990;**301**:266–8.

73   Laor A, Cohen L, Danon YL. Effects of time, sex, ethnic origin and area of residence on prevalence of asthma in Israeli adolescents. *Br Med J* 1993;**307**:841–4.

74   Hagy GW, Settipnae GA. Bronchial asthma, allergic rhinitis and allergy skin tests among college students. *J Allergy* 1969;**44**:323–32.

75   Sibbald B, Rink E, D'Souza M. Is atopy increasing? *Br J Gen Pract* 1990;**40**:338–40.

76* Barbee RA, Kaltenborn W, Lebowitz MD, Burrows B. Longitudinal changes in allergen skin test reactivity in a community population sample. *J Allergy Clin Immunol* 1987;**79**:16–24.

77   Peat JK, Haby M, Spijker J, *et al*. Prevalence of asthma in adults in Busselton, Western Australia. *Br Med J* 1992;**305**:1326–9.

78* Strachan DP. Time trends in asthma and allergy: ten questions, fewer answers. *Clin Exp Allergy* 1995;**25**:791–4.

10 Geography and migration

Jonathan Elford and Yoav Ben-Shlomo

Geographic variations in the risk of coronary heart disease have been widely reported. Such variations may be genetic in origin, influenced by factors acting early in life, later in life or a combination acting throughout the life course. Two epidemiological approaches to investigating geographic variations in disease are considered here—ecological studies and migrant studies. Ecological studies within countries have shown strong associations between past measures of early life conditions as well as current measures of deprivation and cardiovascular disease. Other conventional risk factors showed weak effects or no associations. Current birthweight distribution was also not associated with cardiovascular disease. At an international level, both early life and adult risk factors showed moderate associations, although these were greater for cerebrovascular disease rather than ischaemic heart disease. Migrant studies conducted in the Pacific region, Israel, Kenya, China and Britain showed that people moving from a low blood pressure to a high blood pressure community experienced a rise in blood pressure not seen in those who remained behind. This appeared to occur soon after moving and could not be explained by selective migration. For example, islanders from Tokelau (in the Pacific) who migrated to New Zealand experienced a faster annual rise in blood pressure during follow up than non-migrants, the differential being 1 mmHg/yr for males and 0.4 mmHg/year for females. Factors acting after migration were clearly of aetiological importance for blood pressure. Ecological and migrant studies confirm that factors acting throughout the life course, and not simply at one stage, influence the geographic distribution of coronary heart disease and its risk factors.

10.1 Introduction

International comparisons of cardiovascular disease death rates reveal striking variations between countries. In 1989, among men and women aged 35–74 years, there was a 10-fold difference in age-adjusted coronary heart disease (CHD) mortality between Japan and Scotland (Fig. 10.1). International comparisons of mortality may be hampered by varying practices of death certification, but surveys using uniform clinical procedures have confirmed that vital statistics do reflect genuine differences in the risk of CHD between countries. Geographic differences in the risk of CHD may be genetic in origin, influenced by factors acting early in life, later in life or indeed a combination acting throughout the life course. This chapter considers two epidemiological approaches to investigating geographic variations in disease, ecological studies and migrant studies.

10.2 Ecological studies

Ecological studies examine the correlation between a potential explanatory variable and disease frequency both within and between countries. The distinction between this and other epidemiological study designs is that the unit of analysis is a group rather than an individual, for example factories, cities, counties, or nations.[1]

10.2.1 Strengths and weaknesses of ecological studies

In general, ecological studies are regarded as fairly weak study designs for the following reasons:

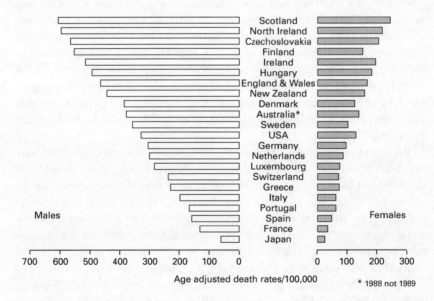

Figure 10.1 Age-adjusted death rates per 100, 000 from CHD among men and women aged 35-74 years in 1989 in selected countries. Source: World Health Organization. *World Health Statistics Annual 1989*. Geneva: WHO, 1990.

(i) explanatory variables are often taken from routinely collected data and may be proxy measures

(ii) the direction of causality between exposure and disease may not be clear

(iii) interpreting any association between exposure and disease is complicated by the 'ecological fallacy' in that what is observed at a group level may not actually occur at an individual level. For example, areas with greater death rates from cardiovascular disease may also have a greater proportion of smokers. However it may actually be the non-smokers who are dying. In addition there is specification bias, that is exposure at a group level is confounded by other risk factors.[2]

These limitations have led most epidemiologists to restrict ecological analyses to simple exploratory studies indicating '. . . the presence of effects worthy of further investigation'.[1]

The importance of factors that determine disease at an individual level may be different from those at a population level.[3] There are two reasons for this.

Firstly, within populations the variation in an exposure may be far less than between populations. This can be illustrated by the weak relationships between sodium intake and blood pressure at an individual level that are far stronger at a group level.[4]

Secondly, at an individual level the relationship between exposure and outcome may be weaker due to the multifactorial nature of disease causation. However, between groups these other factors may be more homogenous and hence the relative importance of a key variable may be accentuated. In addition, some variables may be better characterized at an area level,[5–8] for example environmental exposures such as air pollution. Similarly there may be interactions between individual and area level variables.[7,9] The advent of new techniques, such as multilevel modelling, have enabled these to be explicitly quantified.

The failure to confirm an ecological association at the individual level may reflect the limitations of ecological analyses. However, the failure to replicate an individual-based study at an ecological level does not negate the causal importance of that variable. Assuming this is not merely a measurement error problem, this either suggests the other variables are more important in explaining ecological variations, or that there may be important interactions between different risk factors, which may be more marked at the ecological rather than individual level. For example, a correlation between prevalence of smoking and heart disease mortality would highlight Japan as an outlier as it has a very low rate of heart disease despite having a high rate of smoking.[10] However, smoking is still a risk factor for heart disease amongst Japanese, as seen within individual-based studies.[11]

10.2.2 Variations in cardiovascular disease within countries

Geographical variations in disease rates have been noted in England and Wales since the mid nineteenth century. William Farr reported that life expectancy for boys in Liverpool, inner London, and Surrey were 25, 35, and 44 years respectively (cited in reference 12). Early attempts at ecological correlations often focused on environmental factors, such as air pollution, water hardness and elevation above sea level.[13] Studies noted increasing mortality rates for degenerative disease, such as arteriosclerosis, with ecological measures of social deprivation (cited in 14). These studies were to be replicated several decades later using similar but more sophisticated methods.[15–17]

10.2.2.1 Markers of early life influences

Forsdahl postulated that poverty in adolescence followed by later affluence might result in increased mortality from ischaemic heart disease. He noted strong correlations (males 0.79, females 0.61) between infant mortality from 1896–1925 and adult mortality from heart disease between 1964–67 for the 19 counties in Norway.[18] This work was replicated for counties in England and Wales by Williams and colleagues, who noted, however, that correlations with both past and present infant mortality rates were strong, as areas poor in the past remain poorer today.[19] These studies grouped all infant deaths together.

Subsequent work from the MRC unit in Southampton differentiated between neonatal (within first month) and postneonatal (after first month but within first year) mortality. Their results showed that stroke deaths were more strongly correlated with neonatal mortality; bronchitis, stomach cancer, and rheumatic heart disease with postneonatal mortality; ischaemic heart disease strongly correlated with both.[20] An earlier birth cohort analysis from the USA also suggested that infant mortality from diarrhoea and enteritis was a strong predictor of ischaemic heart disease.[21] Subsequent ecological analyses highlighted the relationships between maternal mortality and both stroke and ischaemic heart disease,[22] as well as infant mortality from bronchitis and pneumonia with subsequent adult mortality from chronic obstructive airways disease.[23] Despite the greater specificity of these findings, the associations did not try to control for any other confounding factors.

A later study which did adjust for contemporary measures of deprivation revealed that associations between infant mortality and adult mortality were greatly attenuated and most were no longer statistically significant except for bronchitis, emphysema, and asthma.[24] The authors concluded that geographical patterns in mortality could be explained by 'continued deprivation throughout life leading to an accumulation of detrimental health effects.'[24]

10.2.2.2 Height: an indicator of childhood conditions?

Height is a measure that indicates both genetic and environmental factors acting from the perinatal period into early adulthood. Using data from the three UK birth cohorts, it is possible to rank counties in England and Wales into five groups based on the mean heights of their inhabitants. A clear trend is seen for both men and women, with taller counties having lower mortality rates from ischaemic heart disease, stroke, and bronchitis, but higher rates of cancers of the breast, ovary, and prostate[26] (see Chapter 3). Similarly, an analysis based on the 1970 and 1946 birth cohorts related measures on maternal and child factors to geographical variations in adult cardiovascular disease.[27] Both maternal and child height showed strong inverse relationships with mortality, but mean birthweight showed no consistent pattern, in contrast to previous ecological analyses. The geographic relationship between height and mortality may, however, be confounded by social class. 'Tall' counties, which tend to be in the south of England, may contain proportionately more people in high socioeconomic groups with lower mortality than short counties, which tend to be in the north.

More direct evidence on the importance of height and hence childhood growth, independent of birthweight, comes from the Ten Towns study. Children from high mortality towns were shorter, and had a higher ponderal index and higher blood pressure, although no differences were noted in cholesterol or post-load glucose measurements.[28] These differences persisted after adjustment for birthweight.

10.2.2.3 Urban and rural differences

Differences in mortality rates between urban and rural areas have been noted in several different countries (reviewed in reference 29). Standardized mortality ratios for coronary disease in England (1950–52)[30] showed lower mortality rates for rural districts as compared with either county boroughs or urban districts, unrelated to the proportion of men in social classes I and II. Conventional risk factors appear inadequate to explain these observations, as modelling differences in smoking, blood pressure, and cholesterol fail to account for the lower mortality rates.[31] The detrimental effects of urbanization has been proposed, but this evidence is based on communities undergoing a transitional phase rather than on stable communities.[32] Rural areas also appear to provide more favourable conditions for early life. Infant mortality rates in 1925 for England show a linear decline from 87 per 1000 births for county boroughs to 72 per 1000 births for other urban districts and 64 per 1000 births for rural districts. Similarly, standardized height ratios measured on school children in 1908–1910 show the opposite gradient with rural children being taller than their urban counterparts (manufacturing towns 97.9, urban county councils 100.5, rural county councils 102.4, total population 100.0).[33] A recent report demonstrated that differences in birthweight and child height still persist today and appear to be independent of socioeconomic status.[34] Temporal data from the US[35] and Norway[36] demonstrate that the rural advantage in adult mortality is rapidly disappearing. It is unclear whether these observations are more consistent with alterations in adult rather than early life factors.

10.2.2.4 Adult risk factors and early life measures

Data from the 1993 Health Survey for England[37] enables one to examine the geographical relationship across Regional Health Authorities in England between the more important adult cardiovascular risk factors, two proxy measures of early life influences (infant mortality in 1925 and birthweight for 1985), current deprivation and prevalent ischaemic heart disease or stroke (see Table 10.1). Ideally data on birthweight from an earlier period would be used but are not available.

Infant mortality in 1925 showed the strongest relationships with both male and female ischaemic heart disease or stroke, closely followed by current Townsend index of socioeconomic deprivation. These results reflect the relative importance of factors acting both in early and later life. Conventional risk factors such as smoking and body mass index showed moderate to weak associations, with cholesterol and fibrinogen showing no or an inverse

Table 10.1 The relationship between cardiovascular risk factors and prevalent ischaemic heart disease or stroke in 14 English Regional Health Authorities

	Male IHD or stroke	Female IHD or stroke
smoking 20+ cigs per day[a]	0.55*	0.28
mean BMI	0.23	0.13
high blood pressure	0.12	0.03
fibrinogen[a]	0.02	0.28
mean cholesterol	−0.03	0.41
birth weight in 1986	−0.26	−0.01
infant mortality rate (1925)	0.78*	0.53*
Townsend deprivation score	0.65*	0.51

* $p < 0.05$
[a] indicates a standardised ratio measure was used
BMI = body mass index

Data taken from 1993 Health Survey for England,[37] 1981 Census, Registrar's General Statistical Review of England and Wales 1925, and unpublished birth statistics (VS2) 1985 kindly provided by the Office for National Statistics

association in men and weak to moderate associations for women. The poor ability of cholesterol to predict geographical variations in ischaemic heart disease mortality has been noted in the British Regional Heart Study[38] and the Scottish Heart Health Study.[39] Birthweight, measured in 1986, surprisingly had a negative correlation and did not show the same pattern as infant mortality rates (see Fig. 10.2), similar to a previous birth cohort analysis.[27] This may either reflect a problem with using mean birthweight, unadjusted for gestational age, or because contemporary birthweight should be compared with future rather than current regional mortality. Alternatively, low birthweight today may reflect different factors from those operating at the beginning of the century which resulted in high rates of infant mortality. If this is the case, then it is possible that the low birthweight–ischaemic heart disease relationship may will differ over time for future cohorts.

10.2.3 Variations in cardiovascular disease between countries

The Seven Countries study was one of the earliest international studies that demonstrated a strong correlation (0.84) between percent of dietary energy from saturated fatty acids and mortality from coronary heart disease.[40] The ratio of monounsaturates to saturated dietary fat, age, body mass index, systolic blood pressure, serum cholesterol and cigarette consumption explained 96% of the variance between countries.[41] Estimates of the strength of the relationship between cholesterol and ischaemic heart disease mortality suggest that a difference of 0.6 mmol/l (about 10% of the average value in western countries) is associated with an average difference of 37% in ischaemic heart disease mortality in 55–64 year olds.[42] A more detailed analysis based on 27 countries and examining lipid sub-fractions noted correlations of 0.67, −0.57 and 0.74 for serum cholesterol, HDL cholesterol and serum cholesterol : HDL cholesterol ratio respectively.[43] Analyses have failed to demonstrate an independent effect of alcohol, fish intake, fibre, and antioxidant vitamins after adjustment for saturated fatty acids.[44]

The large international MONICA study has obtained standardized data on 39 centres from 26 countries.[45] Using cross-sectional data on risk factors and routine mortality, it found much weaker associations between conventional risk factors and ischaemic heart disease with only 25% of the variance explained by smoking, blood pressure, and total cholesterol. These associations may become stronger, as future analyses will be based on prospective events within the cohorts rather than routine data. A further analysis using the MONICA data but also including data on infant mortality rates (1932) for selected countries is shown in Table 10.2. Because China is an extreme outlier, results have been presented both including and excluding it. Smoking shows no significant association with ischaemic heart disease but a strong association with stroke for men. Raised cholesterol, as noted in the previous MONICA

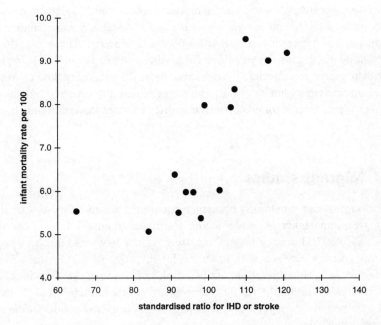

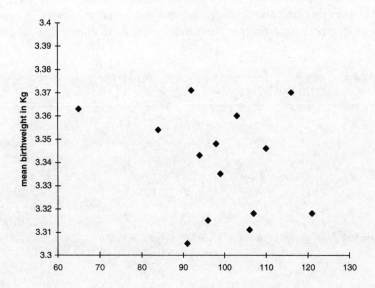

Figure 10.2 Scatterplot showing the association between the standardised prevalence ratio for ischaemic heart disease or stroke and (a) infant mortality rates in 1925 (b) mean birthweight for English Regional Health Authorities.

publication, surprisingly shows no significant associations.[45] Infant mortality shows moderately strong correlations with cardiovascular disease, similar in magnitude to hypertension for cardiovascular disease. However, these associations mask a strongly positive correlation with stroke mortality and a weak or negative correlation with ischaemic heart disease, in marked contrast to the pattern seen within countries. This suggests that any perinatal influences may play a greater role for cerebrovascular disease rather than ischaemic heart disease.

10.3 Migrant studies

Migration provides a naturally occurring experiment which may establish the aetiological importance of factors acting at different points in the life course. If the risk of CHD among people migrating from a low incidence to a high incidence country increases with time, it is highly probable that factors acting later in life, following migration, are of aetiological importance. On the other hand, if migrants retain the risk of their country of origin, then it is likely that genetic characteristics or factors operating early in life exert a greater influence than exposures later on.

Migration also provides the opportunity to test Forsdahl's hypothesis that poverty in early life followed by later affluence increases the risk of CHD.[18] According to this hypothesis, migrants who encounter prosperity in adult life, having experienced relative deprivation during childhood, should face

Table 10.2 The relationship between all cause and cardiovascular disease by several risk factors for 19 countries involved in the MONICA WHO Project

	Males			Females		
	CVD	**IHD**	**Stroke**	**CVD**	**IHD**	**Stroke**
smoking (%)	0.21	−0.05	0.62*	−0.06	−0.01	−0.10
	0.39**	0.10	0.61*	−0.05	−0.03	−0.06
hypertension (%)	0.44	0.19	0.59*	0.56*	0.40	0.47*
	0.44	0.19	0.61*	0.60*	0.39	0.53*
raised cholesterol (%)	0.08	0.14	−0.25	−0.19	0.10	−0.32
	−0.10	−0.03	−0.18	−0.10	0.05	−0.18
infant mortality	0.17	−0.10	0.66*	0.40	0.15	0.38
rate (1932)	0.32	0.01	0.60*	0.31	0.17	0.27
(15 countries)						

* $p < 0.05$
** second row shows correlation coefficients excluding China
Source: reference [45]

an even *greater* risk of CHD than the long term residents of the country they migrate to.

One of the major methodological challenges presented by these studies is that migration may be selective. Migrants may differ from non-migrants and so may not be representative of the population they left. Some of the most comprehensive migrant studies in recent years have examined changes in *blood pressure* on migration rather than CHD incidence or mortality. This chapter considers only blood pressure studies, focusing on those which have attempted to address the issue of selective migration. The appendix at the end of this chapter references other studies that have described changes in CHD incidence and mortality among migrants.

10.3.1 Tokelau Island Migrant Study

Tokelau, a former New Zealand dependency, is comprised of three small atolls in the South Pacific. Following a hurricane in 1966, many Tokelauans migrated to New Zealand. The migration of Tokelauans from their traditional life on the atoll to urban life in New Zealand provided the opportunity to study the effects of migration on their health.

The strength of the Tokelau Island Migrant Study lay in its ability to collect detailed information on Tokelauans prior to migration, as well as after, enabling the authors to investigate any selection effects among migrants.[46,47] A number of published papers examined changes in blood pressure associated with migration.[48–52] Some were longitudinal in nature, initially examining subjects in Tokelau and then re-examining them several years later either in New Zealand (migrants) or in Tokelau (non-migrants).[48–50] Other studies were cross-sectional in nature, comparing Tokelauans who had migrated with those who had not at the same point in time.[51,52]

10.3.1.1 Longitudinal studies

Children

In 1971, of all 518 children aged 5–14 years resident in Tokelau, 502 (97%) were examined. Follow up examinations of 456 (91%) of these children were conducted 5 years later in New Zealand (121 migrants) and Tokelau (335 non-migrants). At baseline, in 1971, there were no significant differences between non-migrants and migrants in mean systolic or diastolic blood pressure, weight, height, or body mass index.

At follow up examination, mean systolic and diastolic blood pressures were higher in male migrants than non-migrants, significantly so at ages 5–9 years. Adjusted for age at follow up the difference between migrants and non-migrants aged 5–9 years was 6.4 mmHg for systolic and 10.0 mmHg for diastolic blood pressure ($p < 0.01$). For girls, younger migrants (5–9 years) had higher mean blood pressure than non-migrants although this difference was only significant for diastolic pressure (62.4 vs. 54.0 adjusted for age, $p < 0.01$). For the older girls, however, the situation was reversed, with non-migrants having a higher mean blood pressure than migrants although this difference was significant only for systolic pressure.[48] The authors suggested that psychosocial factors may have contributed to the different blood pressure patterns among male and female migrants. In particular, anthropologists had observed that the behaviour of non-migrant girls (but not boys) living in Tokelau was particularly constrained by family and social pressures.

Adults

Of 1018 adults aged 15–69 years who were examined in Tokelau in 1968–71, 812 were re-examined approximately 5 years later (1975–77) in New Zealand (280 migrants) or Tokelau (532 non-migrants). At baseline, there were no systematic significant differences between migrants and non-migrants in blood pressure or body mass index. On re-examination 5 years later, blood pressures had risen substantially among male migrants, by an average of 10 mmHg systolic and 7mmHg diastolic. It was found that after adjusting for baseline age, body mass index, blood pressure, and rate of change of body mass index, the blood pressure of male migrants had risen faster than that of non-migrants, by a factor of about 1 mmHg a year for males ($(p < 0.001)$ and 0.4 mmHg/year for females (systolic $p = 0.054$; diastolic $p = 0.02$).[50] No information was available on corresponding increases in blood pressure among long term New Zealand residents.

The authors commented that the lack of systematic differences between migrants and non-migrants at the pre-migration survey ruled out measurable selection bias in these analyses.

10.3.1.2 Cross sectional studies

In a study conducted in the mid-1970s, 856 Tokelauan children living in New Zealand had significantly higher mean systolic blood pressure than 571 children still living in Tokelau (non-migrants), even after adjusting for height and weight ($p < 0.001$).[51] A mean difference in blood pressure of 6.0 mmHg was recorded. Similarly, the prevalence of hypertension was higher among 1181 Tokelauan adults examined in New Zealand than among 807 still in Tokelau (non-migrants) (definite hypertension, males 9.4% vs. 2.6%, females 10.3% vs. 7.6% respectively).[52] It was thought unlikely that the findings of these cross-sectional studies, which were consistent with the longitudinal studies, were the result of non-response, biased assessment, or selection.

10.3.2 Yi Migrant Study - China

The Yi people are an ethnic minority who live principally in remote mountainous areas in southwest China. Isolated from the outside world, they have preserved their own language and traditional life style. Since the 1950s, Yi farmers have migrated to Xichang City and urban 'county seats' within the prefecture. The traditional residents of these urban areas are Han people, the majority ethnic group in China. A survey conducted in 1979–80 (and published only in Chinese) found that among Yi people still living in mountain areas blood pressure was low, and did not increase with age during adulthood, and that hypertension, CHD, and stroke were extremely rare.[53] Two large scale surveys have subsequently been conducted among Yi farmers (non-migrants), Yi migrants, and Han residents, the first in 1986–88,[53] the second in 1989.[54] Both were cross-sectional in design. The main aims were to compare blood pressure patterns (i) among the same ethnic group living in different environments and (ii) among different ethnic groups living in the same environment.

10.3.2.1 1986–88 survey

Between 1986–88 a survey was undertaken among more than 6000 men and women (overall response exceeded 80%), comparing 2327 Yi farmers living in high mountain areas and 2631 Yi farmers in mountainside areas (mean age of both groups 30 years) with 517 Yi migrants and 1143 Han residents in Puge county seat (mean age of both groups 34 years).

For men, mean systolic blood pressure was similar for Yi migrants and Han residents (107.3 and 108.3 mmHg) but significantly lower ($p < 0.01$) among Yi farmers (101.8 and 100.8 for high mountain and mountainside farmers respectively). A similar pattern was seen for diastolic pressure ($p < 0.001$). The differential was reduced, but nonetheless persisted after adjusting for age and body mass index (Yi migrants and Han residents were older and had higher BMI than non-migrants). For women, after adjusting for age, BMI, and altitude, diastolic but not systolic blood pressure was lower among Yi farmers compared with migrants and Han residents. The prevalence of hypertension was higher among Yi migrants and Han residents than among non-migrant farmers. Mean blood pressure rose very little with age after puberty among Yi farmers, but there was a trend of increasing blood pressure with age in Yi migrants and Han residents.[53]

10.3.2.2 1989 survey

Of 16 301 men and women aged 15–89 years eligible for the 1989 study, 14 505 (89%) were examined: 8241 Yi farmers living in remote mountain villages (mean age 31 years), 2575 Yi migrants, and 3689 Han people living in urban county seats (mean age 34 and 35 years respectively). Median length of residence in the county seats by Yi migrants was 10 years.

Although blood pressure rose significantly with age in all three groups, the rate of increase was lowest in Yi farmers (systolic 0.13 mmHg/yr males, 0.06 females) and highest in Yi migrants (systolic 0.33 mmHg/yr males, 0.37 females) and Han people (systolic 0.36 mmHg/yr males, 0.56 females) ($p < 0.01$). After adjusting for body mass index the differences remained significant except for diastolic pressure in women. The age adjusted prevalence of definite hypertension (systolic $\geqslant 160$mmHg and/or diastolic $\geqslant 95$mmHg) in males was higher among Yi migrants and Han people (4–5%) than in Yi farmers (< 1%). A similar pattern was seen in females. The differentials were slightly reduced after adjusting for age, body mass index, heart rate, alcohol use, and smoking but still remained statistically significant ($p < 0.05$).[54,55] Although blood pressure levels rose steadily with alcohol consumption in all three groups, Yi farmers consistently had lower blood pressure than Yi migrants and Han people at all daily alcohol intake levels.[56]

Although the ethnic background of Yi migrants was similar to that of the Yi farmers, their mean blood pressure levels, rate of increase of blood pressure with age, and prevalence of hypertension closely resembled the Han people. Differences between Yi migrants and farmers in blood pressure could only be partially explained by age, BMI, heart rate, smoking, and alcohol use.[54] Compared with Yi farmers, however, Yi migrants ate more sodium, fat, and cholesterol and less potassium, calcium, and magnesium. In fact their diet was similar to that of the Han people. Thus, dietary changes appear to have contributed to the development of raised blood pressure in Yi migrants.

10.3.3 Ethiopian migrants to Israel

Ethiopian Jews traditionally lived in remote rural areas, and only a relatively small number emigrated to Israel in the 1970s and 80s. However, during a dramatic airlift in 1984–85 known as Operation Moses, more than 6500 Ethiopian Jews, having left Ethiopia during a drought, were airlifted to Israel from Sudanese refugee camps.[57] The migration from rural villages in Ethiopia to urban areas in Israel provided the opportunity to examine changes in blood pressure among Ethiopians by duration of residence in Israel and also to compare their blood pressure levels with those of long term Israeli residents.[58–64]

10.3.3.1 Longitudinal studies

In 1984, blood pressure was measured in 483 Ethiopians aged 5 years and above a few weeks after their arrival in Israel (Operation Moses). After 1 year, blood pressure was measured again in 265 of these subjects. Mean blood pressure at baseline among those who were re-examined and those who were not was similar for all but one age group. Average diastolic blood pressure increased by about 4 mmHg in those who were re-examined, a differential which remained after adjusting for age and weight change over the year. Systolic pressures, however, changed only slightly over the year.[58]

Of 87 Ethiopian immigrants in their early twenties who were examined within 3 months of their arrival in Israel, on enrolling in a residential agricultural college, 53 were still living in the college 2 years later. Most of those lost to follow up had been drafted for regular army service, but they were not significantly different at baseline from those who were available for re-examination. Among the 53 immigrants, there was a significant rise in blood pressure over the 2 year period ($p < 0.01$). Mean systolic pressure increased from 118 to 129 mmHg, diastolic from 62 to 71 mmHg. Eleven of the 53 subjects (21%) were found to be hypertensive at 2 years; none were at baseline. Mean BMI did not change during follow up. The authors thought it unlikely that alcohol consumption had increased during the two years, due to its lack of ready availability at the schools, but salt intake could have increased.[59]

10.3.3.2 Cross-sectional studies

Ethiopian immigrants who had recently arrived in Israel had lower mean blood pressure than those who had lived there for 2–3 years.[60–63] For example, mean blood pressure among new Ethiopian immigrants in their early twenties living in a residential college ($n = 87$) was 118.6 mmHg compared with 125.7 mmHg in immigrants ($n = 63$) who had been there at least 2 years.[63] Conversely, Ethiopians who had lived in Israel for 4 years had a blood pressure distribution similar to veteran Israelis of the same age.[64] This suggested to the authors that Ethiopian immigrants to Israel developed the blood pressure patterns of the society to which they migrated. The cross-sectional studies were not as methodologically robust as the longitudinal investigations. Nonetheless, all the studies reported an increase in blood pressure among Ethiopians associated with duration of residence in Israel.

10.3.4 Luo migrants in Kenya

The Luo tribe live in a rural area to the north of Lake Victoria in western Kenya. Seeking work, a number of Luo people have migrated to Nairobi. The migration of Luo people from a rural to an urban area provided the opportunity to examine blood pressure in migrants before and after they moved, by duration of residence in Nairobi, and to compare their blood pressure with non-migrants who remained in the rural areas.[65–68]

10.3.4.1 Longitudinal studies

One hundred Luo migrants to Nairobi (90 men, 10 women, mean age 21 years) were traced who had already been examined on average 10 months earlier, prior to migration. Among the 90 males, mean systolic blood pressure increased from 120.9 mmHg before migration to 127.2 mmHg after (diastolic 59.0 to 65.3) ($p < 0.01$). Mean body weight and mean sodium/potassium ratio also increased. Pre-migration mean blood pressures among the migrants, however, were almost identical to those seen in age-matched rural non-migrants who were examined at the same time. time. Mean body weights were also similar. The authors concluded that while selective migration was a theoretical and sometimes real cause for concern in the interpretaton of migrant studies, it did not appear to play an important role in the Kenya Luo migrant study.[65]

Between 1981 and 1985 rural non-migrants and urban migrants aged 15–34 years were recruited for an investigation of changes in blood pressure over time. Migrants ($n = 63$) were examined shortly after migration and then 3, 6, 12, 18, and 24 months later. Age-sex matched non-migrants ($n = 143$) were examined at the same time periods. Mean systolic blood pressure was significantly higher in migrants than in non-migrants throughout the study ($p < 0.02$). Mean diastolic pressures were also elevated among migrants, although not always significantly. The distribution of both systolic and diastolic blood pressures for migrants was shifted to the right of non-migrants. Selective migration was not a factor since blood pressure measurements in male migrants prior to migration were not significantly different from rural non-migrants. The authors concluded that differences in blood pressure between rural and urban groups were apparent, on average, 1 month after migration.[66]

10.3.4.2 Cross-sectional studies

In a 1980 study, the rate of increase of blood pressure with age was greater among 310 migrants aged 20 years and over living in Nairobi than among 861 rural non-migrants (males 0.56 mmHg vs. 0.14 mmHg per year, $p < 0.001$). Mean blood pressures were similar in migrant and non-migrants until the age of 35 years, but above that age were consistently higher among migrants. After age adjustment, systolic, but not diastolic blood pressure was significantly correlated with duration of urban residence.[67]

10.3.5 Migrants within Britain

For the British Regional Heart Study, approximately 300 men aged 40–59 years were recruited between 1978–80 from one general practice in each of

24 towns throughout England, Scotland, and Wales (7735 subjects in all). Overall, mean blood pressure was higher in the north of England and Scotland than in the south. For example mean systolic and diastolic blood pressures in Guildford (south of England) were 135.9 and 77.6 mmHg respectively compared with 152.4 and 88.5 in Dunfermline (Scotland).[69]

The men were divided into two groups: non-migrants who were born in the town where they were examined for the study ($n = 3144$), and migrants who were born elsewhere in Great Britain ($n = 4147$). Regardless of where they were born, men living in the south of England had lower mean blood pressures than men living in the north of England or Scotland. Furthermore, men born in the south who moved to Scotland had higher mean blood pressure levels than those who stayed in south (systolic 156.7 vs. 141.7, diastolic 88.5 vs. 79.9). Equally, men born in Scotland who moved south had lower mean blood pressure than those who stayed put (systolic 143.1 vs. 147.7, diastolic 80.1 vs. 84.9).[70] Yet, according to Forsdahl,[18] migrants from Scotland to the south of England should have experienced an increased risk of CHD (i.e. raised blood pressure) since they had lived in a relatively deprived area as children and then moved to a relatively prosperous region later in life.

Clearly, geographic variations in blood pressure were strongly influenced by where the men had lived for most of their adult lives rather than by where they were born and brought up. It was thought unlikely that selective migration could account for these findings.[71] The authors concluded that regional differences in blood pressure in Britain were more closely linked to factors acting in adult life rather than those present early in life.

10.4 Conclusions

10.4.1 Ecological studies

Ecological studies have provided useful clues as to important risk factors for disease. Within England, both measures of past early life conditions and current deprivation show the strongest associations. Current measures of birthweight do not, however, show the same patterns, suggesting either that this is an inadequate measure or that the biological relationships between poor fetal growth and cardiovascular disease are different today from those in the past. Internationally, current adult risk factors and past measures of early life influences show associations with cardiovascular disease. In both cases, these appear stronger for cerebrovascular disease and there appears to be no relationship between past infant mortality rates and current ischaemic heart disease. These results highlight the importance of a life course approach since focusing solely on adult or early life factors is unlikely to explain adequately geographical variations in disease.

10.4.2 Migrant studies

The migrant studies conducted among Tokelau islanders, Yi farmers, Ethiopian Jews, and the Luo people, British men all provide compelling evidence that people moving from a low to a high blood pressure community experience a rise in blood pressure not seen in those who remain behind. This was observed in both children and adults, appeared to occur fairly rapidly after moving and could not be explained by selective migration. Nor could corresponding changes in weight fully account for the increase in blood pressure. Although the mechanism for the rise in blood pressure among migrants is not fully understood, the consistency of the findings in different migrant groups highlights the aetiological importance of factors acting *after* migration, in late childhood or adult life, on blood pressure levels. Interestingly, blood pressure studies among migrants provide no evidence to support Forsdahl's hypothesis that poverty early in life followed by later affluence raises the risk of CHD (and in this case blood pressure) to a level over and above that of long term residents in the host population.

Although genetic and early life factors may play a role in determining blood pressure levels and the risk of CHD, migrant studies reveal that factors acting at a later stage in the life cycle can exert an even greater influence. Looking to the future, migrant studies will continue to provide researchers with invaluable evidence for evaluating the impact of factors acting at different stages in the life course on CHD risk.

References

Those marked with an asterisk are especially recommended for further reading

1 Rothman KJ. *Modern Epidemiology*. Little, Brown and Company, Boston/Toronto 1986.
2 Morgenstern H. Uses of ecological analysis in epidemiological research. *Am J Public Health* 1982;**72**:1336–44.
3 Rose G. Sick individuals and sick populations. *Int J Epidemiol* 1985; **14**:32–8.
4 Intersalt Cooperative Research Group. Intersalt: an international study of electrolyte excretion and blood pressure. Results for 24 hour urinary sodium and potassium excretion. *Br Med J* 1988;**297**:319–28.
5 Schwartz S. The fallacy of the ecological fallacy: the potential misuse of a concept and the consequences. *Am J Public Health* 1994;**84**:819–23.
6 Susser M. The logic in ecological: I. The logic of analysis. *Am J Public Health* 1994;**84**:825–9.
7 Susser M. The logic in ecological: II. The logic of design. *Am J Public Health* 1994;**84**:830–5.

8   Macintyre S, MacIver S, Sooman A. Area, class and health: should we be focusing on places or people? *J Soc Pol* 1993;**22**:213–34.

9   Shouls S, Congdon P, Curtis S. Modelling inequality in reported long term illness in the UK: combining individual and area characteristics. *J Epidemiol Community Health* 1996;**50**:366–76.

10   Marmot MG, Davey Smith G. Why are the Japanese living longer? *Br Med J* 1989;**299**:1547–51.

11   Szatrowski TP, Peterson AVJ, Shimizu Y, Prentice RL, Mason MW, Fukunaga Y, et al. Serum cholesterol, other risk factors, and cardiovascular disease in a Japanese cohort. *J Chron Dis* 1984;**37**:569–84.

12   Charlton J. Which areas are healthiest? *Popul Trends* 1996;**83**:17–24.

13   Sauer HI. Epidemiology of cardiovascular mortality-geographic and ethnic. *Am J Public Health* 1962;**52**:94–105.

14   Antonovsky A. Social class and the major cardiovascular diseases. *J Chron Dis* 1968;**21**:65–106.

15   Carstairs V, Morris R. Deprivation: explaining differences in mortality between Scotland and England and Wales. *Br Med J* 1989;**299**:886–9.

16   Townsend P, Phillimore P, Beattie A. *Health and deprivation. Inequality and the North*. London: Croom Helm, 1988.

17   Eames M, Ben-Shlomo Y, Marmot MG. Social deprivation and premature mortality: regional comparison across England. *Br Med J* 1993;**307**:1097–102.

*18 Forsdahl A. Are poor living conditions in childhood and adolescence an important risk factor for arteriosclerotic heart disease? *Br J Prev Soc Med* 1977;**31**:91–5.

19   Williams DRR, Roberts SJ, Davies TW. Deaths from ischaemic heart disease and infant mortality in England and Wales. *J Epidemiol Community Health* 1979;**33**:199–202.

*20 Barker DJP, Osmond C. Infant mortality, childhood nutrition, and ischaemic heart disease in England and Wales. *Lancet* 1986;**1**:1077–81.

21   Buck C, Simpson H. Infant diarrhoea and subsequent mortality from heart disease and cancer. *J Epidemiol Community Health* 1982;**36**:27–30.

22   Barker DJP, Osmond C. Death rates from stroke in England and Wales predicted from past maternal mortality. *Br Med J* 1987;**295**:83–6.

23   Barker DJP, Osmond C. Childhood respiratory infection and adult chronic bronchitis in England and Wales. *Br Med J* 1986;**293**:1271–5.

*24 Ben-Shlomo Y, Davey Smith G. Deprivation in infancy or in adult life: which is more important for mortality risk? *Lancet* 1991;**337**:530–5.

25   Ben-Shlomo Y, White IR, Marmot M. Does the variation in the socioeconomic characteristics of an area affect mortality? *Br Med J* 1996;**312**:1013–4.

26   Barker DJP, Osmond C, Golding J. Height and mortality in the counties of England and Wales. *Ann Hum Biol* 1990;**17**:1–6.

*27 Barker DJP, Osmond C, Golding J, Kuh D, Wadsworth MEJ. Growth in utero, blood pressure in childhood and adult life, and mortality from cardiovascular disease. *Br Med J* 1989;**298**:564–7.

*28 Whincup PH, Cook DG, Adshead F, Taylor S, Papacosta O, Walker M, *et al*. Cardiovascular risk factors in British children from towns with widely differing adult cardiovascular mortality. *Br Med J* 1996;**313**: 79–84.

29 Marks RU. A review of empirical findings. *Milbank Mem Fund Q* 1967;**45**: part 2, 51–108.

30 Martin WJ. The distribution in England and Wales of mortality from coronary disease. *Br Med J* 1956;**1**:1523–5

31 Kleinman JC, DeGruttola VG, Cohen BB, Madans JH. Regional and urban-suburban differentials in coronary heart disease mortality and risk factor prevalence. *J Chron Dis* 1981;**34**:11–9

32 Tyroler HA, Cassel J. Health consequences on culture change-II. The effect of urbanization on coronary heart mortality in rural residents. *J Chron Dis* 1964;**17**:167–77.

33 Greenwood A *The health and physique of school children*.King PS & Son, Westminster. 1913.

34 Reading R, Raybould S, Jarvis S. Deprivation, low birthweight, and children's height: a comparison between rural and urban areas. *Br Med J* 1993;**307**:1458–62.

35 Barnett E, Strogatz D, Armstrong D, Wing S. Urbanisation and coronary heart disease mortality among African Americans in the US South. *J Epidemiol Community Health* 1996;**50**:252–7.

36 Krieger O, Aase A, Westin S. Ischaemic heart disease mortality among men in Norway: reversal of urban-rural difference between 1966 and 1989. *J Epidemiol Community Health* 1995;**49**:271–6.

37 Bennett N, Dodd T, Flately J, Freeth S, Bolling K. *Health Survey for England*. 1st ed. London: HMSO, 1993.

38 Shaper AG, Elford J. Regional variations in coronary heart disease in Great Britain: risk factors and changes in environment. In Marmot M, Elliott P, eds. *Coronary heart disease epidemiology: from aetiology to public health*. 2nd ed. Oxford: Oxford University Press, 1995:127–35.

39 Crombie IK, Smith WCS, Tavendale R, Tunstall-Pedoe H. Geographical clustering of risk factors and lifestyle for coronary heart disease in Scottish Heart Health Study. *Br Heart J* 1990;**64**:199–203

*40 Keys A. *Seven Countries: a multivariate analysis of death and coronary heart disease*. Cambridge, MA: Harvard University Press, 1980.

41 Keys A, Menotti A, Karvonen MJ, Aravanis C, Blackburn H, Buzina R, et al. The diet and 15-year death rate in the Seven Countries Study. *Am J Epidemiol* 1986;**124**:903–15.

42 Law MR, Wald NJ. An ecological study of serum cholesterol and

ischaemic heart disease between 1950 and 1990. *Eur J Clin Nutr 1994;* **48**:305–25.

43 Simons LA. Interrelations of lipids and lipoproteins with coronary artery disease mortality in 19 countries. *Am J Cardiol* 1986;**57**:5G–10G.

44 Kromhout D, Bloemberg PM, Feskens EJM, Hertog MGL, Menotti A, Blackburn H. Alcohol, fish, fibre and anti-oxidant vitamin intake do not explain population differences in coronary heart disease mortality. *Int J Epidemiol* 1996;**25**:753–9.

45 The World Health Organization MONICA Project. Ecological analysis of the association between mortality and major risk factors of cardio-vascular disease. *Int J Epidemiol* 1994;**94**:705–16.

46 Prior IAM, Stanhope JM, Grimley Evans J, Salmond CE. The Tokelau Island Migrant Study. *Int J Epidemiol* 1974;**3**:225–32.

47 Stanhope JM, Prior IAM. The Tokelau Island migrant study: prevalence of various conditions before migration. *Int J Epidemiol* 1976;**5**:259–66.

48 Beaglehole R, Eyles E, Prior I. Blood pressure and migration in children. *Int J Epidemiol* 1979;**8**:5–10.

49 Ward RH, Chin PG, Prior IAM. Tokelau Island Migrant Study, effect of migration on the familial aggregation of blood pressure. *Hypertension* 1980;**2 (Supp 1)**:I-43–54.

*50 Salmond CE, Joseph JG, Prior IAM, Stanley DG, Wessen AF. Longitudinal analysis of the relationship between blood pressure and migration: the Tokelau Island migrant study. *Am J Epidemiol* 1985; **122**:291–301.

51 Beaglehole R, Eyles E, Salmond C, Prior I. Blood pressure in Tokelauan children in two contrasting environments. *Am J Epidemiol* 1978;**108**: 283–8.

52 Joseph JG, Prior IAM, Salmond CE, Stanley D. Elevation of systolic and diastolic blood pressure associated with migration: the Tokelau Island migrant study. *J Chron Dis* 1983;**36**:507–16.

53 He J, Tell GS, Tang YC, Mo PS, He GQ. Effect of migration on blood pressure: the Yi people study. *Epidemiology* 1991;**2**:88–97.

*54 He J, Klag MJ, Whelton PK, Chen JY, Mo JP, Qian MC, Mo PS, He GQ. Migration, blood pressure pattern, and hypertension: the Yi migrant study. *Am J Epidemiol* 1991;**134**:1085–101.

55 He J, Klag MJ, Whelton PK, Chen JY, Qian MC, He GQ. Body mass and blood pressure in a lean population in southwestern China. *Am J Epidemiol* 1994;**139**:380–9.

56 Klag MJ, He J, Whelton PK, Chen JY, Qian MC, He GQ. Alcohol use and blood pressure in an acculturated society. *Hypertension* 1993;**22**: 365–70.

57 Rosen H. Ethiopian Jews: an historical sketch. *Israel J Med Sci* 1991; **27**:242–3.

*58 Goldbourt U, Khoury M, Landau E, Reisin LH, Rubinstein A. Blood pressure in Ethiopian immigrants: relationship to age and anthropometric factors, and changes during their first year in Israel. *Israel J Med Sci* 1991;**27**:264–7.

59   Bursztyn M, Raz I. Blood pressure and insulin in Ethiopian immigrants: longitudinal study. *J Hum Hypertens* 1995;**9**:245–8.

60   Rosenthal T, Grossman E, Knecht A, Goldbourt U. Blood pressure in Ethiopian immigrants in Israel: comparison with resident Israelis. *J Hypertens* 1989;**7 (suppl 1)**:S53–5.

61   Rosenthal T, Grossman E, Knecht A, Goldbourt U. Levels and correlates of blood pressure in recent and earlier Ethiopian immigrants to Israel. *J Hum Hypertens* 1990;**4**:425–30.

62   Goldbourt U, Rosenthal T, Rubinstein A. Trends in weight and blood pressure in Ethiopian immigrants during their first few years in Israel: epidemiological observations and implications for the future. *Israel J Med Sci* 1991;**27**:260–3.

63   Bursztyn M, Raz I. Blood pressure, glucose, insulin and lipids of young Ethiopian recent immigrants to Israel and in those resident for 2 years. *J Hypertens* 1993;**11**:455–9.

64   Green MS, Etzion T, Jucha E. Blood pressure and serum cholesterol among male Ethiopian immigrants compared to other Israelis. *J Epidemiol Community Health* 1991;**45**:281–6.

65   Poulter NR, Khaw KT, Sever PS. Higher blood pressures of urban migrants from an African low-blood pressure population are not due to selective migration. *Am J Hypertens* 1988;**1**:143S–145S.

*66 Poulter NR, Khaw KT, Hopwood BEC, Mugambi M, Peart WS, Rose G, Sever PS. The Kenyan Luo migration study: observations on the initiation of a rise in blood pressure. *Br Med J* 1990;**300**:967–72.

67   Poulter N, Khaw KT, Hopwood BEC, Mugambi M, Peart WS, Rose G, Sever PS. Blood pressure and its correlates in an African tribe in urban and rural environments. *J Epidemiol Community Health* 1984;**38**:181–6.

68   Poulter NR, Khaw KT, Mugambi M, Pearl WS, Sever PS. Migration-induced changes in blood pressure: a controlled longitudinal study. *Clin Exp Pharmacol Physiol* 1985;**12**:211–6.

69   Shaper AG, Ashby D, Pocock S. Blood pressure and hypertension in middle-aged British men. *J Hypertens* 1988;**6**:367–74.

70   Elford J, Phillips AN, Thomson AG, Shaper AG. Migration and geographic variations in blood pressure in Britain. *Br Med J* 1990;**300**:291–5.

71   Elford J, Whincup P, Shaper AG. Selective migration by birthweight. *J Epidemiol Community Health* 1993;**47**:336.

Appendix

Additional references on migration and coronary heart disease

Japan, Hawaii and California

72   Syme SL, Marmot MG, Kagan A, Kato H, Rhoads G. Epidemiologic studies of coronary heart disease and stroke in Japanese men living in Japan, Hawaii and California: introduction *Am J Epidemiol* 1975; **102**:477–80.

73   Worth Rm, Kato H, Rhoads GG, Kagan A, Syme SL.Epidemiologic studies of coronary heart disease and stroke in Japanese men living in Japan, Hawaii and California: mortality. *Am J Epidemiol* 1975;**102**: 481–90

74   Marmot MG, Syme SL, Kagan A, Kato H, Cohen JB, Belsky J. Epidemiologic studies of coronary heart disease and stroke in Japanese men living in Japan, Hawaii and California: prevalence of coronary and hypertensive heart disease and asociated risk factors. *Am J Epidemiol* 1975;**102**:514–25.

Australia

75   Powles JW, Hopper JL, Macaskill GT, Ktenas D. Blood pressure in subjects from rural Greece, comparing individuals migrating to Melbourne, Australia with non-migrant relatives. *J Hum Hypertens* 1993;**7**:419–28.

76   Armstrong BK, Margetts BM, Masarei, Hopkins SM. Coronary risk factors in Italian migrants to Australia. *Am J Epidemiol* 1983;**118**: 651–8.

77   Stenhouse NS, McCall MG. Differential mortality from cardiovascular disease in migrants from England and Wales, Scotland and Italy, and native-born Australians. *J Chron Dis* 1970;**23**:423–31.

Europe

78   Alfredsson L, Ahlbom A, Theorell T. Incidence of myocardial infarction among male Finnish immigrants in relation to length of stay in Sweden. *Int J Epidemiol* 1982;**11**:225–8.

79   Elford J, Phillips AN, Thomson AG, Shaper AG. Migration and geographic variations in ischaemic heart disease in Great Britain. *Lancet* 1989;**I**:343–6.

80   Marmot MG, Adelstein AM, Bulusu L. Lessons from the study of immigrant mortality. *Lancet* 1984;**I**:1455–7.

81   Strachan DP, Leon DA, Dodgeon B. Mortality from cardiovascular disease among interregional migrants in England and Wales. *Br Med J* 1995; **310**:423–7.

11 Socioeconomic differentials

George Davey Smith

Socioeconomic differentials in mortality from many causes of death are seen in adulthood. There has been a long tradition of considering early life influences which contribute to this, but more recently the specific contribution of adverse socioeconomic conditions in infancy and childhood on cardiovascular disease morbidity and mortality in adulthood has been investigated. Risk appears to accumulate over the life course, and independent contributions of childhood and adulthood socioeconomic circumstances to coronary heart disease incidence in adulthood are seen. Since exposures acting across the life course, together with the interactions between socially patterned exposures acting at different stages of life, contribute to disease risk, studies which have data concerning only one period of the life course are inadequate for further advancing our understanding of both disease aetiology and the production of socioeconomic differentials in health.

11.1 Introduction

Differences in life expectancy between social groups have been demonstrated since the early days of industrialization.[1] In 1845 Frederick Engels presented such data, using both area-based and individual indicators of socioeconomic position (Table 11.1).[2] Engels described the wretched housing conditions of the working people, the soul- and body-destroying work, the poor sanitary state of the city environment, and the inadequate diet which had to be contended with. The direct contribution of such factors to poor health seemed obvious to Engels, as it would to any reader of his book today.

Engels was writing at a time when the mortality experience of the inhabitants of some of the great cities was worsening[3] and the decline in overall population mortality rates which had been occurring in Britain had ceased.[4] From the 1860s on, however, mortality rates started to decline, first for children and young adults and then for older adults.[5] Infant mortality rates, interestingly,

Table 11.1 Mortality ratios (number of living people for each death) in Chorlton-on-Medlock, Manchester

Class of street	Class of house		
	1st (Best)	**2nd**	**3rd (Worst)**
1st (Best)	1/51	1/45	1/36
2nd	1/55	1/38	1/35
3rd (Worst)	—*	1/35	1/25

* no data
Source: Engels, 1845[2]

failed to fall until after the turn of the century. Mortality rates have continued to decline with only occasional reversals—for example, among middle aged men and women between 1920 and 1940.[6]

Socioeconomic differentials have persisted against this background of generally improving mortality rates. During the depression of the 1930s, another period when the influence of environmental adversity on poor health and increased mortality risk seemed obvious, Dr G C M M'Gonigle, Medical Officer of Health for Stockton-on-Tees, analyzed the mortality experience of a group of local residents over a 4 year period in relation to family income level.[7] Age-standardized death rates and family income were inversely related. The relationship was not simply one in which the very poor had high mortality: there was a steady gradient between family income and death rate.

From the years around the 1921 census onwards (with a trial run around the 1911 census) routine statistics on social class mortality differences have been produced, providing at international level the best longitudinal series of such data. For middle aged men from the years around the 1921 census to the years around the 1981 census dramatic declines in mortality have occurred for social classes I and II, while for social classes IV and V small and inconsistent decreases in mortality are seen. Increases in both the relative and absolute differentials in mortality between the social class groups have occurred since the early 1950s,[8,9] a pattern which recent data demonstrate has continued throughout the 1980s.[10]

Socioeconomic differentials in many, but not all, causes of death are currently seen in industrialized societies.[11–14] The usual tendency for disease risk to be higher for poorer members of society has encouraged some investigators to interpret socioeconomic differentials in health as in some way reflecting higher levels of susceptibility to disease in general amongst the socioeconomically disadvantaged.[15–18] The differences in the magnitude—and even direction—of associations between social position and various forms of morbidity and mortality offer a challenge to simplistic versions of the 'general susceptibility' hypothesis. This becomes even clearer when social factors acting across the life course are considered.

11.2 Socioeconomic position at different stages of life and mortality

Statistical studies of socioeconomic differentials in health have generally paid most attention to the influence of social position, and related differential exposures, in adulthood. The notion that unfavourable social environments in early life could adversely affect health in adulthood has long been held, however.[2,5,19] Engels considered that the mortality of working class children was clear evidence of unwholesome living conditions. He went on to quote from the report of Dr Loudon to the factories enquiry commission that

> 'The consequence is that many have died prematurely, and others are afflicted for life with defective constitutions, and the fear of a posterity enfeebled by the shattered constitution of the survivors is but too well founded, from a physiological point of view.'

Writing on the state of health in poor areas of the country during the depression of the 1930s, Wal Hannington, leader of the National Unemployed Workers Movement considered that unemployment had an adverse effect on youth through the undernourishment of their mothers during pregnancy.[20] Other, less activist, authors held similar opinions of the long term effects on health of conditions in early life. H M Vernon, investigator for the Industrial Health Research Board, considered that with

> 'the provision of adequate nourishment at all stages of human existence, we should find a further diminution of infant mortality, which has already improved so remarkably in recent years, and . . . we should find considerable improvement in the health and physique of the children. Such improvement would certainly lead to a healthier adult life'[21]

and went on to state that adequate nutrition is

> 'specially important, not only for children but for expectant and nursing mothers, if good physique coupled with good health, is to be attained when the children reach adult life'.

In early epidemiological studies of coronary heart disease concern was shown with socioeconomic position in early life, but this mostly related to the investigation of hypothesized influences of social incongruity—e.g. the possible stress of moving from a disadvantaged background into the (perceived) stressful environment of the professional and managerial world.[22] The interest in possible specific effects of socioeconomic deprivation in early life on later health was instigated by the work of Forsdahl[23,24] (subsequently developed by Barker and Osmond[25]), who demonstrated that areas with high infant mortality rates earlier this century had high coronary heart disease (CHD) rates currently. Forsdahl interpreted this as demonstrating that deprivation in early life, followed by later affluence, worked together to increase coronary risk, in part mediated by elevation of blood cholesterol concentrations.[26]

Several studies have now investigated the association between childhood socioeconomic circumstances and disease risk in adulthood.[27–36] In a cohort of 35–64 year old men recruited from workplaces in the west of Scotland in the early 1970s, mortality over a 21 year period has been related to fathers social class, social class at labour market entry, and social class at the time of screening. Social position at each stage of the lifecourse is related to all cause, cardiovascular disease, cancer, and other mortality (Table 11.2).[37] When analysed simultaneously, father's social class and social class at screening both remained predictors of mortality, while social class at labour market entry became non-predictive. For all-cause mortality the manual to non-manual relative risks were the same for father's social class and current social class. When different cause of death groups are examined, father's social class makes a particular contribution to cardiovascular disease risk, while it is only weakly and non-significantly associated with cancer mortality once social class at

Table 11.2 Mortality by social class at three different stages of the life course

Age adjusted relative rates for manual compared with non-manual social class locations, with individual and simultaneous adjustments for each social class indicator

	Father's social class	First social class	Current social class
All cause			
Individual	1.44 (1.27–1.64)	1.29 (1.16–1.43)	1.40 (1.27–1.55)
Simultaneous	1.28 (1.11–1.47)	1.01 (0.89–1.16)	1.29 (1.14–1.47)
Cardiovascular			
Disease Individual	1.58 (1.32–1.89)	1.35 (1.16–1.56)	1.38 (1.20–1.59)
Simultaneous	1.41 (1.15–1.72)	1.08 (0.90–1.30)	1.20 (1.01–1.43)
Cancer			
Individual	1.26 (1.02–1.56)	1.25 (1.04–1.50)	1.35 (1.13–1.61)
Simultaneous	1.11 (0.87–1.41)	1.04 (0.82–1.31)	1.28 (1.03–1.60)
Non Cardiovascular, Non cancer			
Individual	1.45 (1.07–1.98)	1.18 (0.92–1.53)	1.59 (1.24–2.03)
Simultaneous	1.28 (0.91–1.80)	0.80 (0.58–1.10)	1.67 (1.22–2.28)

Source: Davey Smith G et al, 1997[37]

screening is taken into account. For non-cardiovascular, non-cancer mortality, social class at screening also appears to be the more important socioeconomic marker.

Most,[27–32,36,37] but not all[33,38] studies have revealed an association of childhood socioeconomic circumstances with CHD risk, which is apparently not purely due to adverse social class destinations of those born into poor circumstances. Stroke risk has also been found to be higher in those with less favourable socioeconomic circumstances in childhood.[39] In a Swedish census follow up, men with fathers in manual occupations had considerably higher coronary heart disease mortality risk than those whose fathers were in non-manual occupations.[31] For all-cause mortality the association with father's social class was less clear, with mortality being dependent on adult social class to a considerably greater degree than childhood social class. The particular dependence of CHD risk in comparison with other causes of death on childhood socioeconomic circumstances has also been observed in area-based studies from Finland.[40,41] Analyses of the association between height and cause-specific mortality, in which height is taken, in part at least, to be an indicator of childhood circumstances, demonstrate similar specificity.[42]

Studies which have examined socioeconomic circumstances in early life and later affluence have provided little support for the component of the Forsdahl hypothesis relating to an interaction between childhood deprivation and affluence in adult life.[27,30,36] The suggestion that the effects of early life deprivation are mediated through high blood cholesterol concentrations in adulthood has also received little support.[30,36] In the west of Scotland cohort, cardiovascular disease risk factors were analyzed in relation to childhood and adult social class.[43] Men with manual social class fathers had lower, rather than higher, serum cholesterol concentrations compared with men with non-manual fathers. Behavioural risk factors, such as smoking and exercise, were more dependent on adulthood social position than parental social class. This supports the notion that such activities are powerfully influenced by the social environment experienced during adult life, and that their modification is dependent upon the presence of the social circumstances required for maintaining favourable health-related behaviours. A similar analysis by education and social class supported this finding; smoking behaviour was unrelated to years of education once achieved social class was taken into account.[44] Blood pressure and lung function are associated with both current and parental social class, but more strongly with the former. This suggests that exposures—such as smoking and occupational exposures in relation to lung function, or alcohol and other dietary factors in relation to blood pressure, are more dependent upon adult than childhood social circumstances. However, body mass index and triglyceride levels were dependent on childhood social class rather than current social class: men with manual fathers had higher body mass indices and higher triglyceride levels than men with non-manual fathers, and once fathers' social class was taken into account there was no association of current social class with body mass index and if anything a reverse association for triglycerides: i.e. higher triglyceride levels amongst the men in non-manual rather than manual occupations in adulthood. High body mass index and elevated triglycerides are components of the insulin resistance syndrome. This is compatible with some studies that have indicated that the concomitants of adverse childhood socioeconomic circumstances are associated with an elevated risk of diabetes and impaired glucose tolerance in adulthood.[45,46] The components of insulin resistance syndrome cluster in childhood[47,48] and this clustering tracks into adulthood. This suggests that a common factor, already active in young childhood, underlies the risk of syndrome X from early life onwards.

A Finnish study also failed to find an association between poor childhood socioeconomic circumstances and high cholesterol levels in adulthood.[30] In this study there was no consistent influence of childhood socioeconomic position on smoking behaviour or blood pressure,[39] as is true of a Norwegian study.[26] In the 1946 and 1958 British birth cohort studies, obesity and high body mass index in adulthood were more prevalent among participants with fathers in manual social class occupations.[49,50] Fibrinogen levels have been found to be higher in men and women whose fathers were in manual rather than non-manual occupations,[51] although among Finnish men the association between unfavourable childhood socioeconomic circumstances and fibrinogen was only seen amongst those participants who themselves had low incomes in adult life.[52]

As with the heterogeneity in strength and direction of associations between adult social circumstances and cause-specific mortality, the heterogeneity of the associations between childhood social circumstances and health in adult life argue against general susceptibility (or miasma) accounts of inequalities in health. For breast cancer in women, for example, rates tend to be higher for those in more favourable socioeconomic circumstances.[53] This is reflected in a positive association between height and breast cancer risk in some studies[54] (see Chapter 3, section 3.3.2). Cohort analyses have also suggested that nutrition in childhood, which will be socially patterned, is related to breast cancer risk, with higher calorie intake being associated with increased risk.[55] The long term follow up of children in whom leg length, a sensitive indicator of nutritional status in childhood, was measured in the late 1930s reveals that longer legs in childhood are associated with lower cardiovascular disease mortality in adulthood in males and females, but with higher cancer mortality among males.[56]

Although there is some evidence for the contribution of early life socioeconomic position to respiratory disease, diabetes, and some cancers in adulthood, most investigations have related to cardiovascular disease. The remainder of the chapter will focus on cardiovascular disease, and particularly CHD.

11.3 Was there a social class cross-over in cardiovascular disease?

Currently there are large social class gradients in mortality from all the major cardiovascular diseases. Figure 11.1 displays social class differences in ischaemic heart disease, stroke and all-cause mortality for men of working ages between 1976 and 1989.[10] The socioeconomic distribution of cardiovascular disease mortality is reflected in morbidity rates. In a large survey of over 20 000 people aged 35 and over in Somerset and Avon, England, histories of angina, myocardial infarction, and stroke were all more common amongst individuals living in deprived compared with affluent areas.[57] Socioeconomic position is also related to the early stages of developing cardiovascular disease. For example, low income, manual occupation, and little education are all related to an increased degree of carotid atherosclerosis in a Finnish study.[58]

It has been widely considered that cardiovascular disease used to affect the rich more than the poor. This generalization is, in fact, only true if the category of ischaemic heart disease is considered alone. In the analysis of social class differences in mortality around the 1911 census,[59] for example, non-manual social class men did have high mortality attributed to 'angina pectoris

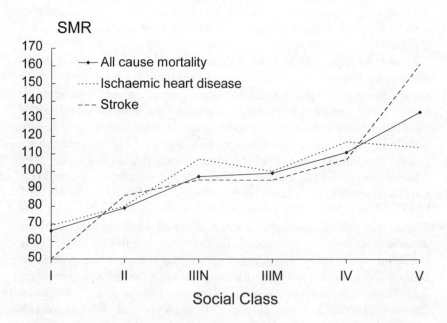

Figure 11.1 Social class differences in mortality of men aged 15–64 between 1976 and 1989 from various causes of death.
Source: Harding, 1995[10]

and arteriosclerosis' (deaths were not attributed to CHD during this period), but for overall overall circulatory disease mortality this was not the case.

Conditions now subsumed into the category 'coronary artery disease' were considered a disease of the affluent classes from the time they were first recognised. Dr Samuel Black of Newry, County Down, in the eighteenth century, described many cases of angina pectoris and contributed to the development of the hypothesis that ischaemia underlay angina pectoris.[60] He described factors which were associated with increased or decreased susceptibility to angina pectoris (Table 11.3). The congruence of Black's views and current day thinking is remarkable. He recognized exercise, being female, and being French as reducing risk, while lack of exercise, obesity, being male, 'full and plethoric habits' and stress were seen to increase risk. He also considered the better ranks of society to be more liable to the disease, whereas the poor were relatively exempt.

The perceived increased susceptibility of 'the better ranks of society' persisted during the first two decades of this century as the full spectrum of coronary artery disease, including myocardial infarction, was recognised. Large social class differences, with the non-manual groups having considerably greater mortality risk than the manual groups, were seen in the analyses around the 1911, 1921 and 1931 censuses.[61] Writing in 1950 Dr Ian Stewart invoked George Orwells *1984*, stating that Orwell saw the workers of 1949 as the 'proles' of 1984 for whom

Table 11.3 Dr Samuel Black's categorisation of factors related to liability and exemption from angina pectoris

Liable
The male sex
The better ranks of society
The psychologically stressed
Those with an ossific diathesis
Those with an accumulation of fat around the heart
Those with full and plethoric habits who live luxuriously
Those with insufficient exercise
The obese

Exempt
The female sex
The poor The laborious
Those who use strong exercise
The foot-soldier
The French

Source: Evans, 1995[60]

'heavy physical work, the care of home and children, petty quarrels with neighbours, films, football, beer, and, above all, gambling, filled up the horizon of their minds. To keep them in control was not difficult.'

The prolcs, however, were the only happy people in Oceana, Stewart goes on, and one can be sure that like their prototypes—the working class of 1949—they were little troubled by coronary disease.[62]

Sir Robert Platt took issue with Stewart's claim that 'the better educated and those who work with their brains are more liable than their fellows to coronary disease'. Platt quoted data from the Registrar Generals *Decennial Supplement* for 1931 showing standardized coronary heart disease mortality rates being:

agricultural workers 32;

coal-miners below ground 40;

banking and insurance officials 183;

Anglican clergy 218;

physicians and surgeons 368.[63]

There was, apparently, a huge (10-fold) gradient in coronary heart disease mortality across these occupational groups. Platt went on, however, to suggest that the likelihood of persons dying between 1930–32 after having seen a consulting cardiologist, would be in the following order:

physicians and surgeons;

Anglican clergy;

banking and insurance officials;

coal-miners below ground;

agricultural workers.

The clear implication was that varying diagnostic practices for members of different social groups, partly due to the types of physicians they consulted, generated the apparent CHD morbidity differentials. Coronary disease would, in the early 1930s, often be recorded as myocardial degeneration and myocarditis. Mortality from these categories was higher among manual than non-manual groups.

In England and Wales the published analyses of social class differences in mortality around each census since 1911 allow for the construction of better time series of socioeconomic differentials in mortality than is possible for other countries.[64] Table 11.4 presents data from these *Decennial Supplements*. Taken at face value, these data demonstrate higher rates of coronary artery disease mortality among the non-manual social class groups for men, with differentials increasing and the gradient becoming more consistent from 1911 to 1931, then the gradient weakening by 1951 and having reversed by 1961. For married women data became available from 1931 onwards, and a gradient of increasing

Table 11. 4 Cardiovascular disease by social class among men 1911-1981: standardised mortality ratios

Diseases of the circulatory system	I	II	IIIn	IIIm	IV	V
1911	89	94	95		96	141
1921	92	101	94		96	117
1931	102	102	96		100	106
1951	123	102	102		86	102
1961	92	92	104		98	121
1971	86	89	110	106	110	118
1981	68	79	100	105	112	145

Heart Disease	I	II	IIIn	IIIm	IV	V
1911	–	–	–		–	–
1921	92	101	93		97	105
1931	98	101	95		102	109
1951	123	102	103		85	101
1961	94	93	105		97	116
1971	86	89	113	107	109	115
1981	69	80	101	105	111	141

Coronary artery disease etc	I	II	IIIn	IIIm	IV	V	% of all heart disease
*1911	161	106	98		92	99	9*
*1921	156	109	93		85	115	14
1931	237	147	96		67	67	14
1951	147	110	105		79	89	70
1961	98	95	106		96	112	87
1971	88	91	114	107	108	111	90
1981	69	81	102	106	110	137	92

* includes 'arteriosclerosis'
1910–1912 data for men aged 25–65, excluding textile workers, miners and agricultural workers.
1921–1923; 1930–1932 data for men aged 20–65.
1970–1972 data for men aged 15–64.
1979, 1980, 1982, 1983 data for men aged 20–64.

mortality risk from a broad CHD category from wives of higher non-manual men to wives of unskilled manual men has been seen over the entire period.[70]

Studies of the validity of death certification data for CHD demonstrate that these can be unreliable.[65] Comparisons of clinical and death certification diagnoses with autopsy data from the 1910s to the 1950s show initially high levels of premortem underdiagnosis of coronary heart disease, with other forms of heart disease, cerebrovascular disease, renal and respiratory disease being frequent erroneous diagnoses for CHD cases.[66,67] If such misclassification were differential with respect to socioeconomic position in the period up until 1960, it could certainly be substantial enough to allow for the generation of the magnitude of social class differences seen. Unfortunately the only study which has explicitly examined misclassification according to social class used data from the mid-1970s.[68] There are two approaches to evaluating the role of misclassification of cause of death. First, registered coronary artery mortality can be combined with mortality from other conditions within which deaths will be misclassified. Second, social class differences in heart disease mortality at younger ages can be examined, since death certification validation studies also demonstrate that missed CHD diagnoses are less common at younger ages.

Combining categories reveals that only for the 1951 *Decennial Supplement* did overall heart disease mortality show any suggestion of a positive social class gradient (Table 11.4), and even here this was due to high rates in social class I compared with the other social class groups. All-cause mortality in the 1951 *Decennial Supplement* also showed unexpectedly high rates for social class I and unexpectedly low rates for social class IV. The Chief Medical Statistican responsible for the 1951 Decennial Supplement considered that misclassification of occupation had caused numerator–denominator bias and later corrected the all-cause data for this.[69] Mortality rates for males aged 20–64 were recalculated as shown in Table 11.5. Corrected data for cause-specific mortality are not available, but it is clear the general pattern of high mortality in social class I and low mortality in social class IV, seen to be erroneous with respect to all-cause mortality, is the pattern seen in the uncorrected data with respect to heart disease mortality.

Combining heart disease with respiratory disease mortality would produce increasing mortality gradients from social class I to social class V for each

Table 11.5 All cause mortality by social class among men. 1951 Dicennial Supplement: standardized mortality ratios, before and after correction

	Social Class				
	I	II	III	IV	V
uncorrected	98	86	101	94	118
corrected	86	92	101	104	118

Decennial Supplement period. Although some deaths categorized as respiratory were certainly CHD deaths, and this misclassification may be differential with respect to social class, using such a combination would represent overcompensation. Following earlier analyses[70 72] a non-valvular heart disease category—which probably corresponds most closely to coronary heart disease—was constructed for earlier periods, and ratios of mortality in social classes IV and V compared with social classes I and II for men in age groups 25–44 and 45–64 have been calculated (Table 11.6). At younger ages there has never been a marked social class I and II excess, which is only seen at all and in a very weak way for the 1951 *Decennial Supplement*, for which misclassification of occupation caused serious problems. It has been suggested that coronary heart disease emerged first among the affluent, with the elevated risk staying with this group as they aged, then emerged among less affluent groups at a later stage.[73] This notion of a generational social class cross-over in coronary heart disease risk is not supported by these data. Thus the young manual men demonstrating increased CHD risk around the 1911 and 1921 censuses would have been middle aged in 1931 and 1951, but a large apparent gradient in an opposite direction is seen in this older age group at these later periods.

In ad hoc US studies using routine data from 1930 to 1960, total heart disease and CHD mortality generally showed either no consistent association with socioeconomic position or an inverse gradient: higher rates among the less affluent,[61,74–79] although there were occasional exceptions which showed weak positive gradients.[80,81] Widespread recognition of coronary heart disease occurred earlier in the US than in the UK, with physicians in the former being more likely to certify this as a cause of death,[82] a difference which may have contributed to the much higher rates of coronary mortality in the US than the UK around the mid-century. This earlier recognition of

Table 11.6 Ratio of non-valvular heart disease mortality among men in social classes IV and V to social classes I and II, by age

	25–44	45–64
1911	1.40	0.71
1921	1.10	0.87
1931	1.03	0.94
1951	0.96	0.85
1961	1.36	1.15
1971	1.75	1.31
1981	2.09	1.57

CHD in the US would leave less possibility for the creation of artefactual socioeconomic differences due to differential underregistration of this cause of death among less affluent groups.

11.3.1 Geographical distribution of coronary heart disease

The geographical distribution of CHD has remained stable, unlike the apparently changing social class differentials. Rates have always been higher in the north west of England than in the south east.[83,84] This gradient is not congruent with the proposed positive association between coronary disease and socioeconomic position seen in the 1931 and 1951 *Decennial Supplements*, since the north west has remained a less prosperous region than the south east over the century.[85] Analyses for England and Wales in the early 1950s found, if anything, an inverse association between percentage of the population in an area in social class I and II and the CHD mortality rate in men.[86] In Baltimore in 1949–51, coronary mortality among men and women was unrelated to the socioeconomic characteristics of their census tract of residence.[87] One reason for the discrepancy between studies relating individual socioeconomic characteristics to certified cause of death and those using ecological indicators of socioeconomic position could be that diagnostic differences between social groups may occur *within* areas—i.e. the professional groups would be more likely to see specialists than the poorer groups—but such differences would not necessarily be seen *between* large geographical areas, all of which would contain a mixture of specialist and generalist physicians.

In the UK and the US urban areas consistently experienced higher CHD mortality rates than rural areas from the 1930s to the 1970s.[88] In the US, but not the UK, the rural advantage has been lost in recent years.[88] In the US stroke mortality has consistently been higher in rural areas. Rural areas are poorer on average than metropolitan areas, so earlier this century rural residence would confound the associations between socioeconomic measures and CHD risk. Thus a mortality follow up of US railroad workers from the early 1950s found higher all-cause and CHD mortality among clerical workers than switchmen or section men, who were manual workers (the former with generally higher responsibility jobs).[89] This finding, for both coronary and non-coronary mortality, is compatible with the urban concentration of clerical workers and more rural residence of section men.

11.3.2 Objective data

Most early information regarding the distribution of CHD comes from routine death certification, in which the problems of differential misclassification according to socioeconomic position are maximized. Studies which obtained comparable data—with objective measures of disease, or with classificatory methods which were standardized across social groups—are required, but are unfortunately limited for the period under consideration. Evidence of coronary artery disease at autopsy is a potentially objective measure, but decedents who are autopsied do not constitute a representative sample of all deaths. Early US autopsy series, covering the period 1910–37, produced conflicting results regarding the socioeconomic distribution of coronary artery disease,[90,91] perhaps reflecting this problem. In Denmark, Iceland and Austria in the late 1930s, autopsy series found no association between the extent of atherosclerosis and the intellectual versus physical nature of work—intellectual workers presumably being in more favourable socioeconomic circumstances.[92] The most extensive relevant study covered deaths in the UK between 1954 and 1956.[93] This study focused on physical activity of work but reported that among non-coronary deaths evidence of ischaemic myocardial fibrosis showed a positive social class gradient. This gradient was abolished by stratifying by occupational physical activity.

Table 11.7 summarizes the results of studies with defined samples and standardized measures of disease prevalence or incidence among men carried out in the UK or the US, with initial recruitment up until 1960. The overall picture is one of no, or an inverse, association between social position and CHD prevalence and incidence. The only exception is the Evans County study. This largely rural population study revealed that higher social status men had a higher prevalence of CHD in 1960, when the investigation was initiated. However, incident CHD showed no association with social position. The anomalous prevalence data, when compared with the other studies with objective measures of disease, could reflect differences in survival and recruitment, or a genuine gradient in this population at the time the study was carried out, perhaps due to the conflating of social position and degree of urbanization in this largely rural area.

In conclusion, the evidence for a marked positive social gradient in CHD earlier this century is considerably weaker than is generally supposed. There is certainly no strong support for the notion that such an association ever existed among women. From the 1930s through to the 1960s the lack of a positive social gradient among men was constantly rediscovered,[94,153] with many authors expressing surprise at the lack of, or inverse, association between social position and CHD that they found. As Mortensen and colleagues wrote in 1959, 'The popular notion that high executive positions are associated with high coronary mortality is likely due to the greater publicity connected with such deaths rather than to statistical facts'.[96]

Table 11.7 US and UK coronary heart disease studies with defined populations and objective measures of CHD

Study name	Period of study entry	Country	Socioeconomic indicator	Coronary heart disease measure	Association between socioeconomic position and CHD	References
Thomas	1954–58	UK	social class	prevalent CHD;	0	137, 138
Stamler	1954–57	US	occupation, education, income	prevalent CHD and 4 year CHD incidence	0	139, 140
Chapman	1949	US	occupation	5 year CHD mortality	0	141
Framingham	1949	US	education	6 year CHD incidence	–	142
Bell Telephone	1935	US	education	30 year CHD mortality prevalence in survivors in 1962	mortality - prevalence -	143
Brown	1956	UK	social class	prevalent CHD; 1 year CHD incidence	all forms 0 myocardial infarction + other forms of CHD -	144,145
Western Electric	1957	US	occupation	4.5 year CHD incidence	0	146

Du Pont	1956	US	occupation, income group	1, and 6 year CHD incidence	1 year - 6 years -	147,148
Albany	1953–54	US	income, education	6 year CHD incidence	–	149,150
Commission on Chronic Illness	1953–55	US	income	prevalent CHD	–	151
Evans County	1960	US	social status, based on income, education and occupation	prevalent CHD; 2 year CHD incidence	prevalence +* incidence 0	152
Lee	early 1950s	US	occupation	5 year cumulative prevalent CHD	–	153

0 = no consistent association
- = inverse socioeconomic gradient
+ = positive socioeconomic gradient
* = statistically significant; otherwise not significant or not reported

11.4 Adult factors contributing to socioeconomic differentials in cardiovascular disease

Several studies have investigated the contribution of particular health related behaviours and physiological risk factors to mortality differentials. One of the first studies with objective data on CHD incidence, which demonstrated higher rates amongst men with lower income,[148] investigated this through comparing blood pressure levels, cholesterol concentrations, obesity, and smoking patterns of higher and lower income groups.[96] Only small differences in these factors were found between income groups and they did not appear able to account for the differences in disease incidence. The risk factor data did not relate to the individuals experiencing coronary heart disease events in this study, however, so a direct assessment of their contribution to socioeconomic differentials could not be made.

The first Whitehall study of London civil servants demonstrated considerable differences in all-cause mortality risk according to two socioeconomic measures—employment grade in the civil service and car ownership.[11] Car ownership was a good indicator of available income in the late 1960s, when this study was established.[97] The observed differences between the top grade civil servants who owned cars and the lowest grade civil servants who did not were 3–4-fold. Smoking behaviour was patterned such that the lower grade and non-car owning civil servants were more likely to smoke than the higher grade and car-owning ones, but the pattern of mortality differentials among men who had never smoked was identical to that of the whole cohort.[98,99]

Cardiovascular disease mortality showed very similar associations with employment grade and car ownership to all-cause mortality. Cholesterol levels were greater among high grade than low grade civil servants in the late 1960s, when this study was established. Differences in cholesterol levels could not, therefore, account for the higher rates of coronary heart disease among the lower grade employees. This can be taken to suggest that differences in dietary fat intake between grades were not responsible for the coronary heart disease mortality differentials. Indeed, simultaneous consideration of a range of risk factors—including smoking, blood pressure, cholesterol levels, and prevalent cardiorespiratory disease—failed to account for the grade differences in cardiovascular and non-cardiovascular mortality.[11]

A prospective study of a third of a million men screened for the Multiple Risk Factor Intervention Trial between 1970 and 1973, with 16 years of mortality follow up, found a strong inverse association between the income level of the area of residence of the men and their risk of mortality from coronary heart disease and stroke.[13] Adjustment for smoking, cholesterol levels, blood pressure, and diabetes somewhat attenuated these associations, but it did not remove them. Prospective studies from Sweden, Finland,

Denmark, and the US, using a variety of indices of social position, have reached essentially the same conclusions,[101–107] for both men and women. It has been suggested that the residual associations seen between social class and coronary heart disease incidence are due to the inaccuracy inherent in using single measurements of risk factors as proxy measures of lifetime exposure.[108] While measurement imprecision in these risk factors renders the exploration of causes of differentials problematic,[109,110] the use of social class alone leads to a marked underestimation of the strength of the relationship between socioeconomic position and mortality.[99] Studies with more accurate classification of socioeconomic circumstances demonstrate much greater differentials than those using cruder measures, such as occupational class.[97,104] Studies with precise measurement of life course socioeconomic position and risk factors are required to take this issue forward.

As a result of the finding that conventional risk factors fail to account adequately for the social distribution of cardiovascular disease, the Whitehall II study was initiated in 1985 to explore additional psychosocial, behavioural, dietary and metabolic factors which could contribute to the socioeconomic differentials in health. The baseline examinations demonstrated that higher grade civil servants, with higher incomes, had lower prevalence of cardiorespiratory disease, among both sexes.[111] Average cholesterol levels were similar in each grade, but concentrations of serum apolipoprotein AI, the main structural protein of HDL cholesterol, showed an association with grade[112] and suggested that characteristic disturbances of lipid metabolism associated with lower occupational status were potentially identifiable. Several of the components of the insulin resistance syndrome—waist–hip ratio, glucose 2 h after an oral load, insulin 2 h after an oral load, triglyceride levels, and (inversely) HDL cholesterol levels—clustered amongst civil servants in low employment grades.[113] Fibrinogen levels, as discussed previously, were also higher amongst the lower grade civil servants.[51]

A study of Finnish men constitutes the most detailed prospective investigation of factors contributing to the socioeconomic gradient in cardiovascular mortality undertaken to date.[114] The risk of all-cause and cardiovascular disease mortality across quintiles of adulthood income showed 2.5–3-fold differences. It was possible to adjust for 22 risk factors: plasma fibrinogen, serum HDL cholesterol, serum apolipoprotein B, blood leukocytes, serum copper, mercury in hair, serum ferritin, blood haemoglobin, serum triglycerides, systolic blood pressure, body mass index, height, cardiorespiratory fitness, cigarette smoking, alcohol consumption, leisure time physical activity, depression, hopelessness, cynical hostility, participation in organizations, quality of social support, and marital status.[114] On adjustment for all these factors the association between social position and cardiovascular disease mortality was greatly attenuated, while the associations between social position and all (fatal and non-fatal) CHD incidence remained substantial. As the authors acknowledge, it is difficult to interpret such analyses, for several reasons. First, some of the factors adjusted for may be markers of existing disease (e.g. blood leukocytes, fibrinogen), and statistical adjustment for these could, in essence, be adjusting for the presence of cardiovascular disease, which is itself produced by social factors. The reduction in relative risks in the lower income groups which occurs on adjustment for these factors cannot be taken as demonstrating the 'explanation' of why the social distribution of cardiovascular mortality exists. Second, some factors, such as height, body mass index, serum triglycerides, may be the outcome of socioeconomic processes which act in early life. Adjusting for them similarly fails to account for the reasons for the social distribution in cardiovascular mortality, since it automatically leads to questions as to how childhood social conditions may influence insulin resistance syndrome and thus coronary disease risk. Finally, the reasons for the social distribution of certain behaviours, such as smoking and exercise, should itself become a target for explanation.[100]

11.5 Early life factors and the social distribution of cardiovascular disease

The apparent difficulty of uncovering socially patterned biological influences in the adult environment which adequately account for the social distribution of cardiovascular disease led Barker[115] to postulate that the environment during fetal and infant life programmes people from socioeconomically unfavourable backgrounds—who are likely to be in similarly relatively unfavourable circumstances in adult life—to be at an elevated risk of cardiovascular disease. Referring to the demonstration that infant mortality earlier this century correlates with cardiovascular disease mortality currently,[25] Barker considered that in a similar way early life factors could influence the social distribution of these (and other) diseases. He concluded that 'the seeds of inequalities in health in the next century are being sown today—in inner cities and other communities where adverse influences impair the growth, nutrition and health of mothers and their infants'.[115]

With respect to CHD this explanation encounters difficulties when considerations turn to the increase in CHD mortality from the beginning of the century to the mid-1970s. The apparent higher rate of CHD among the affluent earlier this century has also been seen to be problematic, although as discussed above the evidence for this has been overstated. Material conditions which would influence early life development have improved through the century.[116] This is mirrored in an almost unbroken decline in infant mortality rate.[116] Barker advanced a two-stage hypothesis to account for the trends in CHD,[117] with the high energy western diet being implicated as the adulthood factor of importance.[115] The need to postulate interactions between early life and later life factors also applies when accounting for the low rates of coronary heart disease in some developing countries, where very poor maternal and infant health existed when the adults of today were born.[118]

Infant mortality rates showed large social class differences earlier this century,[119] which is compatible with current social class differentials in cardiovascular disease mortality. When examining trends the association is less clear. Even given the problems with cause of death classification, it is clear that there have been increasing socioeconomic differentials in coronary heart disease and stroke mortality since 1961.[10,120–122] These have been most marked at younger ages, where semi-skilled and unskilled manual groups have always exhibited higher coronary heart disease rates than higher and intermediate non-manual groups.[123] All age groups from 25–34 to 55–64 show increasing manual to non-manual ratios from 1951 onwards. Thus social class differences in infant mortality during an identified earlier period could only account for the time trends if a steady accelerating increase in differentials since the 1870s can be observed. This is not what the, admittedly imperfect, data suggest. While social class differentials in infant mortality seem to have increased from 1895 to 1911,[124] there was then a stabilization or possibly a decrease in the relative magnitude of the social class differentials, even when the changing size of social class groups is taken into account.[125] These trends are not compatible with the observed recent parallel widening of social class differences in CHD and stroke mortality among all age groups.

The correlations between maternal mortality earlier this century and current CHD and stroke mortality have been taken to indicate the influence of maternal physique and health on the long term cardiovascular disease risk of their offspring.[126] Maternal mortality was higher in the more affluent social groups earlier this century,[127] however, and is thus not congruent with the socioeconomic distribution of cardiovascular disease mortality between the 1960s and the 1980s. The complex causes of maternal mortality make it a problematic ecological indicator of influences which may be detrimental to the intrauterine development of children,[127] and little can be made of this discrepancy.

Another approach to investigating the possible contribution of early life factors to social class differentials in mortality currently is to examine trends in social class differences in height. Height can be taken to be an indicator of early environment, including nutrition (see discussion in Chapter 3, section 3.2.3). Stature displays an inverse socioeconomic gradient and short stature is associated with increased CHD risk. Stature has increased for men and women over the century,[128] which is consistent with declining mortality rates from various causes. It has been argued that trends in height over a longer period underlie changes in life expectancy.[129] Social class differences in height show a slow convergence in men and a slow divergence in women. These do not mirror the changes in social class differentials in cardiovascular disease mortality for successive birth cohorts.

Adult height is related to childhood height, but relative and absolute height differentials are generally greater in childhood than adulthood, reflecting the ability of catch-up growth to compensate for restricted earlier growth, partly through an extension of the growing period. Insults which reduce growth in the first 4 years of life appear to endure into adulthood, however.[130] The long term influences of childhood environment would be better indexed by examining height in childhood rather than adult height. Social class differences in the height of children have persisted through the century.[131] Only limited data exist regarding changes in magnitude of social class differences over time, but they did not appear to greatly increase or decrease from the turn of the century to the mid-1950s.[132] No parallelism with trends in socioeconomic differentials in cardiovascular disease mortality can be demonstrated.

In summary, infant mortality and height, but not maternal mortality, demonstrated social class differences earlier this century which are congruent with present day social class differences in cardiovascular disease mortality. However, *trends* in the socioeconomic differentials of these indicators do not parallel trends in coronary heart disease differentials, except in the case of maternal mortality where the cross-over of social class differences in maternal mortality in the mid-1930s can be considered to be consistent with the widening social class differentials in coronary heart disease mortality which are currently seen. The general lack of parallelism between differentials in these indicators of early development and present day differentials in cardiovascular disease occurrence is similar to the failure of differentials in stroke mortality between greater London and the rest of south east England to parallel differences in infant and maternal mortality between these areas earlier this century.[133] The time course of changes in CHD mortality differentials is congruent with increasing social class differences in cigarette smoking and consumption of micronutrients, but not with changes in fat consumption.[71,134]

11.6 Conclusions

Social class at different stages of the life course is associated with morbidity and mortality risk in adulthood to a variable degree depending upon the outcome of interest. For cardiovascular disease mortality, poor early life social conditions appear to make an important contribution to disease risk in adulthood. However, an index of life course social position, which combines data regarding social position from different stages of life, is more strongly related to cardiovascular disease mortality risk than is any indicator relating to just one point in time.[37]

The interaction of socially patterned exposures at different periods of the life course to health status in adulthood renders the explanation of trends in both overall health status and in social class differentials in health status problematic. To give one example, the socially patterned exposure of low birthweight appears to interact with a socially patterned adulthood factor, obesity, to produce elevated risks for high blood pressure and CHD mortality[135,136] (Fig. 11.2). Countervailing trends at different times would lead to different expectations regarding present day disease risk and social class differentials. For example, reductions in infant mortality and improvements in birthweight happening around the time a cohort was born would be expected to reduce cardiovascular disease risk for this cohort in adult life. If there is an increasing trend in obesity, however, this would be expected to increase the risk, and trends in an opposite direction in factors which interact to elevate risk could lead to expectations in any direction. Since exposures acting across the life course, together with interactions between exposures acting at different times, contribute to disease risk, studies which only have data concerning one period of the life course are inadequate for further advancing our under-standing of both disease aetiology and the production of socioeconomic differentials in health.

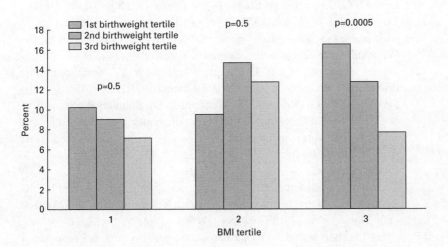

Figure 11.2 Coronary heart disease incidence by birthweight and Body Mass Index in The Caerphilly Study

Source: Frankel et al 1996[136]

References

Those marked with an asterisk are recommended for further reading

1   Woods R, Williams N. Must the gap widen before it can be narrowed? Long-term trends in social class mortality differentials. *Continuity and Change* 1995;**10**:105–37.

2*   Engels F. *The condition of the working class in England.* Penguin, Harmondsworth, 1987 (1st edition 1845).

3   Williams R. Medical, economic and population factors in areas of high mortality: the case of Glasgow. *Sociol Health Illness 1994;***16**: 143–81.

4   Wrigley EA, Schofield RS. *The population history of England, 1541–1871.* Cambridge, Mass: Harvard University Press, 1981.

5   Kuh D, Davey Smith G. When is mortality risk determined? Historical insights into a current debate. *Social History of Medicine* 1993;**6**:101–23.

6   Davey Smith G, Marmot MG. Trends in Mortality in Britain: 1920–1986 *Ann Nutr Metab* 1991;**35 (suppl 1)**:53–63.

7   M'Gonigle GCM, Kirby J. *Poverty and Public Health.* London, Gollancz, 1936.

8   Blane D, Bartley M, Davey Smith G. Disease aetiology and socio-economic mortality differentials. *Eur J Public Health* 1997, in press.

9   Najman JM. Health and poverty: past, present and prospects for the future. *Soc Sci Med* 1993;**36**:157–66.

10   Harding S. Social class differences in mortality of men: recent evidence from OPCS Longitudinal Study. *Popul Trends* 1995;**80**:31–7.

11   Davey Smith G, Shipley MJ, Rose G. The magnitude and causes of socioeconomic differentials in mortality: further evidence from the Whitehall study. *J Epidemiol Community Health* 1990;**44**:260–5.

12   Davey Smith G, Leon D, Shipley MJ, Rose G. Socio-economic differentials in cancer in men. *Int J Epidemiol* 1991;**20**:339–45.

13   Davey Smith G, Neaton JD, Wentworth D, Stamler R, Stamler J. Socioeconomic differentials in mortality risk among men screened for the multiple risk factor intervention trial: part I—results for 300,685 white men. *Am J Public Health* 1996;**86**:486–96.

14   Davey Smith G, Wentworth D, Neaton JD, Stamler R, Stamler J. Socioeconomic differentials in mortality risk among men screened for the multiple risk factor intervention trial: part II - results for 20,224 black men. *Am J Public Health* 1996;**86**:497–504.

15   Syme SL, Berkman LF. Social class, susceptibility and sickness. *Am J Epidemiol* 1976;**104**:1–8.

16   Najman JM, Congalton AA. Australian occupational mortality, 1965–67: cause specific or general susceptibility? *Sociol Health Illness* 1979; **1**:158–76.

17   Susser MW, Watson W, Hopper K. *Sociology in medicine*. Oxford: Oxford University Press, 1985.

18   Marmot MG, Shipley MJ, Rose G. Inequalities in death—specific explanations of a general pattern. *Lancet* 1984;**i**:1003–6.

19   Davey Smith G, Kuh D. Does early nutrition affect later health: Views from the 1930s and 1980s. In: Smith D, ed. *The history of nutrition in Britain in the twentieth century: science, scientists and politics*. Routledge, 1997.

20   Hannington W. *The problem of the distressed areas*. London: Gollancz, 1937.

21   Vernon HM. *Health in relation to occupation*. London: Oxford University Press 1939.

22*   Marks RU. A review of empirical findings. *Milbank Mem Fund Q* 1967; **45**:51–107.

23   Forsdahl A. Are poor living conditions in childhood and adolescents an important risk factor for arteriosclerotic heart disease? *Br J Prev Soc Med* 1977;**31**:91–5.

24   Fosdahl A. Living conditions in childhood and subsequent development of risk factors for arteriorsclerotic heart disease. *J Epidemiol Community Health* 1978;**32**:34–7.

25   Barker DJP, Osmond C. Infant mortality, childhood nutrition, and ischaemic heart disease in England and Wales. *Lancet* 1986;**i**:1077–81.

26   Arnesen E, Forsdahl A. The Tromso heart study: coronary risk factors and their association with living conditions during childhood. *J Epidemiol Community Health* 1985;**39**:210–4.

27   Burr ML, Sweetnam PM. Family size and paternal unemployment in relation to myocardial infarction. *J Epidemiol Community Health* 1980; **34**:93–5.

28   Gliksman MD, Kawachi I, Hunter D, Colditz GA, Manson JE et al. Childhood socioeconomic status and risk of cardiovascular disease in middle aged US women: a prospective study. *J Epidemiol Community Health* 1995;**49**:10–5.

29   Kaplan GA, Salonen JT. Socioeconomic conditions in childhood and ischaemic heart disease during middle age. *Br Med J* 1990;**301**:1121–3.

30   Notkola V, Punsar S, Karvonen MJ, Haapakaski J. Socio-economic conditions in childhood and mortality and morbidity caused by coronary heart disease in adulthood in rural Finland. *Soc Sci Med* 1985;**21**: 517–23.

31   Vågerö D, Leon D. Effect of social class in childhood and adulthood on adult mortality. *Lancet* 1994;**343**:1224–5.

32   Gillum RF, Paffenbarger RS. Chronic disease in former college students. XVII Socio-cultural mobility as a precursor of coronary heart disease and hypertension. *Am J Epidemiol* 1978;**108**:289–98.

33   Hasle H. Association between living conditions in childhood and myo-cardial infarction. *Br Med J* 1990;**300**:512–3.

34   Gliksman MD, Kawachi I, Hunter D, Colditz GA, Manson JE et al. Childhood socioeconomic status and risk of cardiovascular disease in middle aged US women: a prospective study. *J Epidemiol Community Health* 1995;**49**:10–5.

35   Coggon D, Margetts BM, Barker DJP, Carson PHM, Mann JS, Oldroyd KG, Wickham C. Childhood risk factors for ischaemic heart disease and stroke. *Paediat Perinat Epidemiol* 1990;**4**:464–9.

36* Wannamethee SG, Whincup PH, Shaper G, Walker M. Influence of father's social class on cardiovascular disease in middle-aged men. *Lancet* 1996;**348**:1259–63.

37* Davey Smith G, Hart C, Blane D, Gillis C, Hawthorne V. Lifetime socioeconomic position and mortality: prospective observational study. *Br Med J* 1997;**314**:547–52.

38* Lynch JW, Kaplan GA, Cohen RD, Kauhanen J, Wilson TW, Smith NL, Salonen JT. Childhood and adult socioeconomic status as predictors of mortality in Finland. *Lancet* 1994;**343**:524–7.

39* Notkola V. Living conditions in childhood and coronary heart disease in adulthood. *Commentationes Scientiarum Socialium* 1985;**29**:15–119.

40   Valkonen T. Male mortality from ischaemic heart disease in Finland, relation to region of birth and region of residence. *Eur J Popul* 1987;**3**: 61–83.

41   Koskinen S. *Origins of regional differences in mortality from ischaemic heart disease in Finland.* National Research and Development Centre for Welfare and Health Search Report 41. NAWH, Helsinki, 1994.

42   Leon D, Davey Smith G, Shipley M, Strachan D. Height and mortality in London: early life influences, socioeconomic confounding or shrinkage? *J Epidemiol Community Health* 1995;**49**:5–9.

43   Blane D, Hart CL, Davey Smith G, Gillis CR, Hole DJ, Hawthorne WM. The association of cardiovascular disease risk factors with socio-economic position during childhood and during adulthood. *Br Med J* 1996;**313**:1434–8.

44   Davey Smith G, Hart C, Hole D, Gillis C, Watt G, Hawthorne V. Education and occupational social class; which is the more important indicator of mortality risk? (Abstract). *J Epidemiol Community Health* 1994;**48**:500.

45   Lehingue Y. Fetal environment and coronary ischemia risk: review of the literature with particular reference to syndrome X. *Rev Epidem et Sante Publ* 1996;**44**:262–77.

46   Alvarsson M, Efendic S, Grill VE. Insulin responses to glucose in healthy males are associated with adult height but not with birth weight. *Journal of Int Med* 1994;**236**:275–9.

47   Bao W, Srinivasan SR, Wattigney WA, Berenson GS. Persistence of multiple cardiovascular risk clustering related to syndrome X from childhood to young adulthood. *Arch Intern Med* 1994;**154**:1842–7.

48   Raitakari OT, Porkka KVK, Rdsdnen L, Rvnnemaa T, Viikari JSA. Clustering and six year cluster-tracking of serum total cholesterol, HDL-cholesterol and diastolic blood pressure in children and young adults. *J Clin Epidemiol* 1994;**47**:1085–93.

49   Power C, Moynihan C. Social class and changes in weight-for-height between childhood and early adulthood. *Int J Obesity* 1988; **12**:445–53.

50   Braddon F, Rodgers B, Wadsworth MFJ, Davies JMC. Onset of obesity in a 36-year birth cohort study. *Br Med J* 1986;**293**:299–303.

51   Brunner E, Davey Smith G, Marmot M, Canner R, Beksinska M, O'Brien J. Childhood social circumstances and psychosocial and behavioural factors as determinants of plasma fibrinogen. *Lancet* 1996;**347**:1008–13.

52   Wilson TW, Kaplan GA, Kauhanen J, et al. Association between plasma fibrinogen concentration and five socioeconomic indices in the Kuopio ischaemic heart disease risk factor study. *Am J Epidemiol* 1993;**137**: 292–300.

53   Kogevinas E. *Socio-economic differentials in cancer incidence and survival 1971–1981*. Series LS5, London: HMSO, 1990.

54   Vatten LJ, Kvinnsland S. Body height and risk of breast cancer. A prospective study of 23,831 Norwegian women. *Br J Cancer* 1990;**61**: 881–5.

55   Tretli S, Gaard M. Lifestyle changes during adolescence and risk of breast cancer: an ecologic study of the effect of World War II in Norway. *Cancer Causes Control* 1996;**7**:507–12.

56   Gunnell D, Davey Smith G, Frankel S, Nanchahal K, Braddon FEM, Peters TJ. Childhood leg length and adult mortality - follow up of the Carnegie Survey of diet and growth in pre-war Britain (abstract). *J Epidemiol Community Health* 1996;**50**:580–1.

57   Eachus J, Williams M, Chan P, Davey Smith G, Grainge M, Donovan J, Frankel S. Deprivation and cause-specific morbidity: evidence from the Somerset and Avon Survey of Health. *Br Med J* 1996;**312**:287–92.

58   Lynch J, Kaplan GA, Salonen R, Cohen RD, Salonen JT. Socio-economic status and carotid athrosclerosis. *Circulation* 1995;**92**: 1786–92.

59   Stevenson THC. The social distribution of mortality from different causes in England and Wales, 1910–12. *Biometrika* 1923;**15**:382–40.

60   Evans A. Dr Black's Favourite Disease. *Br Heart J* 1995;**74**:676–7.

61*   Antonovsky A. Social class and the major cardiovascular diseases. *J Chron Dis* 1968;**21**:65–106.

62 Stewart ING. Coronary disease and modern stress. *Lancet* 1950;**ii**: 867–70.

63 Platt R. Coronary disease and modern stress. *Lancet* 1951;**i**:51.

64 Pamuk ER. Social class inequality in mortality from 1921 to 1972 in England and Wales. *Popul Stud* 1985;**39**:17–31.

65 Stehbens WE. Review of the validity of national coronary heart disease mortality rates. *Angiology* 1990;**41**:85–94.

66 James G, Patton RE, Heslin AS. Accuracy of cause-of-death statements on death certificates. *Public Health Rep* 1955;**70**:39–51.

67 Registrar General. Statistical Review of England and Wales for the year 1956. Part III, Commentary. London, HMSO, 1958:182–207.

68 Samphier ML, Robertson C, Bloor MJ. A possible artefactual component in specific cause mortality gradients. *J Epidemiol Community Health* 1988;**42**:138–43.

69 Logan WPD. Occupational mortality. *Proc Royal Soc Med* 1959;**52**: 463–8.

70 Heller RF, Williams H, Sittampalam Y. Social class and ischaemic heart disease: use of the male:female ratio to identify possible occupational hazards. *J Epidemiol Community Health* 1984;**38**:198–202.

71 Marmot MG, Adelstein AM, Robinson N, Rose GA. Changing social-class distribution of heart disease. *Br Med J* 1978;**ii**:1109–12.

72 Halliday ML, Anderson TW. The sex differential in ischaemic heart disease: trends by social class 1931 to 1971. *J Epidemiol Community Health* 1979;**33**:74–7.

73 Cassel J, Heyden S, Bartel AG, Kaplan BH, Tyroler HA, Cornoni JC, Hames CG. Incidence of coronary heart disease by ethnic group, social class, and sex. *Arch Intern Med* 1971;**128**:901–6.

74 Britten RH. Mortality rates by occcupational class in the United States. *Public Health Rep* 1934;**49**:1101–11.

75 Lew EA. Some implications of mortality statistics relating to coronary artery disease. *J Chron Disease* 1957;**6**:192–209.

76 Ellis JM. Socio-economic differentials in mortality from chronic diseases. *Social Problems* 1957;**5**:30–6.

77 Kent AP, McCaroll JR, Schweizer MD, Willard HN. A comparison of coronary artery disease deaths in health areas of Manhattan. *Am J Public Health* 1958;**48**:200.

78 Stamler J, Kjelsberg M, Hall Y. Epidemiologic studies of cardiovascular-renal diseases: I. Analysis of mortality by age-race-sex-occupation. *J Chron Disease* 1960;**12**:440–55.

79 Kjelsberg M, Stamler J. Epidemiologic studies of cardiovascular-renal diseases: I. Analysis of mortality by age-race-sex-place of residence, including urban-rural comparisons. *J Chron Disease* 1960;**12**: 456–63.

80 Altenderfer ME. Relationship of per-capita income and mortality, in the states of 100,000 or more population. *Public Health Rep* 1947; **62**:1681–91.

81 Breslow L, Buell P. Mortality from coronary heart disease and physical activity of work in California. *J Chron Disease* 1960;**11**:421–44.

82 Reid DD, Rose GA. Assessing the comparability of mortality statistics. *Br Med J* 1964;**ii**:1437–9.

83 Ryle JA, Russell WT. The natural history of coronary heart disease. *Brit Heart J* 1949;**11**:370–89.

84 Britton M. *Mortality and geography - a review in the mid-1980s*. OPCS Series DS No.9, London: HMSO, 1990.

85 Martin R. The political economy of Britains north-south divide. *Trans Inst Br Geogr* 1988;**13**:389–418.

86 Martin WJ. The distribution in England and Wales of mortality from coronary disease. *Br Med J* 1956;**i**:1523–5.

87 Lilienfeld AM. Variation in mortality from heart disease: race, sex, and socioeconomic status. *Public Health Rep* 1956;**71**:545–52.

88 Pearson TA. Socioeconomic status and cardiovascular disease in rural populations. In: *Report on the Conference on Socioeconomic Status and Cardiovascular Health and Disease*. Washington: US Department of Health and Human Services, 1996:101–8.

89 Taylor HL, Klepetar E, Keys A, Parlin W, Blackburn H, Puchner T. Deaths rates among physically active and sedentary employees of the Railroad industry. *Am J Public Health* 1962;**52**:1697–707.

90 Levy RL, Bruenn HG, Kurtz D. Facts on disease of the coronary arteries, based on a survey of the clinical and pathological records of 762 cases. *Am J Med Sci* 1934;**187**:376–90.

91 Gordon WH, Bland EF, White PD. Coronary artery disease analyzed post mortem with special reference to the influence of economic status and sex. *Am Heart J* 1939;**17**:10–14.

92 Bjornsson J. *Arteriosclerosis: a chemical and statistical study*. Copenhagen: Munksgaard, 1942.

93 Morris JN, Crawford MD. Coronary heart disease and physical activity of work: evidence of a national necropsy survey. *Br Med J* 1958;**ii**: 1485–96.

94 Boas EP, Donner S. Coronary artery disease in the working classes. *JAMA* 1932;**98**:186–9.

95 Pell S, DAlonzo CA. Blood pressure, body weight, serum cholesterol, and smoking habits among executives and nonexecutives. *J Occup Med* 1961; **3**:467–70.

96 Mortensen JM, Stevenson TT, Whitney LH. Mortality due to coronary disease analysed by broad occupational groups. *Arch Industrial Health* 1959;**19**:1–4.

97 Goldblatt P. Social class mortality differences. In: Mascie-Taylor CG, ed. *Biosocial aspects of social class*. Oxford: Oxford University Press, 1990.

98 Davey Smith G, Shipley MJ. Confounding of occupation and smoking: its magnitude and consequences. *Soc Sci Med* 1991;**32**:1297–300.

99 Davey Smith G, Blane D, Bartley M. Explanations for socioeconomic differentials in mortality: evidence from Britain and elsewhere. *Eur J Public Health* 1994;**4**:131–44.

100 Davey Smith G, Morris JN. Increasing inequalities in the health of the nation. *Br Med J* 1994;**309**:1453–4.

101 Salonen J. Socioeconomic status and risk of cancer, cerebral stroke, and death due to coronary heart disease and any disease: a longitudinal study in eastern Finland. *J Epidemiol Community Health* 1982;**36**:294–7.

102 Holme I, Helgeland A, Hjermann I, Leren P, Lund-Larsen PG. Physical activity at work and at leisure in relation to coronary risk factors and social class. *Acta Med Scand* 1981;**209**:277–83.

103 Burling JE, Evans DA, Fiore M, Rosner B, Hennekens CH. Occupation and risk of death from coronary heart disease. *JAMA* 1987;**258**:791–2.

104 Hein HO, Suadicani P, Gyntelberg F. Ischaemic heart disease incidence by social class and form of smoking: the Copenhagen Male Study - 17 years follow-up. *J Intern Med* 1992;**231**:477–83.

105 Pekkanen J, Tuomilehto J, Uutela A, Vartiainen E, Nissinen A. Social class, health behaviour, and mortality among men and women in eastern Finland. *Br Med J* 1995;**311**:589–93.

106 Rosengren A, Wedel H, Wilhelmsen L. Coronary heart disease and mortality in middle-aged men from different occupational groups in Sweden. *Br Med J* 1988;**297**:1497–500.

107 Eaker ED, Pinsky J, Castelli WP. Myocardial infarction and coronary death among women: psychosocial predictors from a 20-year follow-up of women in the Framingham study. *Am J Epidemiol* 1992; **135**:854–64.

108 Pocock SJ, Shaper AG, Cook DG, Phillips AN, Walker M. Social class differences in ischaemic heart disease in British men. *Lancet* 1987;**2**: 197–201.

109 Davey Smith G, Phillips AN. Declaring independence: why we should be cautious. *J Epidemiol Commununity Health* 1990;**44**:257–8.

110 Phillips A, Davey Smith G. How independent are independent effects? Relative risk estimation when correlated exposures are measured imprecisely. *J Clin Epidemiol* 1991;**44**:1223–31.

111 Marmot MG, Davey Smith G, Stansfeld S, Patel C, North F, Head J, White, Brunner E, Feeney A. Inequalities in health twenty years on: the Whitehall II study of British Civil Servants. *Lancet* 1991;**337**:1387–94.

112 Brunner EJ, Marmot MG, White IR, OBrien JR, Etherington MD, Slavin BM, Kearney EM, Davey Smith G. Gender and employment

grade differences in blood cholesterol apolipoproteins and haemostatic factors in the Whitehall II study. *Atherosclerosis* 1993;**102**:195–207.

113 Davey Smith G, Brunner E. Socioeconomic differentials in health: the role of nutrition. *Proc Nutr Soc* 1997;**56**:75–90.

114 Lynch JW, Kaplan GA, Cohen RD, Tuomilehto J, Salonen JT. Do known risk factors explain the relation between socioeconomic status, risk of all-cause mortality, cardiovascular mortality and acute myocardial infarction? *Am J Epidemiol* 1996;**144**:934–42.

115 Barker DJP. The foetal and infant origins of inequalities in health in Britain. *J Public Health Med* 1991;**13**:64–8.

116 Coleman D, Salt J. *The British population: patterns, trends, processes.* Oxford: Oxford University Press 1992.

117 Barker DJP. Rise and fall of Western diseases. *Nature* 1989;**338**:371–2.

118 Ioannidis PJ, Efthymiopoulou GD. International transeconomic trends of arterial diseases in the mid 1970s. *Am J Epidemiol* 1982;**115**:278–97.

119 Watterson PA. Infant mortality by father's occupation from the 1911 census of England and Wales. *Demography* 1988;**25**:289–306.

120 Blane D, Davey Smith G, Bartley M. Social class differences in years of potential life lost: size, trends and principal causes. *Br Med J* 1990;**301**:429–32.

121 Registrar General. *Decennial Supplement, England and Wales 1961, Occupational Mortality tables.* London: HMSO, 1971.

122 OPCS. *Occupational Mortality 1970–1972, Decennial Supplement (D.S. Series number 1).* London: HMSO, 1978.

123 Halliday RF, Williams H, Sittampalam Y. Social class and ischaemic heart disease: use of the male:female ratio to identify possible occupational hazards. *J Epidemiol Community Health* 1984;**38**:198–202.

124 Woods R, Williams N, Galley C. Infant mortality in England, 1550–1950. In: Corsini CA, Viazzo PP, eds. *The decline in infant mortality in Europe 1800–1950.* Florence: UNICEF and the International Child Development Centre, 1993.

125 Pamuk ER. Social-class inequality in infant mortality in England and Wales from 1921 to 1980. *Eur J Popul* 1988;**4**:1–21.

126 Barker DJP, Osmond C. Death rates from stroke in England and Wales predicted from past maternal mortality. *Br Med J* 1987;**295**:83–6.

127 Loudon I. Maternal and infant mortality 1900–1960. *Social History of Medicine* 1991;**4**:29–73.

128 Kuh DL, Power C, Rogers B. Secular trends in social class and sex differences in adult height. *Int J Epidemiol* 1991;**20**:1001–9.

129 Floud R, Wachter K, Gregory A. *Height, health and history.* Nutritional status in the United Kingdom 1750–1980. Cambridge: Cambridge University Press, 1990.

130 Dahlmann N, Petersen K. Influences of environmental conditions during infancy on final body stature. *Pediat Res* 1977;**11**:695–700.

131 Clements EMB. Changes in the mean stature and weight of British children over the past seventy years. *Br Med J* 1953;**2**:897–902.

132 Craig JO. The heights of Glasgow boys: secular and social influences. *Hum Biol* 1963;**35**:524–39.

133 Maheswaran R, Strachan DP, Elliott P, Shipley MJ. Trends in stroke mortality in Greater London and South-East England—evidence for a cohort effect? *J Epidemiol Community Health* 1997;**51**:121–6.

134 Morgan M, Heller RF, Swerdlow A. Changes in diet and coronary heart disease mortality among social classes in Great Britain. *J Epidemiol Community Health* 1989;**43**:162–7.

135 Leon DA, Koupilová I, O Lithell H, Berglund L, Mohsen R, Vegerv, Lithell U, McKeigue PM. Failure to realise growth potential in utero and adult obesity in relation to blood pressure in 50 year old Swedish men. *Br Med J* 1996;**312**:401–6.

136 Frankel SJ, Elwood P, Sweetnam P, Yarnell J, Davey Smith G. Birthweight, body mass index in middle age and incident coronary heart disease. *Lancet* 1996;**348**:1478–80.

137 Thomas AJ, Cochrane AL, Higgins ITT. The measurement of the prevalence of ischaemic heart disease. *Lancet* 1958; 540–44.

138 Higgins ITT, Cochrane AL, Thomas AJ. Epidemiological studies of coronary disease. *Br J Prev Soc Med* 1963;**17**:153–65.

139 Stamler J, Lindberg HA, Berkson DM, Shaffer A, Miller W, Poindexter A. Prevalence and incidence of coronary heart disease in strata of the labor force of a Chicago industrial corporation. *J Chronic Diseases* 1960;**II**:405–19.

140 Berkson DM, Stamler J, Lindberg HA, Miller W, Mathies H, Lasky H, Hall Y. Socioeconomic correlates of atherosclerotic and hypertensive heart diseases. *Ann NY Acad Sci* 1960;**84**:835–50.

141 Chapman JM, Goerke LS, Dixon W, Loveland DB, Phillips E. The clinical status of a population group in Los Angeles under observation for two to three years. *Am J Public Health* 1957;**47 (April Suppl)**: 33–42.

142 Dawber TR, Kannel WB, Revotskie N, Stokes J, Kagan A, Gordon T. Some factors associated with the development of coronary heart disease. Six years follow-up experience in the Framingham Study. *Am J Public Health* 1959;**49**:1349–56.

143 Hinkle LE, Benjamin B, Christenson WN, Ullmann DS. Coronary Heart Disease: 30 year experience of 1,160 men. *Arch Environ Health*;**13**:312–21.

144 Brown RG, Davidson LAG, McKeown T, Whitfield AGW. Coronary artery disease. Influences affecting its incidence in males in the seventh decade. *Lancet* 1957;**ii**:1073–7.

145 Brown RG, McKeown T, Whitfield AGW. Observations on the medical condition of men in the seventh decade. *Br Med J* 1958;555–62.

146 Paul O, Lepper MH, Phelan WH, Dupertuis GW, MacMillan A, McKean H, Park H. A longitudinal study of coronary heart disease. *Circulation* 1963;**28**:20–31.

147 Pell D, DAlonzo CA, Del W. Myocardial infarction in a one-year industrial study. *JAMA* 1958;**166**:332–7.

148 Pell S, DAlonzo CA, Del W. Acute myocardial infarction in a large industrial population. *JAMA* 1963;**185**:831–8.

149 Doyle JT, Heslin SA, Hilleboe HE, Formel PF, Korns RF. A prospective study of degenerative cardiovascular disease in Albany: Report of three years experience - 1. Ischaemic heart disease. *Am J Publ Health* 1957; **47 (Suppl, April)**:25–32.

150 Kinch SH, Doyle JT, Hilleboe HE. Risk factors in ischemic heart disease. *Am J Public Health* 1963;**53**:438–42.

151 Commission on Chronic Illness: *Chronic Illness in a Large City: The Baltimore Study* (Vol. IV of the series, Chronic Illness in the United States), Cambridge: Harvard University Press, 1957.

152 McDonough JR, Hames CG, Stulb SC, Garrison GE. Coronary heart disease among negroes and whites in Evans County, Georgia. *J Chron Dis* 1965;**18**:443–68.

153 Lee RE, Schneider RF. Hypertension and arteriosclerosis in executive and nonexecutive personnel. *JAMA* 1958;**167**:1447–50.

E

Implications for policy and future research

12 Should we intervene to improve fetal growth?

K. S. Joseph and Michael Kramer

Numerous recent studies have demonstrated associations between specific patterns of fetal and infant growth and coronary heart disease. In this chapter, we examine the potential long term health impacts of interventions to improve fetal and infant growth. Although the available evidence does not permit firm inference that reduced fetal or infant growth causes coronary heart disease, our discussion is based on the assumption that the reported associations are in fact causal. The magnitudes of the effect that interventions to improve fetal growth are likely to have on subsequent coronary heart disease were estimated using data from the Hertfordshire cohort. About 33% and 26% of coronary heart disease deaths among women and men, respectively, would be averted if all births weighed between 9–9.5 lbs (3969–4422 g). Most of this decline would occur secondary to increases in the birthweight of babies in the 7–8.5 lbs (3061–3968 g) category. Simulations with more realistic assumptions based on the 1993 Canadian birth cohort show a marginal impact on subsequent coronary heart disease deaths. For instance, a 100 g increase in the birthweight of female and male babies would result in a 2.5% and a 1.9% decrease in coronary heart disease deaths, respectively. Various options for improving fetal growth were reviewed, including interventions to improve maternal nutrition before and during pregnancy, reduce smoking in pregnancy and improve other aspects of prenatal care. The effects of such interventions are likely to be relatively modest, at least in terms of their impacts on subsequent coronary heart disease. For instance, observational studies show that the mean birthweight reduction in smoking mothers is approximately 150 g, while clinical trials evaluating the effects of intervention to reduce smoking in pregnancy have reported mean birthweight increases ranging from 31 to 92 g. Other issues that must be considered before intervening to improve fetal growth include the potential for unintended (adverse) effects. An increased risk of cesarean section and maternal obesity would be important maternal concerns, and possible increases in the occurrence of cancers of the prostate, breast, and ovary would constitute long-term threats to the health of the offspring. We conclude that interventions designed to improve fetal and infant growth would lead to marginal reductions, at best, in the occurrence of adult chronic disease and might have adverse effects. Furthermore, such interventions could detract from the contemporary obstetric focus on preventing preterm, very low birthweight infants by shifting the emphasis to normal weight infants born at term.

12.1 Introduction

Numerous recent studies have shown associations between specific fetal and infant patterns of growth and coronary heart disease (CHD) and other adult chronic diseases. These studies have served as the basis for the hypothesis that physiologic or metabolic 'programming' during gestation and infancy substantially determines the occurrence of various pathological phenomena in later life.[1–12] If the evidence and arguments supporting the programming hypothesis are valid, they carry important implications for both clinical practice and public health policy. As we have argued elsewhere,[13,14] however, onerous methodologic challenges are inherent in this domain of research, including the wide temporal separation between determinant (fetal or infant growth) and outcome (CHD or other chronic disease) and the particular susceptibility of the determinant-outcome relation to confounding. Furthermore, various other studies have failed to corroborate the hypothesis (see reference 13). Causal inferences for the observed associations, therefore, may not be warranted.[13,14]

Because various authorities[15] have embraced the programming hypothesis, however, this chapter speculates on the impact that interventions in pregnancy and early childhood might have on diseases in adult life, assuming that the documented associations are in fact causal. Using data from the Hertfordshire studies, we first estimate the magnitude of coronary heart disease that can be attributed to inadequate fetal growth. In the next section, we review the current literature with regard to the efficacy of interventions for improving fetal growth. The following section deals with the possible unintended effects that such interventions may have on the mother and the infant. In the final section, we discuss the implications for public health policy and clinical practice.

12.2 Magnitude of intervention effects

Table 12.1 provides estimates of the impact of changes in the birthweight distribution on subsequent CHD mortality. Estimates are based on the results of studies of the Hertfordshire cohort.[16] The relative risk for CHD associated with each birthweight category in Table 12.1 was estimated using the

Table 12.1 Estimated proportion of coronary heart disease that would be prevented if all infants in any birthweight category had weights in the 9 to 9.5 pound range, based on results of the Hertfordshire studies.[16] SMR denoted standardized mortality ratio and RR refers to relative risk.

Birth-weight* (pounds)	Women					Men				
	Number	SMR	Crude RR	SMR ratio	EF1† (%)	Number	SMR	Crude RR	SMR ratio	EF1† (%)
≤5.5	307	83	1.8	1.9	3.5	458	102	1.7	1.8	2.7
6–6.5	1068	72	1.6	1.7	8.7	1317	83	1.4	1.5	4.6
7–7.5	1956	67	1.5	1.6	13.2	2991	82	1.4	1.5	10.1
8–8.5	1532	59	1.4	1.4	6.9	3166	75	1.3	1.3	7.8
9–9.5	551	43	1.0	1.0	0.0	1505	56	1.0	1.0	0.0
≥10	171	49	1.1	1.1	0.3	704	66	1.2	1.2	0.9

* Birthweight categories are the same as those defined in the Hertfordshire studies, with weights rounded to the nearest half-pound. This means that, for instance, the birth weight category 9 to 9.5 lb includes birthweights in the range 3,969 to 4,422 g.
† EF1, proportion of CHD deaths that could be potentially prevented if births in any birth weight category attained birth weights in the 9 to 9.5 lb range. The SMR ratio was used as the relative risk estimate in the calculation.

birthweight category 9–9.5 lbs (3969–4422 g since birthweights were rounded to the nearest half-pound) as the reference category. Two approximate estimates are provided based on the published findings:[16] the ratio of crude rates of CHD mortality and the ratio of the standardized mortality ratios. Although neither method of relative risk calculation is ideal, the results are generally similar and are likely to represent fair approximations.

Two hypothetical estimates of the proportion of CHD cases that can be attributed to low birthweight were obtained using these relative risk estimates.[17] These estimates depend on the magnitude of effect (relative risk) associated with the determinant category and the proportion of the population within the determinant category. The first etiologic fraction estimate (EF1) expresses the proportion of CHD deaths attributable to each birthweight category, with birthweights between 9 and 9.5 lbs taken as the reference. These estimates show the proportion of CHD deaths that could be potentially prevented if births in any particular birthweight category attained weights in the 9 to 9.5 lb range. For instance, 3.5% of CHD deaths among women would be averted if babies in the ≤5.5 lbs (≤2606 g) birthweight category attained birthweights between 9 and 9.5 lbs (Table 12.1). If all births weighed between 9 and 9.5 lbs 33% and 26% of CHD deaths would be prevented among women and men, respectively. Most of the impact under this scenario would arise from increases in the birthweight category 7–8.5 lbs (3061–3968 g). We also estimated the proportion of CHD deaths that would be averted if subjects within any birthweight category attained birthweights in the succeeding birth-weight category (EF2). Such an increase in birthweight would lead to an approximately 9% decrease in CHD deaths. These latter estimates assume a mean birthweight increase of approximately 1 lb (454 g).

The scenarios considered in Table 12.2 are more realistic, because available interventions cannot change birthweight distributions as dramatically as assumed in Table 12.1 (see below). The CHD death rate for the 1993 Canadian birth cohort was obtained by applying the birthweight-specific rates of CHD death observed in Hertfordshire to the Canadian birth cohort. The overall rates of CHD death for both the male and female Canadian birth cohorts are virtually identical to those observed in Hertfordshire. This is because the (categorized) birthweight distribution of the Hertfordshire cohort is very similar to that of the 1993 Canadian birth cohort. This identity of birthweight distributions is probably due to selective follow up in the

Table 12.2 Expected rates of coronary heart disease mortality in the 1993 Canadian birth cohort[81] and estimated preventive fractions, assuming the birth weight-specific rates of CHD death as observed in the Hertfordshire cohort[16] (lb denotes pound).

Cohort	Assumption	CHD death rate (per 1000)	Preventive fraction (%)
Women			
Hertfordshire	None	15.8	
Canada 1993 (reference)	None	16.0	
	≤5.5 lb births shifted to birthweight 6 to 6.5 lb	15.9	0.6
	100 g increase in birthweight	15.6	2.5
	200 g increase in birthweight	15.2	5.0
	300 g increase in birthweight	14.8	7.5
Men			
Hertfordshire	None	84.1	
Canada 1993 (reference)	None	85.6	
	≤5.5 lb births shifted to birthweight 6 to 6.5 lb	84.0	1.9
	100 g increase in birthweight	83.9	2.0
	200 g increase in birthweight	82.5	2.6
	300 g increase in birthweight	80.8	5.6

Hertfordshire cohort; for instance, in the Hertfordshire cohort, multiple births and infant deaths (which were more likely to have a low birthweight) were excluded and those who were followed up weighed more than those who were not traced. Exclusion of very low birthweight babies from the Canadian birth cohort does not appreciably alter these estimates. Similarly, altering the birthweight distribution of the Canadian birth cohort (100, 200 or 300 g shifts to the right in the birthweight distribution) does not appreciably reduce the estimated CHD death rates (preventive fractions 2.5%, 5.0%, and 7.5%, respectively, for women and 1.9%, 2.0%, and 5.6%, respectively, for men).

The preventive fractions for some of the other diseases considered in the Hertfordshire studies may be somewhat higher than those estimated for CHD. For instance, if the association between infant weight and adult chronic obstructive lung disease (COLD) mortality[18] is causal, then increases in infant weight will have a slightly greater impact on COLD mortality than will increases in birthweight on CHD mortality.

Thus interventions in early life seem likely to have a small impact, if any, on adult chronic disease. It is useful to compare the magnitude of such an impact with those of alternative interventions currently advocated for reducing the burden of adult disease. For instance, 20-year follow-up results from the Framingham heart study[19] show that CHD mortality declined by 51% across the 50–59 year-old female cohorts of 1950 and 1970. The same estimate for the decline in CHD mortality in the male Framingham cohorts was 44%. More than half of the decline in CHD mortality observed in women and one-third to one-half of the decline observed in men has been attributed to changes in risk factor status (i.e. changes in levels of cigarette smoking, total cholesterol, systolic blood pressure, and diabetes mellitus).[19] Similar estimates have been obtained from other studies.[20,21] Table 12.3, which is based on data from the British Regional Heart Study, presents estimates of the magnitude of impact likely to result from three potential areas for adult intervention. These data show that 51% of CHD deaths would be prevented if the entire population consisted of never smokers. Similarly, 48% and 34% of CHD deaths, respectively, would be prevented if all subjects had cholesterol and systolic blood pressure values in the reference range (these estimates are independent but not mutually exclusive[22]). On the other hand, a single category shift towards the reference category in cholesterol, systolic blood pressure and smoking status would result in an approximately 13%, 12%, and 24% decrease, respectively, in CHD deaths.

Studies such as the Framingham analysis cited above have not considered fetal growth determinants in modelling CHD aetiology. For this reason, it may be more appropriate to consider the results of experimental studies for evaluating the effects of adult intervention (fetal determinants would be balanced in the treatment groups because of randomization). The largest

Table 12.3 Estimated proportion of coronary heart disease events and deaths that would be prevented by changes in risk factor status, based on results of the British Regional Heart Study (data provided courtesy of Lampe F and Whincup P). Estimates calculated using relative risks adjusted for risk factors other than age yield similar results.

Factor (category)	No. of subjects	CHD events	RR (age-adjusted)	EF1*	CHD deaths	RR (age-adjusted)	EF1*
Cholesterol (mmol/l)							
≤5.4	1613	105	1.00	0.0	54	1.00	0.0
5.5–5.9	1384	143	1.59	5.5	89	1.93	8.7
6.0–6.4	1492	167	1.69	6.9	83	1.60	6.1
6.5–7.1	1703	249	2.21	13.8	132	2.20	13.8
≥7.2	1495	297	3.22	22.3	145	2.91	19.3
Systolic BP (mmHg)							
<128	1550	131	1.00	0.0	60	1.00	0.0
128–137	1542	151	1.17	2.4	73	1.23	3.0
138–147	1540	165	1.24	3.4	77	1.22	2.9
148–160	1550	238	1.74	10.4	134	1.99	13.1
≥161	1542	282	1.97	13.6	160	2.16	15.2
Smoking							
Never	1819	124	1.00	0.0	54	1.00	0.0
Ex-	2714	336	1.66	12.9	179	1.89	15.4
Current	3183	508	2.37	31.4	271	2.76	35.6

* EF1, proportion of CHD events/deaths that would be prevented if subjects in any risk factor category attained values in the reference category range (≤5.4 mmol/l of cholesterol, <128 mmHg systolic blood pressure and never smokers were the three reference categories).

of the randomized trials on smoking cessation, the Multiple Risk Factor Intervention Trial (MRFIT), showed a substantial and rapid benefit of smoking cessation on CHD mortality in both the usual care and special intervention groups.[23,24] Subjects who had quit for 1 year after trial initiation experienced a 37% decrease in the risk of CHD mortality. The effect was greater among those who had quit for at least the first 3 years of the trial, with a 62% decrease in CHD mortality compared with persistent smokers.[23] These results are not based on an intention-to-treat analysis, however.

Another randomized trial of diet and anti-smoking advice showed a 47% reduction in the incidence of major CHD events, though the effect was attributed more to changes in serum cholesterol than to smoking cessation.[25] The only randomized trial of anti-smoking advice alone involved a subset of the Whitehall study of civil servants; it showed a 7%, 13% and 11% decrease in total mortality, CHD mortality, and lung cancer, respectively.[26] The study investigators estimated that for every 100 men who had stopped smoking, between 6 and 10 were alive 20 years later as a result.

These estimates of course refer to the impact of changes in smoking status among smokers. Reductions in CHD mortality will be smaller in the overall population and will depend on the prevalence of smoking in the population.

12.3 Interventions to improve fetal and infant growth

Of the various recognized determinants of fetal growth, several offer potential avenues for intervention. These interventions must be considered according to the strength of the evidence that they do indeed increase fetal growth and, if so, the magnitude of the fetal growth effect. In this section, we review the evidence regarding four potential areas for intervention:

(1) nutritional advice and/or supplementation during pregnancy;

(2) nutritional advice and/or supplementation prior to pregnancy;

(3) interventions to reduce smoking during pregnancy;

(4) other aspects of prenatal care (see Table 12.4 for summary).

For each of these, we will focus primarily on the results of controlled clinical trials, as summarized in the latest edition of the Cochrane Collaboration Pregnancy and Childbirth (CCPC) database.[27] In the final subsection, we briefly discuss issues related to improving growth rates in infancy.

12.3.1 Nutrition during pregnancy

Strong evidence from both observational studies and controlled clinical trials indicates that gestational weight gain (which reflects increases in both nutritional stores and nonnutritional components, such as plasma volume and oedema fluid) and energy intake during pregnancy are important determinants of fetal growth. Based on a meta-analysis of the literature published through 1984,[28] each kilogram of total gestational weight gain increases gestational age-adjusted birthweight by approximately 20 g; weight gains below 7 Kg are associated with an approximate doubling of the risk of a growth retarded infant. Moreover, the effect of weight gain on fetal growth appears to be conditional, with greater effects in women with low prepregnancy weight or body mass index, and smaller effects in those who are well-nourished prior to pregnancy.

The importance of energy intake on fetal growth is apparent from the results of the Dutch Famine Study, which demonstrated that extreme restriction of energy intake during the third trimester can have a substantial impact on fetal

Table 12.4 Summary of the results of randomized trials on the effects of intervention for improving fetal growth.[27,30,40–44] CI refers to confidence interval.

Intervention	Ooutcome	Results
Balanced energy and protein supplementation	Birthweight	Mean difference, range=−60 to 263 g; weighted average=30 g (95% CI 1 to 58).
	Intrauterine growth retardation	Weighted odds ratio=0.77 (95% CI 0.58 to 1.01).
	Birth length	Mean difference, range=0.1 to 1.8 cms; weighted average=0.2 cm (95% CI 0.0 to 0.4).
	Head circumference	Mean difference, range=-0.4 to 0.6 cms; weighted average=0.0 cm (95% CI -0.1 to 0.1).
High protein supplementation	Birthweight	Mean difference=-25 g (95% CI -115 to 65).
Smoking reduction/ cessation	Birthweight	Mean difference, range in 5 of 6 trials=31 to 92 g.
	Low birthweight	Odds ratio=0.80 (95% CI 0.64 to 1.00)
Intensive prenatal care	Birthweight	No difference compared with standard
Social support	Birthweight	No difference compared with standard care

growth, with reduction in mean birthweight of approximately 300 g.[29] The effects of interventions to increase energy and protein intakes on fetal growth have recently been assessed in a meta-analysis.[30] Nutritional advice to increase energy and protein intakes has succeeded in increasing pregnant women's energy and protein intakes and gestational weight gain. The effects on fetal growth, however, have been small and statistically non-significant. Actual energy and protein supplementation during pregnancy has resulted in more consistent (and statistically significant) effects on fetal growth, but the magnitude of the effect is again modest, with an increase in mean birthweight of 30 g and a pooled odds ratio for the occurrence of intrauterine growth retardation (IUGR) of 0.77 (95% CI=0.58–1.01).[30] Protein supplementation alone appears to have no beneficial effect on fetal growth independent of the energy content of the supplement.[30]

As to micronutrients, it seems clear that iron intake is unrelated to fetal growth.[31] The data are somewhat less clear with respect to folate[32] and zinc[33] intake, although most of the interest in these micronutrients focuses on their effects on preterm delivery, rather than fetal growth.

12.3.2 Prepregnancy nutrition

The previously cited meta-analysis indicates an extremely strong relationship between prepregnancy weight-for-height (e.g., body mass index) and fetal growth, with each additional kilogram prepregnancy weight increasing gestational age-adjusted birthweight by approximately 10 g.[28] Prepregnancy weight below 50 Kf increases the risk for an IUGR infant by about 80%.[28]

To our knowledge, the only evidence from controlled clinical trials bearing on prepregnancy nutritional status comes from the Taiwan trial of balanced energy/protein supplementation.[34,35] In that trial, supplementation was begun following the birth of a previous child and thus included the entire inter-pregnancy interval in addition to during the index pregnancy. Although this intervention was not compared with an intervention provided during pregnancy only, the magnitude of the overall effect on fetal growth was no greater than in trials in which supplementation was restricted to pregnancy itself.[30]

12.3.3 Interventions to reduce smoking during pregnancy

The previously cited meta-analysis[28] clearly indicates a large effect of maternal cigarette smoking during pregnancy on fetal growth; this effect has been detected in virtually every epidemiological study that has investigated the issue. Moreover, a clear dose–response effect has been observed; larger deficits in fetal growth are associated with additional numbers of cigarettes smoked per day.[28] The mean birthweight reduction in smoking mothers is approximately 150 g, or approximately 11 g per cigarette smoked per day.[28] Smokers have a 2.5-fold increased risk of giving birth to a growth-retarded infant.[28]

Interventions to reduce smoking during pregnancy have included simple advice, counselling, feedback techniques, and other behavioural approaches; the behavioural approaches appear to be the most successful in getting women to quit.[36–40] The increase in birthweight in the intervention group ranged from 31 to 92 g in 5 of the 6 trials included in the CCPC meta-analysis (the sixth trial reported a small difference in the opposite direction).[40] The overall magnitude of the effect of these interventions on fetal growth is not entirely clear, because the results in CCPC are reported according to low birthweight, rather than gestational age-adjusted mean birthweight or IUGR.[40] Nonetheless, considering the comparatively modest effect of smoking on preterm delivery,[28] the pooled odds ratio of 0.80 (95% CI 0.62–1.02) can be taken as a rough proxy of the effect on reduction in IUGR. (It should be noted, however, that the pooled odds ratio and 95% CI for reduction in preterm birth from these smoking reduction strategies is quite similar to the corresponding values for low birth-weight, and thus the specific effect of these interventions on fetal growth is unclear.)

12.3.4 Other aspects of prenatal care

Controlled clinical trials of 'intensive' prenatal care (as a combined package) and/or social support have mostly been aimed at reducing preterm delivery, and the results have been disappointing.[41–44] Nor do the results of these trials suggest that more frequent or longer contact with providers of prenatal care or social support has any beneficial effect on fetal growth. Other than nutritional counselling and/or supplementation and interventions to reduce smoking during pregnancy, the main interventions that could potentially have such a beneficial impact include aspirin or other antiplatelet agents for the prevention of IUGR and pre-eclampsia. The overview of this subject in CCPC indicates a 12–13% reduction in preterm birth or low birthweight;[45] results for gestational age-adjusted mean birthweight or IUGR are not reported in the CCPC overview.

12.3.5 Infant growth

Studies from Guatemala[46,47] on the effect of nutritional supplementation during infancy and early childhood have demonstrated that such supplements can result in substantial increases in growth velocity, at least in a developing country with a high prevalence of childhood malnutrition. During the first year of life, each 100 kcal per day of supplement resulted in a 350 g increase in weight.[47] Similar, though smaller, effects have been reported from studies in Colombia, with supplemented infants gaining an additional 110 g between 9 and 12 months.[48] Recent experimental studies on earlier introduction (4 versus 6 months) of complementary foods have not shown similar beneficial effects, however.[49–51]

The applicability of these studies to infants from developed countries is probably limited, at least among the majority of children. Nevertheless, a decision to intervene in infancy based on the programming hypothesis would have implications for clinical practice and public health policy in developed countries. For instance, studies have shown that infants who are breastfed up to 12 months of age (solid foods introduced after 4 months) are leaner than their formula-fed counterparts, even in populations of high socioeconomic status.[52,53] Among female children, statistically significant differences of 373, 733, and 185 g have been observed at 6, 12, and 18 months of age, respectively.[53,54] Similar though smaller differences have also been observed among male children. A decision to increase infant weight gain (based on the programming hypothesis) would imply reversing the current recommendations regarding breast and formula feeding. This would mean forgoing the beneficial effects of breast feeding in late infancy, especially those on infant morbidity.[54–56] In this context, it is worth noting the strength of the infant weight–CHD association relative to the strength of the birthweight–CHD association; to achieve the same reduction in CHD mortality as a 1 lb (454 g) increase in birthweight, a 2 lb (908 g) increase in infant weight would be required.[16]

12.4 Risks and costs of intervention

12.4.1 Risks for the mother

Perhaps the single most important, immediate consequence of an increase in fetal growth would be a rise in caesarean section rates. Studies have shown that rates of caesarean section for dystocia increase as a function of increasing birthweight.[57] Caesarean section rates for dystocia are more than 4 times as high among deliveries involving babies weighing 4000–4499 g, when compared with those of babies in the 3000–3499 g range. Similar increases have also been seen in the requirements for forceps deliveries for dystocia and also in the need for oxytocin to augment labour.[57]

Overall rates of caesarean section (i.e. irrespective of indication), however, do not show as simple a relation with birthweight. Overall rates of caesarean section are relatively high for mothers delivering babies weighing under 2500 g and a positive dose–response relation between birthweight and overall caesarean section rates is seen only among babies with a birthweight of 2500 g or more.[58] Caution is required in interpreting these findings, however, since reverse causality is inherent in the overall birthweight–caesarean section relation; preterm caesarean section is often used to terminate a pregnancy where fetal wellbeing is compromised and this can be responsible for a lower birthweight. Nevertheless, the birthweight–caesarean section relation above 2500 g implies that an across the board increase in fetal growth will raise the overall rate of caesarean section, because births over 2500 g constitute about 95% of all births.

Increased prevalence of maternal obesity is another potential adverse consequence of attempts to increase fetal growth. Although dietary and nutritional interventions for improving fetal growth are likely to have only modest effects in terms of enhancing fetal growth, the same cannot be said for their impact on mothers. Studies have shown that a significant proportion of maternal weight gain during pregnancy is likely to be retained postpartum, thereby putting some women at risk of obesity.[59–61] A recent study reported that women with high rates of gestational weight gain (greater than 0.68 kg/week) weighed 7.9 kg more than their pregravid weight at 6 months postpartum, compared with a 3.2 and 3.8 kg differences for women with low (less than 0.34 kg/week) and moderate (0.34–0.68 kg/week) rates of gestational weight gain, respectively.[60]

12.4.2 Risks for the offspring

Even if fetal growth is negatively associated with adult cardiovascular end-points, several studies have demonstrated positive associations between birthweight (or other early growth indices) and ovarian,[62] prostate,[63] and breast cancer.[64–66] Calculations based on these studies[62,63] show that ovarian cancer mortality would increase by about 11% and prostate cancer occurrence would increase by about 58% if birthweights increased substantially (as previously assumed; see Table 12.1). The increases are comparable with, if not larger than, the decreases estimated in the case of CHD deaths. It should be noted, however, that this argument presupposes a causal relation between birthweight and the above mentioned outcomes. In fact, the studies on which these estimates are based share the same methodologic problems commonly found in many such studies. For instance, in the studies linking birthweight and prostate cancer,[63] and infant weight gain and ovarian cancer mortality,[62] age was the only potential confounder controlled for.

Direct associations have also been reported between birthweight, on the one hand, and atopy,[67] acute lymphoblastic leukaemia,[68] and late adolescent obesity,[69] on the other. A high weight gain in early life has been associated with an increased risk of Type I diabetes mellitus in another study.[70] These possible unintended effects of intervention, though relatively less frequent than CHD and Type II diabetes mellitus, must be balanced against potential benefits when evaluating the desirability of intervention.

12.5 Implications for public health policy and clinical practice

Birthweight is a confusing target for intervention because it reflects two largely independent processes: gestational duration and rate of fetal growth. Most of the recent emphasis in developed countries has been on efforts to prevent preterm birth, and particularly extreme preterm birth, because of its disproportionate contribution to perinatal mortality and morbidity and long term health and performance.[71–73] Yet these efforts have thus far borne little fruit; with the possible exception of France,[74,75] preterm birth rates have not declined.[76–78] Although Canadian data appear to show reductions in preterm birth,[79] there is reason to believe that these differences are due to changes in methods of ascertaining gestational age.

Interventions to improve fetal growth as a result of the programming hypothesis would focus not on preterm birth, but on term, normal-weight infants. Our estimates (Table 12.1) show that the greatest impact (in terms of subsequent CHD reduction) will accrue if birth weights among normal weight, term babies are increased. In fact, countries such as the US,[77] Canada[79] and England and Wales[80] have witnessed an increase in size of infants born at term. The health benefits of such an increase have heretofore been considered rather marginal. If the fetal origins hypothesis proves correct, a continued trend in this direction may yield small long term reductions in cardiovascular and other adult chronic diseases. It should be noted, however, that efforts to further this trend may entail a substantial shift in focus from the current emphasis on preventing preterm births.

In conclusion, we believe that intervening to improve fetal growth based solely on the programming hypothesis cannot be justified. The reasons for this include the lack of sufficient evidence confirming the causal nature of the programming associations, the marginal potential impact of available interventions, the possible short term and long-term unintended effects of such intervention, and the potentially adverse effects of shifting the current focus from preventing preterm birth to increasing the size of term infants.

References

Those marked with an asterisk are especially recommended for further reading.

1   Barker DJP. The intrauterine origins of cardiovascular and obstructive lung disease in adult life: The Marc Daniels Lecture 1990. *J R Coll Physicians Lond* 1991;**25**:129–33.

2   Barker DJP. The fetal origins of diseases of old age. *Eur J Clin Nutr* 1992; **46 (Suppl)**:S3–S9.

3   Barker DJP and Martyn CN. The maternal and fetal origins of cardio-vascular disease. *J Epidemiol Community Health* 1992;**46**:8–11.

4   Barker DJP. Impact of diet on critical events in development: The effect of nutrition of the fetus and neonate on cardio-vascular disease in adult life. *Proc Nutrition Soc* 1992;**51**:135–44.

5   Barker DJP. Fetal growth and adult disease. *Br J Obstet Gynaecol* 1992; **99**:275–82.

6   Barker DJP. Fetal origins of coronary heart disease. *Br Heart J* 1993; **69**:195–6.

7   Barker DJP, Gluckman PD, Godfrey KM, Harding JE, Owens JA and Robinson JS. Fetal nutrition and cardiovascular disease in adult life. *Lancet* 1993;**341**:938–41.

8   Barker DJP. Maternal nutrition and cardiovascular disease. *Nutr Health* 1993;**9**:99–106.

9   Barker DJP. The intrauterine origins of cardiovascular disease. *Acta Pediatr Suppl* 1993;**391**:93–9.

10   Barker DJP and Fall CHD. Fetal and infant origins of cardiovascular disease. *Arch Dis Child* 1993;**68**:797–9.

11   Law CM, Barker DJP. Fetal influences on blood pressure. *J Hypertens* 1994;**12**:1329–32.

12*   Barker DJP. Fetal origins of coronary heart disease. *Br Med J* 1995; **311**:171–4.

13*   Joseph KS and Kramer MS. A review of the evidence on fetal and early childhood antecedents of adult chronic disease. *Epidemiolog Rev* 1996; **18**:158–74.

14   Kramer MS, and Joseph KS. Enigma of fetal/infant origins hypothesis. *Lancet* 1996;**348**:1254–5.

15   Marginal treatments and complex etiologies (Editor's choice). *Br Med J* 1996;312 (7028).

16*   Osmond C, Barker DJP, Winter PD, Fall CHD and Simmonds SJ. Early growth and death from cardiovascular diseases in women. *Br Med J* 1993;**307**:1519–24.

17   Kleinbaum DG, Kupper LL, Morgenstern H. *Epidemiologic research: Principles and quantitative methods*. Belmont CA: Lifetime Learning Publications. 1982:160–9.

18   Barker DJP, Godfrey KM, Fall C, Osmond C, Winter PD and Shaheen SO. Relation of birthweight and childhood respiratory infection to adult lung function and death from chronic obstructive airways disease. *Br Med J* 1991;**303**:671–5.

19   Sytkowski PA, D'Agostino RB, Belanger A and Kannel WB. Sex and time trends in cardiovascular disease incidence and mortality: the Framingham heart study, 1950–1989. *Am J Epidemiol* 1996;**143**:338–50.

20   Goldman L and Cook EF. The decline in ischemic heart disease mortality rates. An analysis of the comparative effects of medical intervention and changes in lifestyle. *Ann Intern Med* 1984;**101**:825–36.

21   Sprafka JM, Burke GL, Folsom AR, et al. Continued decline in cardiovascular disease risk factors: results of the Minnesota Heart Survey, 1980–1982 and 1985–1987. *Am J Epidemiol* 1990;**132**:489–500.

22   Rothman KJ. *Modern Epidemiology*. First Edition. Toronto: Little Brown and Co., 1986.

23   Ockene JK, Kuller LH, Svendsen KH, and Meilahn E. The relationship of smoking cessation to coronary heart disease and lung cancer in the Multiple Risk Factor Intervention Trial (MRFIT). *Am J Public Health* 1990;**80**:954–8.

24   Kuller LH, Ockene JK, Meilahn E, Wentworth DN, Svendsen KH, Neaton JD. Cigarette smoking and mortality. *Prev Med* 1991;**20**:638–54.

25   Holme I, Hjermann I, Helgeland A and Leren P. The Oslo Study: Diet and antismoking advice: Additional results from a 5-year primary prevention trial in middle-aged men. *Prev Med* 1985;**14**:279–92.

26 Rose G and Colwell L. Randomized controlled trial of antismoking advice: final (20 year) results. *J Epidemiol Community Health* 1992;**46**:75–7.

27* *The Cochrane Database of Systematic Reviews* [database on disk and CDROM]. The Cochrane Collaboration; Issue 2, Oxford: Update Software; 1995. Available from BMJ Publishing Group, London.

28* Kramer MS. Determinants of low birthweight: methodological assessment and meta-analysis. *Bull WHO* 1987;65:663–737.

29 Stein Z, Susser M, Saenger G, Marolla F. *Famine and human development: the Dutch Hunger Winter of 1944–45*. New York: Oxford University Press, 1975.

30 Kramer MS. The effects of energy and protein intake on pregnancy outcome: an overview of the research evidence from controlled clinical trials. *Am J Clin Nutr* 1993;**58**:627–35.

31 Mahomed K. Routine iron supplementation in pregnancy. [revised 28 April 1993] In: Keirse MJNC, Renfrew MJ, Neilson JP, Crowther C, eds. *Pregnancy and Childbirth Module*. In: *The Cochrane Database of Systematic Reviews* [database on disk and CDROM]. The Cochrane Collaboration; Issue 2, Oxford: Update Software; 1995. Available from BMJ Publishing Group, London.

32 Mahomed K. Routine folate supplementation in pregnancy. [revised 28 April 1993] In: Keirse MJNC, Renfrew MJ, Neilson JP, Crowther C, eds. *Pregnancy and Childbirth Module*. In: *The Cochrane Database of Systematic Reviews* [database on disk and CDROM]. The Cochrane Collaboration; Issue 2, Oxford: Update Software; 1995. Available from BMJ Publishing Group, London.

33 Mahomed K. Routine zinc supplementation in pregnancy. [revised 28 April 1993] In: Keirse MJNC, Renfrew MJ, Neilson JP, Crowther C, eds. *Pregnancy and Childbirth Module*. In: *The Cochrane Database of Systematic Reviews* [database on disk and CDROM]. The Cochrane Collaboration; Issue 2, Oxford: Update Software; 1995. Available from BMJ Publishing Group, London.

34 Blackwell RQ, Chow BF, Chinn KSK, Blackwell BN, Hsu SC. Prospective maternal nutrition study in Taiwan: rationale, study design, feasibility and preliminary findings. *Nutr Rep Int* 1973;**7**:517–32.

35 McDonald EC, Pollitt E, Mueller WH, Hsueh AM, Sherwin R. The Bacon Chow study: maternal nutritional supplementation and birthweight of offspring. *Am J Clin Nutr* 1981;**34**:2133–44.

36 Lumley J. Advice as a strategy for reducing smoking in pregnancy. [revised 02 October 1993] In: Keirse MJNC, Renfrew MJ, Neilson JP, Crowther C, eds. *Pregnancy and Childbirth Module*. In: *The Cochrane Database of Systematic Reviews* [database on disk and CDROM]. The Cochrane Collaboration; Issue 2, Oxford: Update Software; 1995. Available from BMJ Publishing Group, London.

37 Lumley J. Behavioral strategies for reducing smoking in pregnancy. [revised 27 September 1993] In: Keirse MJNC, Renfrew MJ, Neilson JP, Crowther C, eds. *Pregnancy and Childbirth Module*. In: *The Cochrane Database of Systematic Reviews* [database on disk and CDROM]. The Cochrane Collaboration; Issue 2, Oxford: Update Software; 1995. Available from BMJ Publishing Group, London.

38 Lumley J. Counselling for reducing smoking in pregnancy. [revised 02 October 1993] In: Keirse MJNC, Renfrew MJ, Neilson JP, Crowther C, eds. *Pregnancy and Childbirth Module*. In: *The Cochrane Database of Systematic Reviews* [database on disk and CDROM]. The Cochrane Collaboration; Issue 2, Oxford: Update Software; 1995. Available from BMJ Publishing Group, London.

39 Lumley J. Feedback as a strategy for reducing smoking in pregnancy. [revised 27 September 1993] In: Keirse MJNC, Renfrew MJ, Neilson JP, Crowther C, eds. *Pregnancy and Childbirth Module*. In: *The Cochrane Database of Systematic Reviews* [database on disk and CDROM]. The Cochrane Collaboration; Issue 2, Oxford: Update Software; 1995. Available from BMJ Publishing Group, London.

40 Lumley J. Strategies for reducing smoking in pregnancy. [revised 02 October 1993] In: Keirse MJNC, Renfrew MJ, Neilson JP, Crowther C, eds. *Pregnancy and Childbirth Module*. In: *The Cochrane Database of Systematic Reviews* [database on disk and CDROM]. The Cochrane Collaboration; Issue 2, Oxford: Update Software; 1995. Available from BMJ Publishing Group, London.

41 Mueller-Heuback E, Reddick D, Barnett B, Bente R. Preterm birth prevention: evaluation of a prospective controlled randomized trial. *Am J Obstet Gynecol* 1989;**160**:1172–78.

42 Heins HC, Nance NW, McCarthy BJ, Efird CM. A randomized trial of nurse-midwifery prenatal care to reduce low birthweight. *Obstet Gynecol* 1990;**75**:341–5.

43 Collaborative Group on Preterm Birth Prevention. Multicenter randomized, controlled trial of a preterm birth prevention program. *Am J Obstet Gynecol* 1993;**169**:352–66.

44 Hodnett ED. Support for caregivers during at risk pregnancy. [revised 20 December 1994] In: Keirse MJNC, Renfrew MJ, Neilson JP, Crowther C, eds. *Pregnancy and Childbirth Module*. In: *The Cochrane Database of Systematic Reviews* [database on disk and CDROM]. The Cochrane Collaboration; Issue 2, Oxford: Update Software; 1995. Available from BMJ Publishing Group, London.

45 Collins R. Antiplatelet agents for IUGR and pre-eclampsia. [revised 04 May 1994] In: Keirse MJNC, Renfrew MJ, Neilson JP, Crowther C, eds. *Pregnancy and Childbirth Module*. In: *The Cochrane Database of Systematic Reviews* [database on disk and CDROM]. The Cochrane

Collaboration; Issue 2, Oxford: Update Software; 1995. Available from BMJ Publishing Group, London.

46 Habicht J-P, Martorell R and Rivera JA. Nutritional impact of supplementation in the INCAP longitudinal study: analytic strategies and inferences. *J Nutr* 1995;**125**:1042S –50S.

47 Shroeder DG, Martorell R, Rivera JA, Ruel MT and Habicht J-P. Age differences in the impact of nutritional supplementation on growth. *J Nutr* 1995;**125**:1051S–9S.

48 Lutter CK, Mora JO, Habicht J-P, Rasmussen KM, Robson DS and Herrera MG. Age-specific responsiveness of weight and length to nutritional supplementation. *Am J Clin Nutr* 1990;**51**:359–64.

49 Cohen RJ, Brown KH, Canahuati J, Rivera LL and Dewey KG. Effect of age of introduction of complementary foods on infant breast milk intake, total energy intake, and growth: a randomized intervention study in Honduras. *Lancet* 1994;**343**:288–93.

50 Cohen RJ, Rivera LL, Canahuati J, Brown KH and Dewey KG. Delaying the introduction of complementary food until 6 months does not affect appetite or mother's report of food acceptance of breast-fed infants from 6 to 12 months in a low income, Honduran population. *J Nutr* 1995;**125**:2787–92.

51 Cohen RJ, Brown KH, Canahuati J, Rivera LL and Dewey KG. Determinants of growth from birth to 12 months among breast-fed Honduran infants in relation to age of introduction of complementary foods. *Pediatrics* 1995;**96**:504–10.

52 Dewey KG, Heinig MJ, Nommsen LA, Peerson JM and Lonnerdal B. Breast-fed infants are leaner than formula-fed infants at 1 y of age: the DARLING study. *Am J Clin Nutr* 1993;**57**:140–5.

53 Dewey KG, Heinig MJ, Nommsen LA, Peerson JM and Lonnerdal B. Growth of breast-fed and formula-fed infants from 0 to 18 months: the DARLING study. *Pediatrics* 1992;**89**:1035– 41.

54 Dewey KG, Peerson JM, Brown KH, et al. Growth of breast-fed infants deviates from current reference data: A pooled analysis of US, Canadian, and European data sets. *Pediatrics* 1995;**96**:495–503.

55 Cunningham AS, Jelliffe DB and Jelliffe EFP. Breast-feeding and health in the 1980's: a global epidemiologic review. J Pediatr. 1991;**119**:659–66.

56 Howie PW, Forsyth JS, Ogston SA, Clark A and Florey CV. Protective effect of breast feeding against infection. *Br Med J* 1990;**300**:11–6.

57 Turner MJ, Rasmussen MJ, Boylan PC, MacDonald D and Stronge JM. The influence of birthweight on labour in nulliparas. *Obstet Gynecol* 1990;**76**:159–63.

58 Parrish KM, Holt VL, Easterling TR, Connell FA and LoGerfo JP. Effect of changes in maternal age, parity, and birthweight distribution on primary cesarian delivery rates. *JAMA* 1994;**271**:443–7.

59 Parham ES, Astrom MF and King SH. The association of pregnancy weight gain with the mother's postpartum weight. *J Am Diet Assoc* 1990;**90**:550–4.

60 Scholl TO, Hediger ML, Schall JI, Ances IG and Smith WK. Gestational weight gain, pregnancy outcome, and postpartum weight retention. *Obstet Gynecol* 1995;**86**:423–7.

61 Boardley DJ, Sargent RG, Coker AL, Hussey JR and Sharpe PA. The relationship between diet, activity, and other factors, and postpartum weight change by race. *Obstet Gynecol* 1995;**86**:834–8.

62 Barker DJP, Winter PD, Osmond C, Phillips DIW and Sultan HY. Weight gain in infancy and cancer of the ovary. *Lancet* 1995;**345**: 1087–8.

63 Tibblin G, Eriksson M, Cnattingius S and Ekbom A. High birthweight as a predictor of prostate cancer risk. *Epidemiology* 1995;**6**:423–4.

64 Thompson JA and Janerich DT. Maternal age at birth and risk of breast cancer in daughters. *Epidemiology* 1990;**1**:101–6.

65 Ekbom A, Thurfjell E, Hsieh C-C, Trichopoulos D and Adami H-O. Perinatal characteristics and adult mammographic patterns. *Int J Cancer* 1995;**61**:177–80.

66 Ekbom A, Trichopoulos D, Adami H-O, Hsieh C-C and Lans S-J. Evidence of prenatal influences on breast cancer risk. *Lancet* 1992; **340**:1015–18.

67 Godfrey KM, Barker DJP and Osmond C. Disproportionate fetal growth and raised IgE concentration in adult life. *Clin Exp Allergy* 1994;**24**: 641–8.

68 Kaye SA, Robison LL, Smithson WA, Gunderson P, King FL and Neglia JP. Maternal reproductive history and birth characteristics in childhood acute lymphoblastic leukemia. *Cancer* 1991;**68**:1351–5.

69 Seidman DS, Laor A, Gale R, Stevenson DK and Danon YL. A longitudinal study of birthweight and being overweight in late adolescence. *Am J Dis Child* 1991;**145**:782–5.

70 Johansson C, Samuelsson U and Ludvigsson J. A high weight gain early in life is associated with an increased risk of Type I (insulin dependent) diabetes mellitus. *Diabetologia* 1994;**37**:91–4.

71 McCormick MC. The contribution of low birthweight to infant mortality and childhood morbidity. *N Engl J Med* 1985;**312**:82–90.

72 Morrison JC. Preterm birth: a puzzle worth solving. *Obstet Gynecol* 1990; **(Suppl) 76**:5S–12S.

73 Radetsky P. Stopping premature births before it's too late. *Science* 1994;**266**:1486–8.

74 Papiernik E, Bouyer J, Dreyfus J, et al. Prevention of preterm births: a perinatal study in Haguenau, France. *Pediatrics*1985;**76**:154–8.

75 Bréart G, Blondel B, Tuppin P, et al. Did preterm deliveries continue to decrease in France in the 1980s? *Paediatr Perinat Epidemiol* 1995;**9**: 296–306.

76 Ng E, Wilkins R. Maternal demographic characteristics and rates of low birthweight in Canada, 1961 to 1990. *Health Rep* 1994;**6**:241–252.

77 Kessel SS, Villar J, Berendes HW, Nugent RP. The changing pattern of low birthweight in the United States, 1970 to 1980. *JAMA* 1984;**251**: 1978–82.

78 Division of Nutrition, National Center for Chronic Disease Prevention and Health Promotion. Increasing incidence of low birthweight—United States, 1981–1991. *Morb Mortal Wkly Rep* 1994;**43**:335–9.

79 Arbuckle TE and Sherman GJ. An analysis of birthweight by gestational age in Canada. *Can Med Assoc J* 1989;**140**:157–65.

80 Alberman E. Are our babies becoming bigger? *J Roy Soc Med* 1991;**84**: 257–60.

81 *Births and deaths*, 1993. Health Statistics Division. Statistics Canada. Catalogue No. 84-210-XPB. Ottawa, 1996.

Appendix

The etiologic fraction[17] associated with a multi-category risk factor was estimated using the formula

$$EF = 1 - (1 / (\Sigma \, p_i \, (RR_i)))$$

where EF = the estimated etiologic fraction.

  p_i = the proportion of the population in the exposed category i.

  RR_i = the relative risk associated the exposure category i.

The preventive fraction[17] associated with any multi-category protective factor was estimated using the formula

$$PF = 1 - (\Sigma \, p_i \, (RR_i))$$

where PF = the estimated preventive fraction.

  p_i = the proportion of the population in the exposed category i.

  RR_i = the relative risk associated the exposure category i.

13 Conclusions

Yoav Ben-Shlomo and Diana Kuh

There is a growing body of evidence that patterns of early growth and other factors acting across the life course play an important role in the origin and development of a wide array of common chronic diseases. Knowledge of the determinants of fetal growth, and of the biological processes which mediate the effects of the social environment, is limited. The research emphasis is now moving away from measures of general growth impairment towards specific patterns of growth retardation during gestation. Links between growth and development in childhood and later disease are also being demonstrated. The relative importance of early as compared with later life influences is yet to be fully determined, but there is growing evidence that they have an interactive effect on disease risk. Thus the possibility exists of intervening to break biological and social chains of risk at several stages of life, and of targetting those particularly at risk at times when change is most likely. Prospective studies beginning at birth or in childhood will provide further evidence as they mature about the importance of factors acting across the life course. Public health policy should adopt a truly life course strategy with attention towards the mother, baby, child, adolescent, and adult.

13.1 Introduction

The purpose of this book has been to review the literature on possible factors acting at different stages of the life course which, via biological or social processes, affect the development of chronic disease risk in individuals and populations. Most of the chapters have focused disproportionately on preadult exposures as this is the area where there has been the most exciting epidemiological developments over the last few years.

The work of David Barker and his colleagues at the MRC Environmental Epidemiology Unit in Southampton, England,[1] has been particularly influential in several different ways. First, it has established the concept of programming firmly within the domain of chronic disease epidemiology. Second, it has re-awakened researchers to the importance of early life factors on adult chronic disease, which had been ignored for over half a century with the exception of a few researchers such as Anders Forsdahl.[2] Third, it has revitalized the historical cohort design and demonstrated the enormous value of following up individuals from old, often forgotten, records of birth and child growth. Fourth, it has attracted the attention of researchers in a wide number of related disciplines. For example, from the beginning this work has been explicit in interpreting measures such as infant mortality and birthweight as mere proxy measures for more complex physiological phenomena. The clear demonstration of how much more there is to discover about the determinants of fetal growth and development has acted as an important trigger for work by experimental physiologists, embryologists, neonatologists, and others. Social epidemiologists and medical sociologists have also been presented with a challenge. The mere descriptions of associations between socioeconomic measures and disease no longer suffice; there is a need to delineate potential biological and social pathways and mediators.

13.2 What can we conclude?

The contributors to this book have demonstrated that there is evidence that early life factors affect the subsequent development of cardiovascular, respiratory and allergic diseases, diabetes, hypertension, breast and some other cancers. This is not to deny the importance of adult risk factors; indeed, Whincup and Cook conclude (in Chapter 6) that adult rather than fetal factors are more important in the development of hypertension. What is clear is that factors acting throughout the life course need to be considered; Strachan's chapter on respiratory diseases (Chapter 5) is an eloquent expression of such an approach. The idea that early life may determine one's future health trajectory is not new, yet until fairly recently the development of cardiovascular epidemiology followed a logical but narrow path that chose to ignore these ideas (Chapter 2).

The inclusion of early life factors enriches our understanding of the development of adult chronic disease both because of the additional independent risk they may confer, and because of the *interactive* nature of factors acting at different stages of the life course (Chapter 3). For example, the evidence that overweight adults with the lowest birthweight have the highest risk of hypertension or diabetes helps further to explain the variation that occurs in the relationship between adult exposure and outcome and to target the most at risk group.

Although the broad direction of change in early life circumstances this century is congruent with declining all cause adult mortality rates, early life factors seem to play a less important role than adult factors in accounting for trends in specific chronic diseases (see Chapters 9–11); although, as Davey Smith points out in Chapter 11, the interaction of exposures at different points of the life course renders the explanation of trends rather problematic. Trends in cigarette smoking and the consumption of micronutrients provide a better explanation than trends in early life factors for the increasing social class differentials in coronary heart disease (Chapter 11). The cohort-related rise and fall in chronic obstructive pulmonary diseases is clearly related to the uptake of cigarette smoking (Chapter 9). Several authors concur in concluding that, despite evidence for early life factors, control of obesity and the cessation of smoking are still the most effective means of reducing individual and population chronic disease risk.

13.3 What future research is required?

13.3.1 Further use of historical cohorts

Consistency of research findings is regarded as a necessary criteria of causality.[3] There are now various studies which have demonstrated associations between birthweight or adult height and a number of chronic diseases or adult risk factors, suggesting that preadult exposures play a role in the development of disease risk. A few studies with measures of body proportions at birth have raised the possibility that the type of fetal growth retardation and the timing of undernutrition may be particularly important in establishing future risk. A few others have shown relationships between weight at 1 year or leg length in childhood and later ischaemic heart disease which suggest that account should also be taken of postnatal growth. There is a need to replicate these findings by assembling other cohorts where measures of prenatal and postnatal growth have been previously recorded. Preferably such cohorts would be drawn from different populations living under different conditions, providing a further tests of the consistency of the research findings and, where possible, disentangling the usual confounding nature between early and later life exposures.[4] Several studies are already being conducted in India and China by Barker and his team.

Historical cohorts will continue to contribute valuable research findings, especially where individuals are subsequently followed up again in a prospective fashion so that repeat measures of adult outcomes can be obtained and processes of ageing, for example in cognitive function, can be examined in relation to the measures recorded in early life. More detailed clinical examination of the adults whose body proportions at birth are known will also enhance our understanding of the underlying biological mechanisms. For example one study, described in Chapter 4, has already shown that thinness at birth predicts defects in muscle fuel utilization.

13.3.2 Studies of the life course

Historical cohorts do not have the necessary repeat measures of development and exposure to study the process of insult accumulation and interactions acting throughout the life course. Prospective longitudinal studies beginning at birth[5-7] or in childhood[8-10] can fill some of the missing gaps. These studies can test hypothesized 'chains of risk' by examining the sequence of events, and assess whether later exposures are a direct consequence of earlier events or simply related through a common third factor (Chapter 8). Although they are relatively 'immature' in terms of the age of their participants, these studies are likely to provide a rich source of material not only as replication studies but also for testing new hypotheses at different stages of the life course. The accumulation of risk for adult blood pressure, lung function and respiratory disease is already being investigated in the 1946 cohort.[5,11-13] Results highlight significant biological and social factors operating at all stages of the life course. For example, high blood pressure in midlife was related not only to low birthweight, particularly among those with central obesity, but also to growth and the social environment in childhood and psychosocial factors operating from adolescence. Studying the complex models of risk accumulation presents a challenge to current analytical methods. Recently developed methods for repeat measures, measurement error, and multilevel exposures are becoming essential tools for the analysis of studies of the life course.

13.3.3 Determining biological mechanisms

Those interested in programming have not hesitated to speculate on the potential mechanisms which may account for the link between proxy measures of fetal development and later disease. Although these ideas have often been *post hoc*, they have drawn on previous animal research and, by indicating its possible relevance for the development of chronic disease in humans, have helped to rebuild a valuable bridge between scientific disciplines. These ideas will necessarily be developed in future animal work where interventions can be controlled and pathological outcomes observed in a relatively short time period. For example, the relationship between disproportionate growth retardation and arterial smooth muscle composition could possibly be tested within an appropriate animal model.

Proxy or direct measures applicable to human subjects will also be required. The importance of placental blood flow for fetal development can be investigated with specialized ultrasound techniques. Similarly, measures of the uterine milieu are necessary to measure the impact of maternal characteristics and the subsequent fetal response (Chapter 7). In childhood, measurement of early precursors of atheroclerosis, such as arterial reactivity,[14] will enable researchers to detect subclinical abnormalities at a younger age, when confounding by later adult factors may be unimportant. The ability to examine tracking of biological measures is useful in both determining the timing of any exposure but also its degree of reversibility by later life influences. For example, children in the upper decile of the blood pressure distribution may shift downwards because of alterations in either diet or weight.

Linking physiological parameters, such as growth, with metabolic, endocrine, or cellular events is perhaps less daunting than understanding the biological consequences of social phenomena, such as social hieracrchies.[15] Progress has been made in the areas of psychoneuroendocrinology, but as yet human data are limited. For example, life events or social networks have been linked with markers of immune reactivity and possible cancer etiology.[16] Understanding these biological consequences may elucidate potential interactions between earlier events and later exposures.

The rapid development in human genetics has already contributed to a greater understanding of chronic disease. Previous work has tended to focus on the relationship between genetic polymorphisms and disease end-points such as hypertension,[17] rather than on birthweight. The degree to which programming may reflect genetic rather than environmental factors still remains unclear. As discussed in Chapter 4, genetic influences on birthweight may have been previously underestimated. Studies on half-sibs and genetically mixed populations with similar environmental exposures will help disentangle the relative contribution of genetic factors.

Ultimately, the clearest evidence regarding causality, reversibility, and the public health importance of early life factors will come from studies which first test the effectiveness of interventions to modify the pattern of human fetal growth and then test, at follow ups throughout life, whether any modifications have the expected effect on measures of postnatal growth and development and markers of disease risk.

13.4 The impact of programming on researchers, funding bodies, media, and lay public

In utero programming has been described as a major paradigm shift away from current conventional wisdom concerning cardiovascular disease etiology.[18] Despite initial methodological criticisms of the research undertaken by Barker and his colleagues, the replication of their findings in several other populations, including those in non-UK settings, has caused other epidemiologists to reconsider the importance of early life factors on chronic disease and examine the programming hypothesis within new cohorts. As Latour argues,[19] the emergence of scientific facts is a collective process, dependent on its use by other scientists, and key players in this process attempt to enrol others by the development of alliances and networks. Barker's early collaborators were biological scientists in other MRC funded units.[20,21] He has also forged worldwide alliances with fetal physiologists whose training and interests make them natural allies in support of the programming hypothesis.

The development and growth of any new hypothesis is dependent on its nurturing through adequate funding. The Medical Research Council (MRC), Wellcome Foundation and British Heart Foundation have all provided extensive research funding. The MRC recognized as major scientific achievements the findings that 'adult blood pressure is directly related to impaired growth in the womb' and that 'inadequate nutrition in early life . . . is associated with the later development of impaired glucose tolerance and non-insulin dependent diabetes' (p.69).[22] In 1993–4 they established a major scientific initiative into the fetal and infant origins of adult disease. The Royal Society Wellcome Medal, awarded to Barker in 1995, provides further evidence of his support from biological scientists.

The scientific editorship of the *British Medical Journal* has given wide coverage to publications from Barker's research team; their supportive editorial marked a significant step in acceptance of early life ideas as scientific facts.[18] They also published a book of these collected papers[23] and a book written by Barker to provide a more accessible account of his ideas.[1]

The findings of the new early life theories have also attracted the attention of the wider public. There has been an increasing number of articles in the quality British press and, more recently, wider coverage in more popular newspapers and magazines for women and parents. A noticeable shift has taken place in the tone of the articles, as Latour[19] would predict: the information is now presented less as revolutionary science or ground breaking research attributed to one scientist and more as well established facts in the public domain for which there is an apparent scientific consensus. British television's *Horizon* documentary in 1992 devoted to Barker's reseach ('A diet for a lifetime') has also helped to popularize the findings. Groups like Maternity Alliance, whose interests straddle the academic and policy debates, are using the findings to call for policy change.[24]

13.5 Policy implications

If early life factors affect later disease risk, either through programming or through other mechanisms, there are implications for current preventive health policies. As yet, there has been little discussion of what these might be.

Scientists generally argue that more research is necessary into the possible reversibility or modification of disease risk in later childhood and adult life. Barker has suggested that to ensure appropriate levels of fetal and infant nutrition, preventive strategies should shift their emphasis to improving the health and nutrition of girls and young women, and mothers during pregnancy and lactation, if necessary at the expense of improvements in the nutrition of children.[1] Such a shift in strategy is a potentially dangerous development, as poor childhood nutrition and growth are also associated with a greater risk of heart disease.[25] Health education based on a life course approach to adult disease would target infants, children, and adults.

Both the English and Scottish departments of health have recognised the potential importance of programming for policy[26,27] but fall short of any specific recommendations. Similarly, the recent British Government working group on variations in health also recognized the importance of a life course approach to disease aetiology, which explicitly included biological programming as well as 'cumulative exposure to social advantage or disadvantage, and variation in behaviours, over the lifespan.' (p18).[28]

In Chapter 12, Joseph and Kramer concluded that intervening to improve fetal growth based solely on the programming hypothesis cannot be justified, even if the reported associations are assumed to be causal. They argue that interventions designed to improve fetal and infant growth would lead to only marginal reductions in the occurrence of coronary heart disease and might have other adverse effects.

Despite such evidence, shifts in public policy may occur in response to research findings which suggest that early life factors have an impact on future adult health. This could happen if these findings were used as evidence of part of a wider social problem,[29] for example, as part of a growing concern about the wellbeing of children in developed countries. It is almost 100 years since the physical condition of children become a social problem, resulting in what were considered to be radical social reforms for mothers, infants, and children.[30-32] It is almost 50 years since Bowlby's work helped to create the conditions under which the emotional health of children came to be a social problem and led to a major change of direction in welfare services.[33,34] Both these developments occurred because the time was ripe politically for change, not least because they followed periods of considerable social upheaval. Today there are signs that public anxiety is growing again about the state of children in a number of countries. There is concern both for the wellbeing of individual children, and for the cost to society of increased health care and treatment for socially disruptive young people. The widening social and economic inequalities and other adverse signs that all is not well with the health of children today are being publicized.[35-48] The scientific findings presented in this book may be used as part of the evidence for why the health of children, and their social and economic circumstances, should be given greater political priority.

13.6 The future of chronic disease epidemiology

Interest in programming and early life factors in the development of chronic disease arose from a dissatisfaction with the conventional adult life style model. This model, developed during the postwar period, forms part of what Susser calls 'black box' epidemiology, or conventional risk factor epidemiology, the main purpose of which is to relate individual exposure and outcome in statistical models with little or no attention to the underlying biological mechanisms or the wider social context. Some critics of this approach have advocated the need for further scientific reductionism; '. . . a purpose-built chain of necessary causes—with each link of evidence well tested, and cemented to its neighbours by bonds of strong inference'.[49] Other critics have pointed to the current neglect of socioeconomic factors and the population perspective and called for an 'ecosocial' model, which conceptualizes the '. . . determinants of disease distribution as economic and social relationships forged by a society's political and economic structure'.[50] Susser and Susser have suggested that a synthesis of both macro and micro levels of analysis is required; replacing the 'black box' with 'chinese boxes' where one box sits within another and hence integrates both 'causal pathways at the societal level . . . with pathogenesis and causality at the molecular level'.[51]

We have advocated in this book a life course approach to chronic disease aetiology which studies the interaction of social and biological processes which have long term effects on disease risk. These chains of risk may arise from programming at critical periods during gestation and infancy or accumulate more incrementally throughout life. A life course approach responds to the critics of 'black box' epidemiology because it incorporates various different spatial levels, from the molecular to the global. In addition it emphasizes a temporal level of analysis and the interactions between past and current life experiences. It argues that to understand the pattern of current exposures, and their impact on adult chronic disease, requires knowledge of how past events have shaped both the risk of subsequent exposure and the responsiveness of physiological systems and behavioural patterns.

A life course approach to chronic disease aetiology is in its infancy, but healthy growth and development seem assured. Further epidemiological evidence will come from imaginative historical cohort studies and maturing longitudinal studies using more sophisticated biological, social and statistical models. It will also come from new biological research. These developments will lead to greater understanding of, and a wider interest in, the ways that experiences throughout the life course affect the development of many of the adult chronic diseases that are already prevalent in developed countries, and becoming increasingly prevalent in the developing world.

References

Those marked with an asterisk are especially recommended for further reading

1* Barker DJP. Mothers, babies, and disease in later kife. London: BMJ Publishing Group, 1994.

2 Forsdahl A. Living conditions in childhood and subsequent develop-ment of risk factors for arteriosclerotic heart disease. The cardiovascular survey in Finnmark 1974–75. *J Epidemiol Community Health* 1978; 32:34–7.

3 Bradford Hill A. The environment and disease: association or causation? *Proc R Soc Med* 1965;**58**:295–300.

4 Davey Smith G, Phillips A. Declaring independence: why we should be cautious. *J Epidemiol Community Health* 1990;**44**:257–8.

5 Wadsworth MEJ, Kuh DJL. Childhood influences on adult health: a review of recent work in the British 1946 national birth cohort study, the MRC National Survey of Health and Development. *Paediat Perinat Epidemiol* 1997;**11**:2–20.

6 Power C. A review of child health in the 1958 cohort: National Child Development Study. *Paediat Perinat Epidemiol* 1992;**6**:91–110.

7 Butler NR, Golding J, Howlett BC (eds) *From birth to five: a study of the health and behaviour of a national birth cohort.* Oxford: Pergamon 1985.

8 Whincup PH, Cook DG, Adshead F, Taylor S, Papacosta O, Walker M, Wilson V. Cardiovascular risk factors in British children from towns with widely differing adult cardiovascular mortality. *Br Med J* 1996; **313**: 79–84.

9 Berenson GS, MacMahan CA, Voors AW, Webber AS, Srinivasan SR, Frank GC, Foster TA, Blonde CV. *Cardiovascular risk factors in children: the early natural history of atherosclerosis and essential hypertension.* New York: Oxford University Press, 1980.

10 Lauer RM, Connor WE, Leaverton PE, Reiter MA, Clarke WR. Coronary heart disease risk factors in school children: the Muscatine study. *J Pediatr* 1975;**86**:697–706.

11 Wadsworth MEJ, Cripps HA, Midwinter RA, Colley JRT. Blood pressure at age 36 years and social and familial factors, cigarette smok-ing and body mass in a national birth cohort. *Br Med J* 1985;**291**: 1534–8.

12 Mann SL, Wadsworth MEJ, Colley JRT. Accumulation of factors influencing respiratory illness in members of a national birth cohort and their offspring. *J Epidemiol Community Health* 1992;**46**:286–92.

13 Kuh DJL. *Assessing the influence of early life on adult health.* PhD thesis. London University, 1993.

14   Celermajer DS, Sorensen KE, Gooch VM, Spiegelhalter DJ, Miller OI, Sullivan ID, Lloyd JK, Deanfield JE. Noninvasive detection of endothelial dysfunction in children and adults at risk of atherosclerosis *Lancet* 1992; **340**:1111–5.

15   Sapolsky RM. *Stress, the ageing brain, and the mechanisms of neuron death*. Cambridge, Massachusetts: MIT Press, 1992.

16   Kiecolt-Glaser JK, Glaser R. Psychoneuroimmunology and health consequences: data and shared mechanisms. *Psychosom Med* 1995;**57**: 269–74.

17   Caulfield M, Lavender P, Farrall M, Munroe P, Lawson M, Turner P, Clark AJL. Linkage of the angiotensinogen gene to essential hypertension. *N Engl J Med* 1994; **330**:1629–33.

18   Robinson RJ. Is the child father of the man? *Br Med J* 1992;**304**:789–790.

19* Latour B. *Science in action*. Milton Keynes: Open University Press, 1987.

20   Barker DJP, Meade TW, Fall CHD, et al. Relation of fetal and infant growth to plasma fibrinogen and factor VII concentrations in adult life. *Br Med J* 1992;**304**:148–52.

21   Hales CN, Barker DJP, Clark PMS, et al. Fetal and infant growth and impaired glucose tolerance at age 64. *Br Med J* 1991;**303**:1019–22.

22   Medical Research Council. *Corporate Plan*. London, Medical Research Council, 1992.

23   Barker DJP, ed. *Fetal and infant origins of adult disease*. London: BMJ Publishing Group, 1992.

24   Dallison J and Lobstein T. *Poor expectations. Poverty and undernourishment in pregnancy*. London: NCH Action for Children and the Maternity Alliance, 1995.

25   Gunnell DJ, Davey Smith G, Frankel S, Nanchahal K, Braddon FEM, Pemberton J, Peters TJ. Childhood leg length and adult mortality—followup of the Carnegie (Boyd Orr) Survey of diet and health in prewar Britain (abstract). *J Epidemiol Community Health* 1996;**50**:580–1.

26   Department of Health. *Health of the Nation. A strategy for health in England*. Cm 1986; HMSO, London, 1992.

27   Kendall R. From the Chief Medical Officer. *Health Bulletin* 1993;**51**: 351–2.

28   Department of Health. *Variations in Health. What can the Department of Health and the NHS do?* A report produced by the Variations Sub-Group of the Chief Medical Officers Health of the Nation Working Group. London: HMSO,1995.

29* Bartley M. *Authorities and partisans*. Edinburgh: Edinburgh University Press, 1992.

30   Kuh D, Davey Smith G. When is mortality risk determined? Historical insights into a current debate. *Social History of Medicine* 1993;**6**:101–23.

31   Dwork D.*War is good for babies and other young children. A history of the infant and child welfare movement in England 1898–1918.* London: Tavistock Publications, 1987.

32   Lewis J. *The politics of motherhood: child and maternal welfare in England 1900–1939.* London: Croom Helm, 1980.

33   Bowlby J. *Maternal care and mental health.* World Health Organisation Monograph Series no.2. Geneva: World Health Organisation, 1951.

34   Bowlby J. *Child care and the growth of love.* Harmondsworth: Penguin, 1953.

35   Silver GA. Ending the reign of dogma: designing a child health policy for America.The Duncan W Clark Lecture. *Bull N Y Acad Med* 1989; **65**:255–77.

36   Cornia GA. *Child poverty and deprivation in industrialized countries: recent trends and policy options.* Florence: UNICEF International Child Development Centre: Innocenti Occasional Papers, No.2., 1990.

37   Mistral G. *Beyond rhetoric: a new American agenda for children and families: final report of the National Commission on Children.* Washington, D.C.: Government Printing Office, 1991.

38   George V, Howards I. *Poverty amidst affluence. Britain and the United States.* Aldershot: Edward Elgar, 1991.

39   Fuchs VR, Reklis DM. America's children: economic perspectives and policy options. *Science* 1992;**255**:41–6.

40   Starfield B. Effects of poverty on health status. *Bull N Y Acad Med* 1992;**68**:17–24.

41   Wadsworth MEJ, Kuh DJL. Are gains in child health being undermined? *Dev Med Child Neurol* 1993;**35**:742–5.

42   Allukian M. Forging the future: the public health imperative. *Am J Public Health* 1993;**83**:655–9.

43   Fulginiti VA. Poverty, health, and children: a second look. *American J Dis Child* 1993;**147**:507–8.

44*   Hewlett SA. *Child neglect in rich nations.* New York: Unicef, 1993.

45   McKee M. Poor children in rich countries. Markets fail children. *Br Med J* 1993;**307**:1576–7.

46   Joseph Rowntree Foundation. *Inquiry into income and wealth.* York: Joseph Rowntree Foundation, 1995.

47   Oppenheim C and Harker L. *Poverty: the facts.* London: Child Poverty Action Group, 1996.

48   Wadsworth MEJ. Family and education as determinants of health. In: Blane D, Brunner E, Wilkinson RJ, eds. *Social organisation and health.* London: Routledge, 1996;152–70.

49   Charlton BG. Attribution of causation in epidemiology: chain or mosaic? *J Clin Epidemiol* 1996;**49**:105–7.

50   Krieger N, Zierler S. What explains the public's health? - A call for epidemiologic theory. *Epidemiology* 1996;**7**:107–9.

51* Susser M, Susser E. Choosing a Future for Epidemiology: II. From black box to Chinese boxes and eco-epidemiology. *Am J Pub Health* 1996; **86**:674–7.

Index

abdominal obesity 79, 83, 85, 90–1
  mother's 160
accumulation of risk 6–7, 17, 47, 170,
    184–5
adolescence 6–7, 174, 179
  growth in 60–1
  health related behaviour and
      181–2
adult life style 3–4, 23–7
adult risk factors 3–4, 21–2, 79,
    110–13, 126–9, 132, 182–3,
    208–9, 225–8, 246–7, 258–60,
    281–3, 297–8
  see also alcohol; blood pressure;
      cholesterol; diabetes;
      exercise; smoking;
      socioeconomic environment
age
  at first birth 63
  blood pressure and 123–5
  see also adolescence; childhood;
      fetal growth; infancy
alcohol 26, 127, 180–2
  blood pressure and 127
  see also behaviours
allergic diseases 101–14
  allergic sensitization 108–9
  atopy 102–3
  early life factors and 102–3,
      108–9
  family size and 109

occupation and 111
temporal trends in 212–13
see also asthma
α_1-antitrypsin 110
American Heart Association 20, 25
anaemia, iron-deficiency, see
    maternal factors
asthma 102–3, 105
  adult risk factors and 110–13
  early life risk factors and 105–8
  lung function and 105
  temporal trends in 202–3, 212–13
atherosclerosis
  early onset and 28, 62–3, 69
  post-mortem evidence of 25, 28,
      62, 255
  infant feeding and 28

Barker, David 5–6, 29, 47, 50, 53, 91,
    131, 133, 161, 260–1, 296–7,
    300–1
  see also Medical Research Council
behaviours, health related 170–1
  development of 180–2
  see also alcohol; diet; exercise;
      smoking
beta cell function, defects in 84–9
  birthweight and 87–8
  malnutrition and 86–7
  weight in infancy and 87